Bringing Leadership to Life in Health: LEADS in a Caring Environment

Graham Dickson • Bill Tholl
Editors

Bringing Leadership to Life in Health: LEADS in a Caring Environment

Putting LEADS to work

Second Edition

Springer

Editors
Graham Dickson
Royal Roads University
Victoria, BC
Canada

Bill Tholl
Canadian Health Leadership Network
Ottawa, ON
Canada

ISBN 978-3-030-38535-4   ISBN 978-3-030-38536-1   (eBook)
https://doi.org/10.1007/978-3-030-38536-1

This Springer imprint is published by the registered company Springer Nature Switzerland AG
The registered company address is: Gewerbestrasse 11, 6330 Cham, Switzerland

Foreword

If there is one thing Canada does better than any country in the world, it is study the shortcomings of its health system. From the 1961 Royal Commission on Health Services, led by Supreme Court Justice Emmett Hall, through to the 2019 Ontario Premier's Council on Improving Healthcare and Ending Hallway Medicine, headed by Dr. Rueben Devlin, there have been dozens of learned analyses of how medicare could be improved.

There is much to be done, but the recommendations for reform have been remarkably consistent over the decades:

– Bolster primary care to create a strong foundation and a medical home for every Canadian;
– Move health services out of institutions into the community wherever possible;
– Create a coherent human resources plan to ensure care can be delivered when and where it is needed;
– Invest not just in sickness care but in social services that bolster health, things like income supports, affordable housing, and accessible education;
– Expand the services covered by publicly funded insurance beyond hospital and physician services, most notably by providing universal coverage of prescription drugs;
– Place greater emphasis on the quality of care.

These ideas are usually greeted with enthusiasm, but we never quite get around to making the changes, at least not on a large scale. There are excuses, of course, like lack of money, political priorities, fear of public backlash, and the objections of interest groups but, at the end of the day, the failure to move from ideas to implementation and the penchant for short-term thinking are usually blamed on a lack of leadership.

Because of Canada's laggardness, health system reform is more urgent than ever. So it is refreshing to see that we are finally taking healthcare leadership seriously, as evidenced by the embrace of the LEADS framework, which is now the foundation for leadership in 70 per cent of the country's health organizations.

In the first edition of this book, Graham Dickson and Bill Tholl laid out the five domains of the LEADS framework—Lead self, Engage others, Achieve results, Develop coalitions, and Systems transformation—in a manner that made it compelling and actionable. In this, the second edition, they flesh out what it takes to be a good leader and engage in transformational change, provide some powerful anecdotes of how LEADS can make good leaders better leaders, present a richer evidence base that reflects the increased academic interest in health leadership, and offer some useful comparisons to other jurisdictions. While "patient-centred" and "family-centred" are the buzzwords *du jour*, what those terms mean in practice is brought to life in a series of vignettes peppered throughout the book.

The second edition includes contributions from a number of invited authors, including a powerful chapter on leadership lessons from Indigenous teachings, as well as analysis of how the LEADS philosophy can help promote equity and diversity.

There is a consumer revolution coming to healthcare, along with game-changing technological innovations like artificial intelligence. We can no longer content ourselves with the crisis management approach that has been the norm for so long. In this brave new world, leadership will no longer be about authority and enforcement, but about taking responsibility and having an impact.

Transformational change will require transformational leaders at all levels of the health system, from the bedside to the cabinet table.

The pressures are intense and multifaceted: meeting the ever-growing healthcare needs of an aging population; building and maintaining a health workforce; and bending the cost curve to keep care affordable, individually and collectively. To make matters worse, politicians in Canada have a tendency for micro-managing, instead of getting out of the way and letting professional managers manage.

Yet there continue to be leaders with great potential drawn to public service because they believe in the importance of universal healthcare. The challenges they face—political, social, financial, and practical—cannot be overstated.

One of the invited authors cites the commonly used analogy that Indigenous healthcare transformation is "like driving a bus that's on fire down a road that's in the process of being built." In many ways, that vivid image applies to the health system writ large as well, and the fire will only get more intense as financial constraints increase, and long-overdue structural reforms begin.

Ultimately, healthcare is a people business. The best leaders are those who can communicate and mobilize, and acknowledge that we need the right mix of private and public funding and delivery, and that we obsess too much about the cost and volume of care delivered and too little about value.

We need leaders who can speak those uncomfortable truths to power and who are willing to make the all-important leap from vision to action, and LEADS can help embolden and fortify them.

As Dickson and Tholl state succinctly: "Leadership in health care is about accomplishing three key functions: integrating care for patients and families, creating healthy and productive workplaces and changing the system to respond to environmental pressures and population needs."

And, as the real-life examples presented in the Second Edition attest, good leadership can make an appreciable difference not only to the bottom line but those who ultimately matter most, patients.

André Picard, health columnist, The Globe and Mail.

Preface

Leading healthcare system change is among the most complex, dynamic, and important challenges facing society in 2020. As the co-chairs of two national organizations dedicated to bringing the highest quality of leadership to Canadian health care, we know that the best evidence and knowledge of what good leadership is, and how it works, is a necessary condition for addressing those challenges. Dickson and Tholl demonstrate that a distributed approach or team effort is required, from informal caregivers through front line providers to the C-suite. This book is for everyone who wants to be a better leader and for all of us who are committed to better leadership and followership in the healthcare system.

The 2014 edition of the book introduced us to an easily accessible and memorable common vocabulary of health leadership called LEADS: an acronym for Lead self, Engage others, Achieve results, Develop coalitions, and System transformation. Over the past five years, we have witnessed a growing evolution of health leadership. The 2020 edition chronicles how our knowledge of good leadership has grown and how the LEADS framework, when put into practice, can address modern health leadership challenges. It also explores efforts in other international jurisdictions to use similar frameworks to generate change and purports to learn from their efforts.

The Canadian College of Health Leaders (through LEADS Canada) and the Canadian Health Leadership Network (through its 40+ network partner organizations) have enjoyed a front row seat in this evolution of health leadership. Our two organizations work together to advance leaders and leadership through LEADS. We have been pleased to have been integrally involved in the progression of LEADS and in helping Dickson and Tholl chronicle the many ways that LEADS is being put to work. We believe that the content of this book—and the LEADS framework itself—is vital to the membership of both our organizations. We encourage you to leverage up the LEADS advantage in your leadership practice and strongly endorse the book.

Calgary, AB   Feisal Keshavjee
Halifax, NS   Chris Power
Victoria, BC   Kathy MacNeil

Acknowledgments

Not unlike leading health systems change, writing a collaborative book on health leadership is not for the faint of heart. All the challenges of distributed leadership are at play. Resiliency and mutual respect are required. Clear articulation of individual roles is needed. Expect the unexpected and look to others to help when required. And at the end, in keeping with our car pool metaphor in Chap. 8, give credit to all who helped us get to the destination.

We have been inspired and encouraged by many along the way. We want, first and foremost, to thank our publisher Springer for its support and encouragement from the outset. Springer shared our enthusiasm around the timing for a second edition. Specifically, we are indebted to our editors at Springer (Melissa Morton, Krishnan Srinivasan and Vignesh Iyyadurai Suresh) for their invaluable guidance and ongoing support. Our own editor, the intrepid Jane Coutts, was up to the task of bringing LEADS 2.0 to life and to ensuring that we kept the reader in mind throughout the writing and editing process. She was relentless in her quest for error-free editing and we could not have been better served.

In contrast to LEADS 2014, this second edition focuses on how LEADS is being put to work in practice, both as a talent management and leadership development framework and as a change leadership model. Beginning with the Achieve results domain, we were looking to ensure that we met the twin objectives of writing the second edition of *Bringing Leadership to Life in Health*. The first objective was to assess and evaluate the mass of new research and evidence in support of health leadership as a prerequisite to service integration, organizational health and productivity, and health system change. We set as a goal to only use references published or released after the first edition, except where they are truly seminal. The second objective was to effectively chronicle the many ways in which LEADS had been *put to work* in practice across as broad a range of leadership challenges as possible.

Moving to the Engage others domain of the "E" in LEADS, we want to begin with heartfelt thanks to our respective spouses, Sue Dickson and Paula Tholl. Their patience and unflagging support through the many turns and bumps along the path to publishing is appreciated. We also want to thank our LEADS 2nd Edition Advisory Group for helping frame the overall plan for the book and for helping us settle on the five invited chapters. The group of five included: Kelly Grimes, Brenda Lammi, Dr. Ivy Bourgeault, Sharon Bishop, and Dr. Owen Adams. They also helped us identify and reach out to our invited coauthors for each of the invited chapters:

Stewart Dickson, Dr. Don Philippon, Kelly Grimes, Brenda Lammi, Stevie Colvin, Sharon Bishop, Cathy Cole, Heather Thiessen, Brenda Andreas, Dr. Alika Lafontaine, Caroline Lidstone-Jones, Dr. Elizabeth Hartney, Dr. Karen Lawford, and Dr. John(y) Van Aerde.

We were also committed to identifying those who could bear witness to the various ways that LEADS was being put to practice in the real world of health leader-ship. We were able to identify over 30 mini-case studies or stories and want to thank all those who were able to share their stories to the benefit of others. The list of key informants runs the gamut of health leaders, from deputy ministers and CEOs to mid-level, front-line and informal leaders.

We want to specifically acknowledge and thank all of the following Canadian colleagues: Dr. Arun Garg, Suann Laurent, Dr. Susan Drouin, Dr. Suzanne Squires, Alison Connors, Dr. Peter Vaughn, Lorrie Hamilton, Christine Devine, Amy Porteous, Isabelle Bossé, Hugh MacLeod, Phil Cady, Ellen Melis, Sandra Ramelli, Kathryn Adams, Stephanie Donaldson, Terri Potter, Dr. Gillian Kernaghan, Dr. Carolyn Pullen, Julie Sutherland, Brad Dorohoy, Sheila Betker, Peter Martin, Lauren Ettin, Dr. Karen Cohen, Glenn Brimacombe, Gabriele Cuff, Yabome Gilpin-Jackson, Cam Brine, and Jaci Edgeworth. In terms of our international collabora-tors, we want to thank Stephen Hart (NHS England), Carolyn MacLeod (NHS Scotland); Desmond Gorman (New Zealand), Don Dunoon, David Sweeney, Dr. Neale Fong, and Dr. Elizabeth Shannon (Australia), and Eric de Roodenbeke (International Hospital Federation).

Turning to the Develop coalitions domain, we also want to thank the two organi-zations that have, more than any others, helped us to learn from the practical appli-cation of LEADS over the past five years. The Executive Director of the Canadian Health Leadership Network (Kelly Grimes), the Vice-President of the Canadian College of Health Leaders and leader in charge of LEADS Canada (Brenda Lammi), and the CEO of the Canadian College of Health Leaders (Alain Doucet) have been incredibly supportive of taking on this project and helping us maintain a focus on the practitioners of health leadership.

In terms of System transformation, the "S" in LEADS, we would like to thank the innumerable LEADS champions in health organizations across Canada and abroad, who have taken LEADS to heart and embedded it in their quest for better leadership. Canada's healthcare system has seen dramatic changes in how it is organized and administered, with a continuation in centralization of accountabili-ties and authorities at a province-wide level. And, of course, Canada is not alone in witnessing transformational change to healthcare planning and administration; our colleagues in the UK, Australia, and New Zealand join us in the goal of better leadership to serve our populations. We have seen an acceleration in the adoption of accountable health organizations and dramatic developments in our understand-ing of new technologies and what they can do to improve health leadership, health, and health-care outcomes.

Finally, in terms of the Lead self domain, this is our second major undertaking together as coauthors. We continue to learn from one another and build on our respective experiences in bringing LEADS to life both personally and professionally. Our friendship and our commitment to advancing the cause of better leadership for healthcare have continued to grow through this demanding and rewarding process.

All that said, and with the help of so many, we realize there is a high likelihood that errors of commission and omission remain, for which we take full responsibility.

February, 2020   Graham Dickson, PhD
                                                                        Bill Tholl OC, MA

Contents

From Concept to Reality: Putting LEADS to Work

Graham Dickson and Bill Tholl

The *LEADS in a Caring Environment* framework defines health leadership through five domains:

Lead self;
Engage others;
Achieve results;
Develop coalitions; and
Systems transformation.

Leadership is the collective capacity of an individual or group to influence people to work together to achieve a common constructive purpose: the health and wellness of the population we serve.

Dickson and Tholl [1]

Introduction

Our LEADS journey began more than 10 years ago, and more than five years have passed since we published the first edition of this book: *Bringing Leadership to Life in Health: LEADS in a Caring Environment.* Over the past five years, the challenges leaders face have changed markedly in Canada and elsewhere and literature on

G. Dickson (✉)
Royal Roads University, Victoria, BC, Canada
e-mail: graham.dickson@royalroads.ca

B. Tholl
Canadian Health Leadership Network, Ottawa, ON, Canada
e-mail: btholl@chlnet.ca

© Springer Nature Switzerland AG 2020
G. Dickson, B. Tholl (eds.), *Bringing Leadership to Life in Health: LEADS in a Caring Environment*, https://doi.org/10.1007/978-3-030-38536-1_1

health leadership has exploded; yet the fundamentals of LEADS-based leadership have withstood the tests of change and time. And as we show in the ensuing chapters, the five domains and 20 capabilities of the LEADS framework, which we call the DNA of health leadership, have been reaffirmed in the living labs of health organizations, put to use in ways we could not have imagined back in 2014.

So why write a second edition and how does it differ from the original? First and foremost, we believe leadership is an ongoing, life-long learning process. After five years of watching LEADS evolve, it was time for us to reflect on what we've learned about putting LEADS to work and share it with you. In many ways the evolution of LEADS is a live case study, as you will read in the coming pages.

Another reason for this update on LEADS is that the challenges of leading change in health care are even more daunting in 2020 than they were just five years ago. Ideological, technological and demographic pressures create demand for transformational leadership in all sectors, but it's arguable health care is more vulnerable than any other to the vagaries of political processes. For example, since 2014 we have seen provincial regionalization of health care delivery migrate to larger and larger organizations: Saskatchewan, Nova Scotia and Manitoba all went from multiple smaller health regions to one province-wide system. Services were also centralized in Ontario.

This edition was also a response to an important change we see emerging, as governments increasingly shift their focus to the overall experiences and needs of the people they are intended to serve. People-centred care is a priority in every developed country and appears in every health authority's strategic plan.

In Australia, as part of that agenda, the central government has introduced a national electronic health record scheme and activity-based funding, two changes aimed at triggering broader people-centred health system changes [2]. These include promoting greater integration of services, using technology to improve patient care, promoting patient and community involvement, bringing primary care closer to home and improving mental health care [3].

In the NHS England a significant emphasis has been put on changing entrenched, bureaucratic top-down leadership practices to include distributed leadership approaches that are aimed at creating more compassionate, caring health care workplace cultures in hospitals and primary care trusts; which in turn, serve the public better [4–6]. In NHS Scotland, "health and social care…is transforming to meet the needs of patients and communities" [7].

In Canada, similar rhetoric is used to justify a multiplicity of change demands: electronic medical records, new models of funding, physician engagement, etc. All provincial governments seem to be focusing on developing "closer-to-home" care models, engaging patients, families and communities in the provision of care. But as Aesop said, "When all is said and done, more is said than done." We saw a need to leverage LEADS to move beyond words and take concrete action to put patients and their families first. In this edition we have expressly added patients and informal caregivers into the lineup of health leaders (see Chap. 13 and the self-assessments at the end of each of the domain chapters).

Governments' focus on health care is inevitable: it is *the* big-ticket item in public budgets. Health issues can eat up a lot of political capital in a hurry, as you will see in some of the vignettes featured in this book. As Jeffery Simpson pointed out in his book *Chronic Condition*: "Medicare is the third rail of Canadian politics. Touch it and you die. Every politician knows this truth" [8].

Then, too, the pace of technological change is unrelenting. Our ability to share health information in a digitized world has increased exponentially, straining individual capacity to process information. And yet the information keeps coming: we are witnessing a revolution in the very nature of medical care and struggling to understand how genomics [9, 10], proteomics [11, 12], artificial intelligence [13, 14], and robotics [15, 16] will change how health care is delivered and at what price. According to a 2015 Canadian task force report on health care innovation: "Precision medicine heralds a new era for diagnosing, treating and preventing disease that will move away from a 'one size fits all' strategy to a more individualized approach based on a patient's genetic makeup" [17]. These breakthroughs and other technological advances are already challenging health leaders ethically, economically and legally as never before.

The shift in demographics that Western nations are going through has long been foreseen, but is none the less challenging. The aging of the population is filling an acute care system built in the 1960s with patients suffering complex co-morbidities [18], necessitating transformation of the system into one geared to the needs of older patients. As Monique Bégin, the former federal health minister who led the charge to pass the Canada Health Act (1984) wrote in her memoir: "Today's (health) system has to rethink and accommodate seniors' needs at home and in various types of institutions that are totally different from hospitals. It has to reform its culture from within and it is not first and foremost more funding that will assist" [19].

The impact of this trifecta of turmoil—ideology, technology and demography—on health leaders makes leveraging LEADS more important than ever for individuals and for the whole system. As the scope, breadth and pace of change accelerate, so does the need for effective leaders at *all* levels.

Another reason to update the book is that since 2014 we have seen exponential growth in the use of LEADS in three ways we had not anticipated. It has become *the* common vocabulary of leadership for much of Canada, been adopted as a common learning platform and is increasingly being used as a model for change leadership. At the same time, academic interest in health leadership and its role in overall system and organizational performance [20] has greatly expanded. As a result, we have a much bigger body of research to draw on and better understanding of potential uses for LEADS we want to share.

Finally, since 2014, we have seen increased evidence, albeit still limited, of the value for money in investing in better leadership development programs and ways to better measure its impact on organizational performance [21–23]. We see, for example, that NHS England has continued to invest significantly in leadership development [24] and NHS Scotland has developed a unique national approach to grow leadership in that country [25]. In Canada an estimated 80% of Canadian health institutions now have a leadership framework in place and 69% of those health care institutions have adopted LEADS as their preferred leadership learning platform [26]. This further attests to the value for money in investing in health leadership. So we see this book as establishing a baseline against which to measure progress over the next five years. We say more about international efforts in Chap. 11.

Bringing Leadership to Life in Health: A Primer on LEADS

The *LEADS in a Caring Environment* capabilities framework defines high-quality, modern health leadership. As we explain in Chap. 3, LEADS is a leadership framework by health, for health. The acronym represents the five domains of leadership:

- **L**ead self;
- **E**ngage others;
- **A**chieve results;
- **D**evelop coalitions; and
- **S**ystems transformation.

Each of the domains comprises four measurable, observable capabilities of exemplary leadership. We explain each of the five domains in detail in Chaps. 5–9, along with some of the approaches, techniques and tools supporting use of the framework. In this edition we also feature more case studies, stories and vignettes in each of these domain chapters to help you better understand how LEADS capabilities are being put to work in Canada, Australia and the United Kingdom. So, if you're practice-oriented and want to skip the theoretical foundations for leadership and LEADS, we encourage you to jump directly to Chap. 5: Lead self.

If you want to better understand the challenges of leadership in complex systems like health care, how to grow your leadership capacity, and better understand the changing policy environment shaping how LEADS is being deployed, move on with us through Chaps. 1–4.

Putting LEADS to Work: A Retrospective on a New Perspective

When we wrote the first edition, we used the tag line: "A New Perspective." This was because LEADS was a novel concept and was still in the early stages of the standard "introduction, adoption and diffusion" process of change [27]. As we will explain, we are now well into the adoption upswing and, we believe, entering the rapid diffusion phase of putting LEADS to work as a by health, for health framework.

Back in 2014, the health sector in Canada was largely importing leadership concepts and tools from the leadership articles written by business, for business, with few references relative to health care leadership. LEADS was a new and untested concept. The goal was to integrate relevant constructs of business leadership with health care organizations' competency frameworks and describe leadership in the context and language of health care. The initial efforts to create a toolbox to support development of the LEADS capabilities were quite limited and LEADS support systems were only beginning to take shape (see Chaps. 3 and 11).

Use of LEADS and of the tools in its toolbox has grown significantly over the past five years. LEADS has been put to work in all 10 provinces in Canada, is in use in New South Wales and in other parts of Australia and has influenced leadership development in Israel, Belgium and India.

Importantly, LEADS is not only being used for purposes such as self-assessments and 360 assessments or to help focus teams with a common vocabulary of leadership, or to help in developing personal learning plans. Now it's also helping leaders build bridges with boards, as a basis for developing graduate school curricula, as a foundation for engagement surveys in health workplaces, to shape interviews and as a guide to enhancing workplace health. These and other uses are described in the book. There is even, as we detail in Chap. 11, an infrastructure overseen by LEADS Canada to certify LEADS consultants and facilitators who help build LEADS-based leadership capacity across Canada and globally.

This emphasis on LEADS is not to suggest that other countries like England and Scotland should use LEADS; they have national frameworks and leadership talent management initiatives of their own. Certainly, Canada can learn from them as we outline in Chap. 11, and they from Canada. However, for a country beginning that trek, the LEADS journey has important lessons that can help shape its approach.

What has Changed: Key Ideas

This second edition is built around five cross-cutting ideas, outlined here to help you work through the book. They are:

1. The Centrality of Lifelong Learning for Self, Organization and Systems

LEADS is all about lifelong learning. You will never graduate with a LEADS degree as a fully developed leader because getting better is a continuous process. At the same time, the LEADS framework works for people no matter where they are on the ladder of leadership. It encourages you to lead from who you are and where you are. LEADS is not limited to individuals. We see organizational and systems learning as an analogue to personal learning. Peter Senge's work on systems thinking and the learning organization, begun in the 1990s [28, 29], has been widely embraced and the notion of organizations as learning systems has also been applied to health systems. The theme of learning permeates all chapters in this book.

2. Sharing How LEADS has Been Put to Work in Practice

One of the basic differences between this book and the earlier edition is captured by the title of this chapter, "From Concept to Reality." There are over 30 case studies and vignettes in this edition, each with its own set of insights into *Putting LEADS to Work* (our subtitle). They come from leaders throughout health care—patients, providers, policy makers and administrators. This variety of perspectives helps drive home how LEADS has become more than just a useful leadership framework or learning platform and is now also seen as a way to stay grounded professionally and personally. Many people we interviewed for the book referred to "living LEADS" and spoke of trying to model LEADS in the community as well as in the workplace.

Based on the case studies presented here, when LEADS is put to work—as a way of thinking, acting and developing leadership—it enhances people-centred care and improves overall system performance. We know that without active leadership in turbulent times, complexity can devolve into chaos. It's the job of health care leaders to ensure complex change does not become chaotic but remains focused on improving health and health care for all. In Chaps. 9 and 10 we discuss the limits of linear, reductionist principles of leadership and how we can put LEADS to work to lead change in a sector increasingly characterized by volatility, uncertainty, complexity and ambiguity (known as a VUCA environment). LEADS could almost have been purpose built for the VUCA world of the twenty-first century.

3. Sharing Our Deeper Understanding of Contextual Leadership

All leadership is a function of time, place and circumstance [30]—that's not new. But, as we discuss in depth in the following chapters, every leader works in a different context that demands customized action. We discuss the environmental, structural and personal contexts that shape leadership as they relate to each of the five LEADS domains.

The second dimension of our discussion on context is to compare the use of LEADS in Canada to other countries' leadership frameworks and talent management strategies to explore approaches Canada might learn from. Each country we profile—Australia, the UK (NHS Scotland and NHS England) and New Zealand—has dedicated significant resources to managing leadership talent. They, like Canada, believe their priorities for reform—integrating services, creating healthy workplaces and making structural reforms—will not be realized without better, more sophisticated and distributed leadership.

4. Sharing Different Perspectives on the Caring Ethos of LEADS

Over the past five years, as the challenges of leading in health care have become more complex, LEADS has helped health leaders stay focused on why they chose to work in a caring environment. We have numerous stories in this book about the importance of caring to individual health leaders, and five invited chapters that focus on the topic.

Another aspect of caring is working to ensure equity, diversity and inclusiveness for everyone in the health care system: providers, patients, families and our diverse communities as a whole. The goal is to have enough leaders of different backgrounds in the health system to understand and reflect the broad range of people it serves. LEADS can help with that by enabling leadership that is attentive to equity, diversity and inclusiveness. To guide us in that effort, we invited Dr. Ivy Bourgeault to offer her insights on linking equity, diversity and inclusiveness to the LEADS domains and capabilities [31]. Ivy's perspective is highlighted in each of the five domain chapters.

5. Sharing and Updating Our Curation of Health Leadership Literature

When we began this journey, there was only limited literature on leadership in the social sector overall and virtually none specifically about health care. Today, there is much more peer-reviewed and grey literature [18, 32–35]. Virtually all of the sources we quote in this edition were published in the past five years, a testament to how our understanding is growing of the critical role leadership plays in health care.

What Hasn't Changed: Enduring Ideas

While much has changed, the core values and beliefs of the LEADS framework remain. This edition, like the original, is still about helping all leaders better themselves and achieve better results by understanding the growing evidence in support of LEADS-based leadership development and talent management. It's based on the premise each of us is a leader and we are all CEOs of self. The book is intended to help you be a better leader, whatever age or stage you're at in your leadership journey and in whatever role you find yourself in health care.

What else remains unchanged? LEADS is still predicated on the belief leaders are both born and made. Everyone is born with some predisposition toward being able to lead and given the opportunity, can develop those innate talents through hard work, learning from experience and reflecting on what they learn. Both books show how through LEADS, you too can become the leader you want to be (Chaps. 4 and 5 are devoted to this theme).

Another returning idea is the fundamental belief that leadership is less a function of the power or authority (what's called hard power) you may have by virtue of your position, and far more a function of your influence inside and outside the formal hierarchy (soft power). In our view, those functions in modern health organizations and systems are threefold: one, to integrate service for patients and families; two, to create healthy and productive workplaces so people can deliver optimal service; and three, to successfully implement desired health reform policies and practices. These functions are, of course, interdependent but it is important to recognize them also as distinct.

Many prevailing ideas of leadership are artifacts from a bygone era when hierarchy, privilege, gender and restricted access to information determined who had power and who did not. To us, someone who uses authority without showing respectful, enabling behaviour may be less powerful than someone in an informal role who treats people with respect and supports their efforts. Barbara Kellerman makes this point eloquently in her book, *The End of Leadership* [36]. In this edition of our book, we recommend the use of self-directed learning tools to help you leverage your influence (see Chap. 4). For on line access to new LEADS-based tools please visit our website at: http://www.leadsglobal.ca/.

One of the most frequently asked questions over the past five years when we were speaking about LEADS was where's the leadership going to come from to transition health care into the twenty-first century? The answer is clear to us: it has to come from all of us. LEADS is designed to help you develop the capabilities you need to do your part to transform health care. Our hope—and the hope for the system—is this edition of LEADS will help you become the best leader you can be, developing your full potential to meet ever-changing leadership challenges.

Summary

Health leadership is vital for achieving the health care we need. Ensuring services are people-centred, creating healthy workplaces where providers can thrive and give their best care and reforming the systems that deliver that care are the job of leadership. All of us—formal and informal leaders, from diverse backgrounds and in different roles—must work together to get that job done. The LEADS framework is a guide to the leadership needed to do it.

Let's now look a little more closely at the inspiration behind LEADS and the phenomenon we call leadership, in Chap. 2.

References

1. Dickson G, Tholl B. Bringing leadership to life in health: LEADS in a caring environment. London: Springer; 2014.
2. Braithwaite J. Health reform in Australia: activity based funding, my health record, AI big data, nursing system. Tokyo: Canon Institute for Global Studies; 2018. https://www.canon-igs.org/event/report/180412_Braithwaite_presentation_part2_JP.pdf. Accessed 2 Sep 2019.
3. Chapter 2: Healthier Australians. Shifting the dial: 5 year productivity review. Canberra: Australian Government Productivity Commission; 2017. https://www.pc.gov.au/inquiries/completed/productivity-review/report. Accessed 2 Sep 2019.
4. The Health Foundation. About the Francis Inquiry; 2019. https://www.health.org.uk/about-the-francis-inquiry. Accessed 8 Aug 2019.
5. The NHS long term plan—a summary. London: NHS; 2019. https://www.longtermplan.nhs.uk/wp-content/uploads/2019/01/the-nhs-long-term-plan-summary.pdf. Accessed 2 Aug 2019.
6. People-centred care. London: Health Education England; 2019. https://www.hee.nhs.uk/our-work/people-centred-care. Accessed 2 Sep 2019.
7. Project Lift. Scotland: NHS; 2019. https://www.projectlift.scot/about/. Accessed 31 Jul 2019.
8. Simpson J. Chronic condition: why Canada's health care system needs to be dragged into the 21st Century. Toronto: Penguin Canada; 2012.
9. Cheifet B. Where is genomics going next? Genome Biol. 2019;20(1). https://genomebiology.biomedcentral.com/articles/10.1186/s13059-019-1626-2. Accessed 2 Sep 2019.
10. Cooper DN, Mitropoulou C, Brand A, Dolzan V, Fortina P, Innocenti F, et al. Chapter 10-The genomic medicine alliance: a global effort to facilitate the introduction of genomics into healthcare in developing nations. In: Lopez-Correa C, Patrinos GP, editors. Genomic medicine in emerging economies: genomics for every nation. London: Academic; 2018. p. 173–88.
11. Gregorich ZR, Ge Y. Top-down proteomics in health and disease: challenges and opportunities. Proteomics. 2014;14(10):1195–210.
12. Koriem KM. Proteomic approach in human health and disease: preventive and cure studies. Asian Pac J Trop Biomed. 2018;8(4):226–36.
13. Jiang F, Jiang Y, Zhi H, Dong Y, Li H, Ma S, et al. Artificial intelligence in healthcare: past, present and future. Stroke Vasc Neurol. 2017;2:e000101. https://doi.org/10.1136/svn-2017-000101.
14. Topol EJ. High-performance medicine: the convergence of human and artificial intelligence. Nat Med. 2019;25:44–56.
15. Cresswell K, Cunningham-Burley S, Sheikh A. Health care robotics: qualitative exploration of key challenges and future directions. J Med Internet Res. 2018;20(7):e10410.
16. Weber AS. Emerging medical ethical issues in healthcare and medical robotics. Int J Mech Eng Rob Res. 2018;7(6):604–7.

17. Naylor D, Girard F, Mintz J, Fraser N, Jenkins T, Power C. Unleashing innovation: excellent health care for Canada. Report of the advisory panel on health care innovation. Ottawa: Health Canada; 2015. http://tinyurl.com/qx2cf8z. Accessed 2 Aug 2019.
18. Peerrella A, McAiney C, Ploeg J. Rewards and challenges in caring for older adults with multiple chronic conditions: perspectives of seniors' mental health case managers. Can J Commun Ment Health. 2018;37(1):65–79.
19. Bégin M. Ladies, upstairs! Montreal: McGill-Queen's University Press; 2019.
20. Dickson G. Top ten reading series, Canadian Health Leadership Network; 2019. http://chlnet.ca/top-ten-reading-lists. Accessed 2 Sep 2019.
21. Canadian Health Leadership Network. Leadership development impact assessment toolkit. Ottawa: CHLNet; 2019. http://chlnet.ca/login with authorized username and password. Accessed 20 Aug 2019.
22. Jeyaraman M, SMZ Q, Wierzbowski A, Farshidfar F, Lys J, Dickson G, et al. Return on investment in healthcare leadership development programs. Leadersh Health Serv (Bradf Engl). 2018;31(1):77–97. https://doi.org/10.1108/LHS-02-2017-0005.
23. West M, Eckert R, Armit K, Loewenthal L, West T, Lee A. Leadership in health care: a summary of the evidence base. London: Faculty of Medical Leadership and Management, Center for Creative Leadership and the King's Fund; 2019. https://www.kingsfund.org.uk/sites/default/files/field/field_publication_summary/leadership-in-health-care-apr15.pdf. Accessed 5 Sep 2019.
24. National Health Services. Leadership development. Integrated urgent care/NHS 111 workforce blueprint. NHS England and Health Education England; 2019. www.england.nhs.uk/wp-content/uploads/2018/03/leadership-development.pdf. Accessed 9 Sep 2019.
25. Project Lift. Scotland: NHS. https://www.projectlift.scot/. Accessed 31 Jul 2019.
26. Canadian Health Leadership Network Breakfast Session. Does Canada have the leadership capacity to innovate? Benchmark 2.0. Toronto: National Health Leadership Conference; 2019. http://chlnet.ca/wp-content/uploads/NHLC-CHLNet-Breakfast-Session-2019-V02.pdf. Accessed 20 Aug 2019.
27. Assenova VA. Modeling the diffusion of complex innovations as a process of opinion formation through social networks. PLoS One. 2018;13(5):e0196699. https://doi.org/10.1371/journal.pone.0196699.
28. Senge P. The fifth discipline: the art and practice of the learning organization. New York: Random House; 2006.
29. Kleiner A, Senge PM, Roberts C. The fifth discipline fieldbook. Danvers, MA: Crown Publishing Group; 1994.
30. Edmonstone J. Developing leaders and leadership in health care: a case for rebalancing. Leadersh Health Serv (Bradf Engl). 2011;24(1):8–18.
31. Dr. Ivy Lynn Bourgeault, a Professor, University of Ottawa, is the Project Lead for an initiative aimed at improving diversity, equity and inclusion of women, indigenous women, and women of different ethnic backgrounds in health care. Empowering Women Leaders in Health. Ottawa: Canadian College of Health Leaders; 2019. https://www.cchl-ccls.ca/site/empowering_women. Accessed 2 Sep 2019.
32. Cikaliuk M. Pre-phase preliminary intelligence gathering report: LEADS in a caring environment capabilities framework. [unpublished research report]. Canadian Health Leadership Network and the Canadian College of Health Leaders: Ottawa; 2017.
33. Clay-Williams R, Ludlow K, Testa L, Li Z, Braithwaite J. Medical leadership, a systematic narrative review: do hospitals and healthcare organisations perform better when led by doctors? BMJ Open. 2017;7:e014474. https://doi.org/10.1136/bmjopen-2016-014474.
34. Pihlainen V, Kjvinen T, Lammintakanen J. Management and leadership competence in hospitals: a systematic literature review. Leadersh Health Serv (Bradf Engl). 2016;29(1):95–110. https://doi.org/10.1108/LHS-11-2014-0072.
35. Alilyyani B, Wong CA, Cummings G. Antecedents, mediators, and outcomes of authentic leadership in healthcare: a systematic review. Int J Nurs Stud. 2018;83:34–64.
36. Kellerman B. The end of leadership. New York: HarperCollins; 2012.

Illuminating Leadership and LEADS

2

Graham Dickson, Stewart Dickson, and Bill Tholl

> *Many people spend time studying the properties of animals, or herbs; how more important it would be to study those of people, with whom we must live or die.*
>
> Baltasar Gracian

The Foundations of Modern Leadership

Ancient Greece and Rome are famous for their leaders [1]; Chinese philosophers Lao Tzu, Confucius and Mencius all had thoughts on leadership [2]. Chanakya, an ancient Indian philosopher mused on leadership. Machiavelli's masterpiece of political philosophy *The Prince* is often quoted (rarely flatteringly) [3].[1] Shakespeare's

---

[1] In an interview with the *New York Times*, Pulitzer Prize–winning author Jared Diamond was asked which book he would require President Obama to read if he could. His answer? Niccoló Machiavelli's *The Prince*, written 500 years ago. He argued that while Machiavelli "is frequently dismissed today as an amoral cynic who supposedly considered the end to justify the means," he is, in fact, "a crystal-clear realist who understands the limits and uses of power."

Stewart Dickson, MA, is a Regional Treaty Negotiator (Skeena) for the Ministry of Indigenous Relations and Reconciliation, in the British Columbia Public Service. Stewart contributed to the writing, design, editing and voice of the chapter, and conducted research and interviews with key informants to support its ethnographic elements.

G. Dickson (✉)
Royal Roads University, Victoria, BC, Canada
e-mail: graham.dickson@royalroads.ca

S. Dickson
Ministry of Indigenous Relations and Reconciliation, Victoria, BC, Canada
e-mail: stewart.g.c.dickson@gmail.com

B. Tholl
Canadian Health Leadership Network, Ottawa, ON, Canada
e-mail: btholl@chlnet.ca

© Springer Nature Switzerland AG 2020
G. Dickson, B. Tholl (eds.), *Bringing Leadership to Life in Health: LEADS in a Caring Environment*, https://doi.org/10.1007/978-3-030-38536-1_2

plays examine power through the examples of individuals who strive for it [4]. The seventeenth century [5] Spanish philosopher Baltasar Gracián, who wrote this chapter's opening quote, was yet another writer on leadership.

In a rich tradition going back some 2500 years, the leadership styles of people ranging from Roman emperors to Vladimir Lenin, from Mahatma Gandhi to Margaret Thatcher, have been dissected at length. Much of this literature focuses on the "great man" model of leadership, where character is destiny [6].

However, such accounts fail to recognize the collective leadership of the many. In *War and Peace* Leo Tolstoy argued leadership from the unnamed masses was the engine of success, pointing out that historians give Napoleon credit for the success of the French army in Russia, but in reality, it was commanders and front-line soldiers who exercised the leadership needed to defeat the Russian army. Tolstoy captured that in this amusing vignette of the morning of a great battle:

> *Napoleon wakes up early on a misty summer morning and stands outside his tent, surveying the placement of his armies in the valley below. To his surprise, he sees a Russian regiment moving to flank a division of French troops. He immediately calls a senior general to his side, telling him to get on his horse and ride out to alert the French commander in the field of this maneuver. The general snaps a salute, saying "Of course, my emperor," and runs off to his horse. He quickly realizes the risks of carrying out the order: he could easily be shot delivering the message. So he grabs a bottle of wine and some baguettes, and heads out into the forest for a picnic. Two hours later, having rubbed dust and grime into his uniform, he rides his horse back into camp and says to Napoleon, "Message delivered, Sir!" In the meantime, the French commander in the field, having received intelligence from his sentries, responds to the Russian threat and defeats them as per Napoleon's plans* [7].

After thousands of years of contemplation and writing, there are numerous theories to explain leadership and how it works (see Appendix). Dinh and colleagues [8] described a number of these, including these traditional approaches:

- Trait theory seeks to identify the character traits of a successful leader.
- Behavioural theory posits that it's a leader's behaviour that allows him or her to be successful.
- Situational theory suggests the effectiveness of a leadership style depends on the goals of the organization at the time as well as the nature of the task presented to the leader.

Contextual leadership theories are similar to situational, describing leadership effectiveness as a function of how a leader's behaviour interacts with context. Some newer ideas academics are exploring include: authentic leadership, servant leadership, substitutes for leadership, spirituality and leadership, cross-cultural leadership, complexity leadership, abusive/toxic leadership, change leadership and e-leadership.

Work on LEADS has been informed by an awareness of all these theories and it's perhaps not surprising that since the first edition was released, we've often been told there's nothing fundamentally new about the LEADS framework: "I've heard this all before." Our response has been relief—we'd be concerned if something fundamental was missing. How those multiple theories of leadership come together in a modern, public service-oriented health system has been our first concern as we researched and defined how leadership is understood and put to work in practice through the LEADS framework.

This chapter reviews the understanding of leadership that underpins the LEADS framework and explores various contexts that shape our concept and definition of leadership and generate some of the philosophy behind the LEADS framework. We also use those concepts to define modern health leadership, the definition that gave rise to LEADS.

The Foundations of Leadership

Leadership has been likened to a fog: you can see it and feel it, but you can't grab hold of it. But if we can see it and feel it, why can't we define it? And if we can't define it, how can we possibly develop it?

Simpson and Jackson in their book *Teacher as Philosopher* [9] suggest one way of understanding the implicit meaning of a word is to examine its use in conventional talk, the day-to-day discourse of society. By looking at references to leaders and leadership in advertising slogans we get a sense of its meaning in private-sector discourse. Table 2.1 gives some examples:

Table 2.1 References to leaders and leadership in advertising slogans

Advertiser	Statement	Implied meaning
Cadillac	*The Penalty of Leadership; The Mark of Leadership* (one of the most famous print ads of all time, written in 1915)	Cadillac is the finest vehicle in the automotive world. As a consequence, Cadillac must deal with the pressure of expectations and the potential mean-spirited whispers from those who cannot measure up.
ESPN	*The World-Wide Leader in Sports*	ESPN is the most comprehensive, most polished, and most knowledgeable sports entertainment company. They are the experts.
Seiko Watch Company	*At the Leading Edge of Time*	Seiko is first in the field; its advancements are unequalled. The ad plays on the split-second requirements of competitive sport.
Toshiba	*Leading Innovation*	Toshiba is in the forefront of innovation, and sets standards others should aspire to.
SpecGrade LED	*Sustainable lighting leading the way in the fight against global poverty*	SpecGrade is helping community residents to reverse the cycles of poverty by providing low-cost sustainable lighting products. It sees what other manufacturers have not seen: the potential for using lighting to solve social issues.
Mercedes Benz	*Mercedes Benz Leadership goes beyond just staying ahead*	Mercedes Benz is visionary; not complacent. It's pushing boundaries.
Shell Ultra Helix	*Shell Ultra Helix is leading the way for a new standard in motor oil protection*	Hard working company at the cutting edge is producing new products meeting the highest standards of safety.

The ads are trading on several conventional beliefs about leaders and leadership:

1. *Leaders go first:* People who lead enter new territory—sometimes of thought, sometimes of action. They face challenges or uncertainties and take the initiative to address them.
2. *Leaders face uncertainty and danger:* Exercising initiative means taking risks; leaders have the courage to face them, and confidence in their ability to overcome them.
3. *Leaders have vision and can communicate it compellingly:* Leaders see things others don't, have information or understanding others lack and can engage people in sharing a vision.
4. *Leaders are capable and credible:* Leaders have substance and focus; they know their business and personify quality.
5. *Leaders innovate to provide service to clients:* Leaders are creative and find new solutions to old problems.
6. *Leaders have followers:* Leaders differentiate themselves from others and attract followers who share a willingness to shoulder the risk, initiate action or find a solution.

Learning Moment
Sometimes taking a risk is as simple as risking discomfort in changing one's own behaviour.

At one point one of your co-authors, Graham, was asked by a senior official of British Columbia's Ministry of Education to be its official representative to the BC Federation of Labour, the BC Business Council, and the BC Chamber of Commerce. I was flattered as the government of the time was promoting workplace learning and I was to facilitate their support for a new skills policy for Kindergarten—Grade 12 education.

I went back to my office and did my usual: read papers, researched what each of these organizations did, and planned what I would say when they approached me. I worked out strategies for engagement. However, after 2 weeks, no one from any of the organizations had contacted me or even acknowledged my new role.

"Sam," I said to the man who appointed me, "I don't think this is going to work. It's two weeks since you appointed me to this role and not one person has bothered to pick up the phone and call me." Sam looked at me over his glasses, took them off his head and waggled them at me. "Graham," he said, "Leaders cross the street first."

That was a blinding glimpse of the obvious: rather than reaching out to them I had waited for them to come to me. Given I am an introvert at heart I simply indulged my comfort zone. Taking a risk—in this case—was simply reaching out to make contact.

> **Reflective Questions**
> - Do you have default attitudes and behaviour? What are they?
> - How do they limit your ability to respond to some leadership challenges?
> - Can you think of some current situations where changing an aspect of your habitual behaviour might lead to a resolution?

Looking at how words are used in private-sector advertising doesn't capture every aspect of leadership and leaders; there are some different expectations and realities in public-sector leadership. Because Canada and other developed countries are multi-cultural societies, we looked at the use of the word *leadership* as it pertains to public service in a variety of cultures [10].

There are few accessible records of Canada's Indigenous peoples using the term leadership (in a literal translation), but the concept of leadership is well established. Popularly the notion of a leader is closely tied to that of an elder, someone whose wisdom about spirituality, culture and life is recognized and affirmed by the community [11]. Not all elders are old; sometimes the Creator chooses to imbue a young person with the wisdom of an elder. First Nations communities will normally seek the advice and assistance of elders on a wide range of issues. (We explore Indigenous health leadership in detail in Chap. 14.)

On the west coast of British Columbia, home to the Nisga'a peoples, formal leadership was traditionally held by a hereditary chief, or *Sim'oogit*. This position was passed on through matrilineal succession. From birth, future hereditary chiefs were taught leadership qualities, which were honour (personal integrity), respect (esteem for, or a sense of the worth or excellence of something), and compassion (tenderness, a desire to alleviate suffering). A *Sim'oogit* would also wear a headdress during sacred ceremonies as a reminder to "move with caution and purpose as [they] are a leader" [12]. It is interesting to note that in Nisga'a, the word to lead or chair an event is *diyee*, which captures the idea of guiding, or giving direction.

In Australia, Aboriginal and Torres Strait Islander peoples have different values and criteria for leadership than wider Australian society [13]. There are no words in the native language directly translatable to the English word, but their notions of governance speak to it: a leader is someone to whom other people listen, a person who can create consensus. Leadership is only conferred conditionally and has to be constantly earned. Leadership is also seen *as a process* rather than a position, with the leader on the same plane as those who confer authority on him or her through consensus.

In Hindi, the word for leadership is *netrtva*, pronounced *neh-tu*. It means to guide and exercise initiative. In Punjabi, the word leadership itself is used, direct from English. However, *pardhaan* is the word for leader in a temple. A *pardhaan* leads people in prayer and performs temple duties. Also, in Punjabi, a leader can be called a *surpanch*, which is an elected leader of a village. In traditional Chinese the characters for leadership are: 領導 [pronounced *ling dao*] meaning to direct, to shepherd and to guide. By putting a scroll with this word on the wall of your home, or office you are suggesting you are deliberately honing your leadership skills or hold a position of leadership.

In German, the word for leader is *fuhrer,* synonymous with guide, operator and pilot. In Italian, the word for leader is *capo* (from the Latin word *capit,* meaning head, also the root of the English word captain). The Italian word for leadership, *direzione,* is synonymous with giving direction and guidance, as well as management. In France, the word for leader is *chef*—meaning boss, overseer or superintendent.

It's notable that these multicultural examples capture the importance of guiding and offering wisdom—harkening to the type of leadership people want in a public-service context. They suggest a widespread foundation for Richard Lewis's contention "each society breeds the type of leader it wants, and expects him or her to keep to the path their age-old cultural habits have chosen" [14].

Other key ideas of leadership found in various cultures are:

1. *Service to the people:* In Nisga'a heritage, leaders alleviate suffering. In the indigenous cultures of Australia, leaders listen to the people. Captains and pilots guide others safely on journeys. Implicit in all is the ideal of compassionate, just, and fair service on behalf of others.
2. *Leaders are expected to have moral character:* Leadership qualities are described in terms of honour, respect, compassion, righteous self-esteem and a hard-working character.
3. *Leadership can be developed:* Young Nisga'a future leaders are taught leadership qualities from birth.
4. *Leaders have wisdom:* Implicit in the culture of First Nations is the belief in leading from a place of wisdom: that is, depth of understanding and humanness based on spirituality, culture and life, as affirmed by the community.
5. *Leaders are resilient:* Successful public-service leaders experience sudden shifts in political ideology. Having the inner strength to snap back from inevitable setbacks in advancing service to the public is essential.

Comparing public-service and private-sector concepts of leadership shows they share some attributes but differ on others. Both public- and private-sector leadership link to notions of initiative, foresight, excellence and professionalism, but the public sector definition of leadership does not include the element of risk that characterizes entrepreneurship valued in the private sector.

One other trend is obvious as well: in public-service leadership, the assumption that leadership qualities are genetic and passed on from one generation to the next has faded. For the most part, leaders must establish their own credentials, are elected to (or selected for) positions based on their ability to lead effectively and are held accountable—formally and informally. In today's world of instant social media judgment and feedback, leaders can be constantly under attack for perceived flaws—while people who are not in positions of power but possess natural leadership talent can exert enormous influence, enough sometimes that if a leader is ineffective, someone else will quickly be identified to do the job.

Let's look at how context can affect leadership.

Leadership and Context

Regardless of who a leader is, what will work is not only a function of their leadership behaviour, but also of situation, time, and circumstance. A leader's choice of self-, interpersonal or strategic leadership is not just a function of how he or she acts, but also the degree to which s/he interacts with the context in which the action is done. Recent theories of leadership increasingly focus on context as an important factor in leader effectiveness [15, 16].

Formal health leaders work in large, multi-level organizations or in some cases, larger systems (nation-wide, state-wide, or region-wide amalgams of organizations working together to create health and wellness). Different contexts demand a suite of different leadership actions and styles, customized to the unique situation and particular organization.

Context has two dimensions. The first is the structural context—the organization's design, size, scope, the leader's breadth of responsibility and role, time constraints. Barak Oc states "…characteristics of the task, team, organization, and social network as well as physical distance and time pressure play an important role in shaping the leadership outcomes, more so than the leadership process itself" [15, 16]. Health care leaders, then, must strive to know the multiple contexts in which a decision is made, and its potential impact on both individual contexts and the organization as a whole.

The second dimension of context is people—their emotion, energy, politics, team chemistry and organizational culture and climate. To address this dynamic Tse and colleagues [17] attempted to integrate how feelings and emotions of leaders and followers interact with people factors at five levels: self; between persons; interpersonal; team; and organizational levels. In our research [18], we learned health care leaders should constantly assess their own feelings and emotions, their impact on people with similar levels of responsibility, and on those with different levels of responsibility, on teams and on the organizational climate overall. Better strategic decisions result when leaders are armed with that information.

Let's look now at multiple aspects of context that will shape our definition of modern health leadership.

The Democratic Context

The context of modern democracy demands leadership that is exercised in a different way than it was thousands or even dozens of years ago. Below are some aspects of modern democracy that influence what kind of leadership is most likely to succeed:

- *A highly educated population:* Canada, the United Kingdom and Australia—like most developed nations—have the most educated populace they have ever had. Educated people want to exercise critical thinking, debate issues and use knowledge and evidence to make decisions.
- *The knowledge explosion:* Knowledge is growing at an exponential rate. Leaders don't need to search for knowledge, their task is to assess its truth, relevance and meaning.
- *Professionalism and expertise:* Leaders need to recognize the challenge of professionalism, which gives preferential credibility to a group's expertise and inclines members to be more influenced by their peers than their leaders.
- *Gender and cultural equity:* Women, as the #MeToo movement shows, are demanding the patriarchal power traditionally wielded by males be dismantled and replaced by leadership that is more caring. Indeed, we are now seeing a stepped-up effort initiated by the United Nations to engage more actively with the #HeForShe movement, enjoining men to not just be better mentors for women but also sponsors. Similarly, societies that might earlier have been ethnically monochrome are benefitting from a multiplicity of different cultures and traditions. The involvement of people from all cultures in leadership is vital to modern societies.
- *The revolution in communication technology:* In 2014, we wrote that we live in what Thomas Friedman calls a flatter, faster world, where information is almost universally available [19]. That's even more true today, as the explosion in social media use and the advent of bots sends information travelling at warp speed. Evidence suggests "when you are exposed to a given piece of information multiple times, your chances of adopting this information increase every time" [20].
- *Choice, customization and increased expectations:* There has been a dramatic growth in the choice of treatments in health care. Technological advancements and artificial or augmented intelligence (AI) make it possible to customize care, while public demand has complicated the choices health care leaders face and makes their decisions staggeringly more complex.

- *Economic capacity:* Since 2013, governments in Canada and abroad have been much more preoccupied with "bending the cost curve" of health care spending. Even though economic capacity has been marked by the longest bull market in decades and sustained growth from 2011 to time of publishing, stringent controls on health care expenditures have been maintained [21].
- *Politics of approval:* For two decades, reality shows have dominated prime-time television. One pundit has said we're so good at portraying reality on TV that audiences are hungering for "authentic" reality from their leaders.

These and other factors are why leadership is as stimulating as it is challenging, and different every day. Just as we explored tenets of leadership from a macro per-spective to better understand the impact of culture and context, it's important to consider the micro level as well: the organization you work in.

The Organizational Context: Leadership and Culture

Do our large and growing health delivery organizations have cultures that de-emphasize leadership and accept compliance? Max Shkud and Bill Veltrop, change architects and authors, contend that a major problem that organizations face today "is the widening gap between their existing leadership capacity and the exploding demands of our increasingly complex and rapidly changing world. To return to the computer metaphor, the 'old leadership operating system' is no longer able to keep up—to respond with sufficient agility and intelligence to the growing barrage of challenges and opportunities in the environment" [22].

Shkud and Veltrop have classified organizational culture based on the degree to which leaders and others distribute the qualities of leadership throughout the orga-nization's culture (see Fig. 2.1). The resilience scale on the right hand of Fig. 2.1 suggests that as you move from toxic organizational cultures to generative cultures, your resilience as individuals and organizations increases. In a volatile, uncertain, complex and ambiguous (VUCA) environment, the need for high levels of resil-ience is heightened.

Edgar Schein, an organizational development guru from MIT, defines cul-ture as "a pattern of basic assumptions invented, discovered, or developed by a given group as it learns to cope with its problems of external adaptation and internal integration…," or more simply, culture is "the way we do things around here" [23].

The primary determinant of an organization's culture is the formal leader's influ-ence on it [24]. A recent study found evidence that autocratic leadership at high levels in organizations makes it more likely managers further down in the hierarchy will behave similarly [25].

	Philosophy	Beliefs	Attitudes	Relationships	
Generative	Do for all in a way that best serves all	Organizations are consciously evolving social organisms	We are for each other *and* for the whole	Co-creative Evoking genius Mutually nourishing	+5
Sustainable	Do unto others as you would have them do unto you	Organizations are living systems	We are all in this together	Caring Appreciative High integrity	+3 +1

·········· **THE GREAT CULTURE CHASM** ··········

					+1
Compliant	Do unto others in a way that is fair	Ideal organization is a well oiled machine	You scratch my back...	Respectful Purposeful Honest	-1
Dysfunctional	Do it to others before they do it to you	People are the problem	I will use you	Disrespectful Dishonest Discounting	-3
Toxic	Do others in before they do you in	Might makes right	I will defeat you	Attacking Blaming	-5

Resilience Scale

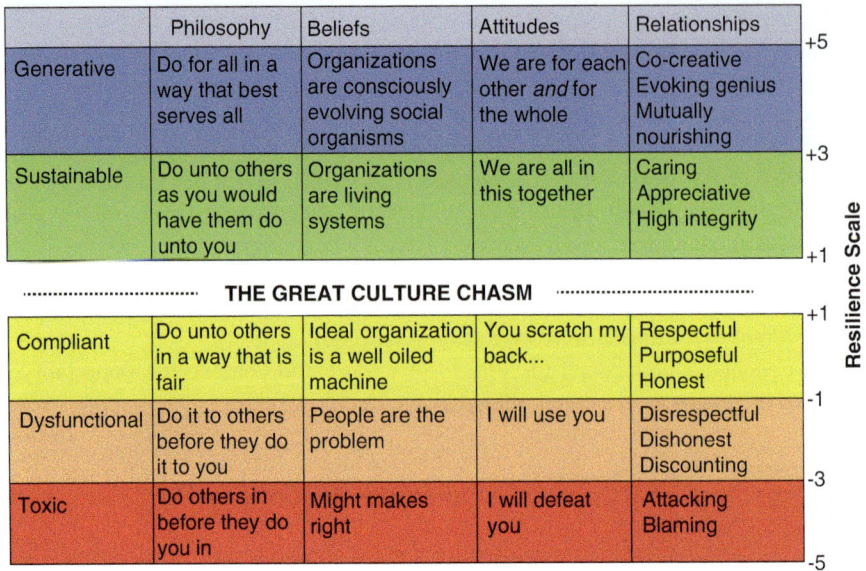

Fig. 2.1 Shkud and Veltrop [22]: A typology of organizational culture as a function of mores and distributed leadership

In Fig. 2.1 the bottom three cultures—toxic at the bottom, moving up through dysfunctional to compliant—emerge from a hierarchical and mechanistic structure, where leadership resides only in formal authority. The formal leader-follower power structure is accepted by leaders and followers alike.

The top two cultures progress from a sustainable culture—where the idea leadership is everyone's function is accepted, and organizational structures are adapted to that notion—to a generative culture, an ideal state in which formal and informal leaders co-create the future. Note the descriptions of compliant, sustainable and generative cultures reflect the sense of moral purpose we ascribe to LEADS: those three cultures are in line with high quality leadership practice.

We interpret the great culture chasm, shown in Fig. 2.1, as Shkud and Veltrop's name for the shift from compliant cultures, with formal leadership only, to cultures where leadership is shared by many. To be compliant is to obey rules and acquiesce—in other words, to be a follower. Indeed, health care's traditional top-down management model and heavily regulated operations have enforced followership, ensuring it's a learned characteristic.[2]

---

[2] Consider the number of compliance requirements in health care such as accreditation; clinical protocols; legal issues from patient/resident/client care, privacy, conflict of interest and possible/actual litigation, to labour and employment issues, workplace safety and the regulation of health care providers.

For that reason, the great culture chasm is a central factor in this book. When we encourage people at every level of an organization to develop their own leadership capabilities, we're asking them to overcome the huge gap between the behaviour and action of a follower (which is likely how they were trained) and behaving and acting in ways aligned with distributed leadership. It takes a significant mental, and cultural transition to move from being a well-trained follower to embracing leadership. It can be done: it takes courage.

The Need for More Courage

A recent study by Deloitte in Canada argues that the culture gap and the difficulty of transitioning from compliance to leadership is due to a lack of courage [26]. The study defines courage as "…doing the right thing—the hard thing—for the greater good, despite being filled with fear, doubt or uncertainty. Courage is taking a stand when it's difficult, not when it's easy."

Leading on behalf of health and wellness is the right thing, the hard thing, and to initiate and bring about significant reform requires courage. The Deloitte study says only 10 per cent of businesses in Canada are courageous. The leaders we revere in Canadian health care were courageous. If Tommy Douglas or Monique Begin had not made bold decisions, we would not have universal health insurance or a Canada Health Act. Today, however, it's not just political leaders who need to show courage, it's everyone working in health care.

Fear limits the ability to lead. Courage, coupled with confidence, hope and conviction must drive leadership and actions. The Deloitte study helps set the direction for those who wish to lead by identifying five elements for operationalizing courage:

1. *Start with yourself.* You can grow courage through deliberate action. What fears do you possess? Why? How might you mitigate them, overcome them?
2. *Do what is right.* Demand of yourself that your actions reflect your beliefs.
3. *Be provocative and challenge the status quo.* Champion meaningful reforms. Force yourself to speak up when naysayers block change.
4. *Take calculated risks.* Be a shi*f*t disturber: where the *f* stands for finesse. Grow your political skills.
5. *Unite to include.* Relationships are the true currency of leadership: talk with others, make inclusion a priority, and build through the power of networks.

Defining Leadership in Health

Now that we've touched on the long history of thought on leadership, and explored factors that shape it, it's time to talk about our definition of leadership, keeping the above notions in mind, as well as the multitudinous concepts and theories of leadership that abound in the academic literature [27].

The key ideas we've been exploring suggest leadership includes:

- taking initiative or going first and facing the risks that go with that;
- influencing through position, character or wisdom; and
- taking responsibility for pursuing a shared purpose or goal.

We've also discussed how leadership is a product of its context. All these factors feed into our definition of leadership in health: "*Leadership is the collective capacity of an individual or group to influence people to work together to achieve a common constructive purpose: the health and wellness of the population we serve.*" (First edition).

To further understand what our concept of leadership is, let's explore what it isn't.

What Leadership Isn't

Leadership is often assumed to reside in formal leadership or authority roles—that is, it's limited to managers and executives. While leadership has strong connections to administration and management, it's also a quality that can be found in anyone who rises to a challenge and uses his or her skills to engage others in solving the problem. Leaders need management and administration skills to solve problems, but those skills alone do not constitute leadership. Further, being appointed to an important job does not automatically endow someone with leadership qualities. A manager with excellent technical skills can still be unable to influence performance, build morale or drive change.

Another concept closely related to leadership is power. If the power differential between a formal leader and those he or she leads is great [28], the leader may be able to wield such authority over people that they have no option but to obey. There's no guarantee in a traditional hierarchy that power is exercised in the best interests of the people it serves. Hierarchical power also promotes a cultural belief that only those with formal authority can use judgment and make decisions; everyone else must simply follow.

That's why influence is a key word in our definition of leadership: it evokes a different type of power. Martin Luther King put it this way: "Power, properly understood, is the ability to achieve purpose…power is not only desirable but necessary in order to implement the demands of love and justice…power without love is reckless and abusive…" [29]. In contrast, our word for power with love is influence. The Oxford Dictionary defines influence as: "The capacity to have an effect on the character, development, or behaviour of someone or something, or the effect itself." As put by Kuhel, "There are two distinctive types of leadership. One is power or line authority and the other is influence… influence is consistently successful, while power wreaks havoc" [30].

In physics, power is the exercise of energy, the capacity to do work. In our definition of leadership, the work is getting people to work together on generating health and wellness. But getting people to work together, or to generate health and wellness are both moral enterprises in their own right, so leadership in health care is inherently moral.

When we were creating the LEADS framework, this principle of moral purpose guided how we expressed many of the domains and capabilities and led us to describe leadership that embraces caring as the foundation of its work.

Contrast this to Robert Greene's [5] description of power where leadership is amoral: some do what it takes to be a winner, for winning's sake. Greene goes so far as to say the exercise of power is a game, in which all humans strive for power over others, and feel worthless and miserable if they don't have it. In this struggle, he says, everything "must appear civilized, decent, democratic and fair. But if we play by those rules too strictly, if we take them too literally, we are crushed by those around us who are not so foolish." Greene argues no leader should ignore the idea that leadership is built on a worldview where winning or losing for personal gratification are the be all and end all. We disagree and think it's fundamentally important that health care leaders resist and rise above that kind of leadership.

Contrary to Greene's perspective, Martin Luther King said there is nothing essentially wrong with power, but as in law, the intent behind the use of power is crucial to its correctness. "The collision of immoral power with powerless morality constitutes the major crisis of our times" [30]. Health leaders need to recognize their intent in using power: What is motivating you? Whose interests are being served?

Finally, Greene offers a caution to those who believe, as we do, in caring leadership: appealing to people's better nature is a good guideline but won't work with everybody. There are people who are pathological and enter the world with one goal—to win the power game at all costs. Appealing to their better nature is interpreted by them as a weakness to be exploited. These leaders—narcissists, sociopaths—are the enemies of caring leadership.

They're also enemies to followers, because they are often "toxic" leaders who wield power like a personal weapon and create deeply unhealthy workplaces.

So just as management and power are often mistaken for leadership, it's important to understand leadership goes beyond exercising power and performing technical skills. In the following sections we will explore some of the central tenets that form the basis of this definition of leadership and how it's enacted through the LEADS Framework.

Self, Interpersonal and Strategic Leadership

Figure 2.2 shows three forms of leadership. The first is self leadership, beginning with looking inwards to know why you lead and then to act in concert with that

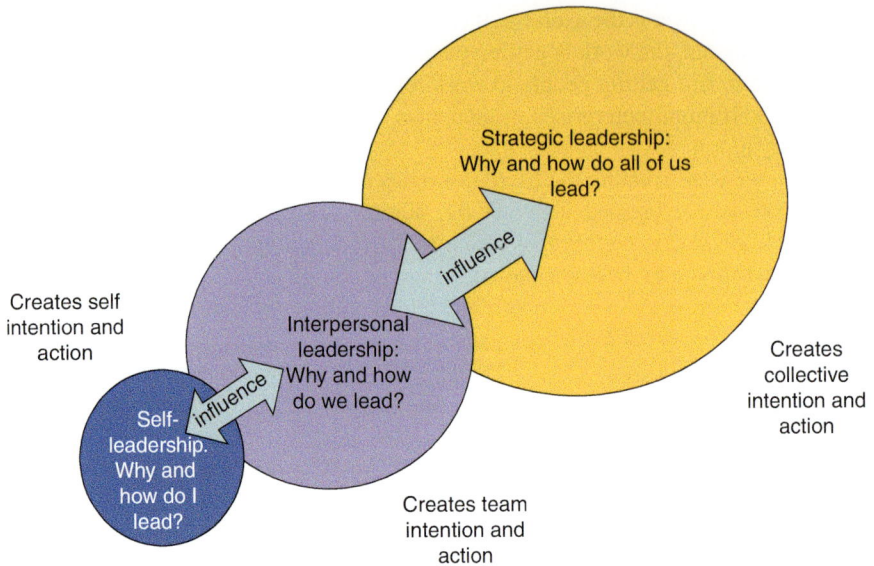

Fig. 2.2 Self, interpersonal and strategic leadership

motivation. Inner leadership is anchored by one's core values, attitudes and beliefs. The second is *interpersonal leadership*, exercising your influence by interacting directly with others. Interpersonal leadership is operational regardless of where the leader fits in the hierarchy or community.

The third, *strategic leadership,* refers to actions that shape the direction and efforts of people beyond the interpersonal orbit of the leader. Those actions can influence organizations or larger systems in which the organization sits. Laws, policies and clinical protocols are all expressions of strategic leadership. When personal, interpersonal and strategic leadership are aligned, the overall impact of leadership is magnified, making it easier to achieve both individual and organizational goals. When they are misaligned, significant energy and power can be wasted through friction between them.

True leadership is a flow of energy between leaders and followers. In self leadership, that flow is internal, starting with undertaking your worthiest challenge—leading yourself. As Bill Ury said in his most recent book *Getting to Yes With Yourself,* "…the better we are able to get to yes with ourselves, the better we will be able to get to yes with others" [31]. This concept links to the Lead self and Engage others domain of LEADS.

Leaders must act according to their values, beliefs, and moral purpose. When those are expressed through deliberate actions to affect structure or culture, energy will flow across the organization or system and encourage everyone to act in a manner consistent with both individual and collective purpose. These notions permeate the Achieve results, Develop coalitions and Systems transformation domains of LEADS. This is strategic leadership.

Distributed Leadership

In Chap. 1 we said leaders are different from others. Indeed, the others are described as "followers" in conventional language. This distinction implies a stratification of leaders and followers, which suggests a hierarchical organization, but if that's the case, how can we say leadership can come from anyone—patients, workers, politicians, the public?

We can say it because, you'll recall, our definition of leadership suggests it's a natural trait, which can be developed like abilities in athletics, painting, music or science. Second, research into leadership has defined it and helped make the knowledge and skills behind it clear so more people will be able to develop the skills to be effective leaders, particularly in a well-educated society. Third, because the complexity of health care has grown so significantly, no one person can have all the expertise needed to solve every problem and issue that emerges. That makes distributed (or shared) leadership essential for finding and implementing solutions.

But if leadership is distributed, and everyone can become a leader, who is a follower? In a distributed leadership model, no one person is always leader. Dr. John Van Aerde (author of Chap. 15) says effective followers and leaders are often the same people, playing different parts at different times. Sometimes a person in a formal leadership position must step back and let someone else lead, because they're the most appropriate person with the will and skill to do so.

The qualities that make effective followers are pretty much the same qualities found in effective leaders—demonstrating character, listening carefully, monitoring and evaluating progress as you go and serving the greater good. Leaders in organizations with distributed leadership engage others by engaging them in a problem where a novel solution, a fresh perspective, is needed.

Ultimately, if we believe social responsibility is a component of leadership, then the democratization of leadership in health organizations is inevitable. We can't assume, however, the transition from authoritative, hierarchical leadership to distributed leadership will be easy. Look at the following study that provides an example of putting LEADS to work:

> As part of a doctoral study, Kirsty Marles used the Health LEADS Australia framework to engage the leadership team of an extended care home in Adelaide to transition from traditional hierarchical leadership to distributed leadership.
> Much of the three-year transition was a process of sense-making, giving leaders the opportunity to talk about what the concepts inherent in distributed leadership mean, reflect on whether or not their learned leadership behaviour—what they called traditional leadership in a bureaucratic setting—was in fact an appropriate way to behave in light of their

growing understanding of distributed leadership, and then taking on the responsibility of changing that behaviour, which they found very challenging to do.

The study documents the team's struggles and demonstrates that shifting from traditional models of hierarchical, top-down leadership to a shared model is a very difficult mental process [32].

Summary

The concept of leadership is undergoing a fundamental transformation in our wired world. Based on both the literature and the use of the word leadership in common language, and within the work of healthcare, we defined health care leadership as: *the collective capacity of an individual or group to influence people to work together to achieve a common constructive purpose: the health and wellness of the population we serve."* And in keeping with Chap. 1, health leadership has three functions. They are to integrate service for patients and families, create healthy and productive workplaces so people can deliver optimal service and successfully implement health reform policies and practices.

Leadership has a moral imperative that must be reflected in both the means and ends of its action. That moral imperative also dignifies the construct of distributed leadership, whereby influence and power is shared amongst many rather than exercised by few. We postulate that leadership plays out in three different arenas of action: personal leadership (leading self), interpersonal leadership (leading others in your span of direct contact) and strategic leadership (leading large departments, organizations, or systems).

The responsibility for new and better leadership is therefore everybody's business, throughout the health system and over the lifecycle of a leader. Increased complexity has created the demand for a common vocabulary of leadership—which is what LEADS offers. It also demands inherent courage in putting LEADS to work, which is the substance of this second edition.

That was the goal of the LEADS project when it began. Through reading this book, by adopting LEADS as your leadership vocabulary and using personal mastery as your approach to development, you can realize your potential as a modern health leader. By then putting LEADS into practice—as those profiled in the vignettes and personal stories in this book have done—you can find the courage needed to truly change your health system for the benefit of the patients, families and citizens you serve.

Appendix: Leadership Theories

This appendix contains short one or two sentence descriptions of the leadership theories most mentioned in recent literature and referenced in Chap. 2. Theories are categorized by theme and by the frequency they were referenced in the literature (adapted from Dinh et al., 2014 [33]). The theories are presented in two categories: *Established Theories*; and *Emerging Theories*. Only the theories with greater than 4% of the total frequency of mention are described in this Appendix.

Category: Established Leadership Theories

Sub-category	Theory	% Frequency	Description
Neo-charismatic theories		39	*Neo-charismatic* theories are those that pertain to attributes of leadership that engage followers in a variety of ways that include emotional bonding, agreement on task, and visioning a future. These sets of theories are based on the emotional appeal of the leaders and the extraordinary commitment of the followers. It encourages leaders and followers to become aware of their own personality types and of the people around them in order to be more effective in their workplace. The weakness of this approach is that there are few skills to learn
	Transformational leadership	20	*Transformational leadership* theory is about how leaders inspire followers by transcending their own self-interests for the good of the organization. Transformational leadership is defined as a process in which a leader increases followers' awareness of what is right and important to motivate followers to exceed performance expectations. Four important characteristics of transformational leadership include: effective communication, inspirational traits, trustworthiness, and teamwork
	Charismatic leadership	10	*Charismatic leadership* theory says that followers make attributions of heroic or extraordinary leadership abilities when they observe certain behaviors from the leader
	Transactional leadership	5	*Transactional leadership* theory posits that leaders involve, motivate and direct followers primarily through appealing to their own self-interest. The power of transactional leaders comes from their formal authority and responsibility in the organization. The main goal of the follower is to obey the instructions of the leader

Sub-category	Theory	% Frequency	Description
Leadership and Information Processing		26	***Leadership and information processing*** theories pertain to cognitive approaches to information processing and decision making processes in leadership including attribution theories, leader and follower cognitions (e.g., perceptions), the connectionist approach, and implicit leadership theories. This thematic category also answers questions like "what do I think leadership means?" and "what do I think is important" in being an effective leader?
	Leader and follower cognition	13	***Leader and follower cognition*** theory posits that leadership is determined by the mental models of both leaders and followers. It suggests that these mental structures are built up in part from experience; and by exploring these cognitive models we can understand how leaders and followers can work together better
	Implicit leadership	7	***Implicit leadership*** theory is a cognitive theory based on the idea that individuals create cognitive representations of the world and use these preconceived notions to interpret their surroundings and control their behaviours. These assumptions guide an individual's perceptions and responses to leaders. The term implicit is used because they are not outwardly stated and the term theory is used because it involves the generalization of past experiences to new experiences
	Attribution theories	4	***The attribution*** theory of leadership suggests that a leader's judgment about his employees (or the follower's judgment of the leader) is influenced by their attribution of the causes of the other individual's performance. Attribution theory attempts to explain behaviours by indicating a cause. More specifically the theory looks at how the leader or follower assesses the meaning of a particular event based on the motives for finding the cause as well as his or her understanding of the environment

Sub-category	Theory	% Frequency	Description
	Information processing and decision making	3	*The information processing and decision making* theory suggests that how leaders process information and their personality are both related to leadership effectiveness, and the relationship is moderated by leader behavior. In this theory, leaders, process information by two interacting, bi-directional systems; that is, the rational (analytical) and experiential (intuitive) systems, and the outcome influences how followers interpret events, make decisions, behave, and feel
Social Exchange/ Relational Leadership Theories			*Social exchange* theories of leadership say that human relationships and social behavior are rooted in an exchange process. In any leader-follower relationship, people weigh the risks and rewards. When those relationships become too risky for either leader or follower, the ability of the leader to influence the follower diminishes accordingly
	Leader-member exchange (LMX)	21	The *leader–member exchange (LMX)* theory is a relationship-based approach to leadership that focuses on the two-way relationship between leaders and followers. It suggests that leaders develop an exchange with each of their subordinates, and that the quality of these leader–member exchange relationships influences subordinates' responsibility, decisions, and access to resources and performance
	Relational leadership	4	*Relational leadership* theory focuses on the idea that leadership effectiveness has to do with the ability of the leader to create positive relationships within the organization. This theory suggests that the leader acknowledges the diverse talents of group members and trust the process to bring good thinking to the socially responsible changes group members agree they want to work toward

Sub-category	Theory	% Frequency	Description
Dispositional/ Trait Theories		20	***The Dispositional/Trait Theories*** category includes theories that looked at individual differences in leaders and investigated specific traits, abilities or clusters of abilities that contribute to leadership effectiveness. It includes the traditional trait approach, as well as other newer approaches, i.e., nature of managerial traits, managerial attributes, skills and competence, situational relevance of skills, and leader motive
	Trait theories	16	***Trait*** leadership theories aim to outline integrated patterns of personal characteristics that reflect a range of individual differences inn leaders; and yet foster consistent *leader* effectiveness across a variety of group and organizational situations
Leadership and Diversity		11	The focus of the ***Leadership and Diversity*** category is on domestic and cross-cultural issues of leadership
	Leadership and diversity	7	***Leadership and Diversity*** theories investigate the experiences of women and minorities in leadership positions, and of diverse followers within domestic borders, e.g., the benefits of more women leaders, the challenges facing women in leadership roles
	Cross-cultural leadership	4	The ***cross-cultural leadership*** thematic category includes articles comparing the leadership processes of one culture to another; or looking at leadership in non-US populations to discern if European/US leadership theories applied in such settings/culture, country & attributes of leadership, universality, cultural & institutional changes, differences in Leadership across cultures, leadership in the multinational firm, and the GLOBE Project
Follower- Centric Leadership Theories		9	***Follower-centric leadership*** theories prioritize the follower in the leader–follower pairing
	Followership theories	7	***Followership theories:*** Specifically, this sub-category includes research that investigate follower attributes related to the leadership process (e.g., identity, motivation, and values), the active roles follower play in leader–follower dynamics, romance of leadership, and follower outcomes

Sub-category	Theory	% Frequency	Description
Behavioural Theories		8	The ***behavioural leadership*** theories sub-category focuses on research into the nature and consequences of participative, shared leadership, delegation, empowerment of leadership, studies on task-oriented behavior and initiating structure, and people or relations-oriented and individualized consideration behavior, critical incidents, the high-high leader, leadership behavior taxonomies, and specific task behaviors
	Participative, shared leadership: delegation and empowerment	5	***Participative, shared leadership*** theories include ***distributed*** leadership and ***collective*** leadership. Shared leadership practice is not related to the knowledge and skills of only one leader, but a participative perspective in which individuals and situations interact with each other. The important part in shared leadership is not the formal position or role of individuals, but their knowledge and competencies regarding the topic. In ***distributed*** leadership, individual expertise is the central concept: collective work as well as collective learning by working on goals through communication and interaction is prominent, rather than individual work
	Leadership skills/ competence	4	The ***leadership skills/competence*** approach takes into account the knowledge, skills and abilities that the leader has. A leader can learn certain skills and/or competencies and become more effective. The focus is on the leader him or herself, rather than the situation or context; although this theory may encompass situational variety in determining what skills are needed. More recent literature emphasizes the concept of capabilities: bundles of competencies that must adapt to situation and circumstance

Sub-category	Theory	% Frequency	Description
Contingency Theories		7	The ***contingency theory*** sub-category encompasses research into how the here the leader adjusts to the situation or adjusts the situation to fit him- or herself. This included the Lease Preferred Co-worker (LPC) contingency model, path-goal theory of leadership, leadership substitution theory, situational leadership theory, multiple linkage model, cognitive resources theory, applications for adaptive leadership, life cycle theory of leadership, and normative decision model, and flexible leadership theory
,	No one theory received more than 1% mention		***Other theories*** include: path and goal theory, situational leadership theory; contingency leadership theory, leader-substitute leadership theory, etc.
Power and Influence of leadership		7	The focus of the ***power and influence*** thematic category is on the concepts of power and influence, power types and sources, consequences of position and personal power, impression management and influence, coding scheme tactics, and political skills. The focal level of analysis for these influence and political tactics is dyadic, group and organizational as opposed to institutional, regional, and societal
	Power and influence of leadership	4	The ***power and influence of leadership*** approach explores the practice of power and influence, considers different leader frames of reference that affect how leaders think about and use power, looks at some sources and types of power, and outlines ways leaders exercise power and influence
	Political theory and influence tactics of leadership	3	The ***political theory and influence tactics of leadership*** research explores how leaders in a formal political context exercise power and influence through political activity

Category: Emerging Leadership Theories

Sub-category	Theory	% Frequency	Description
Strategic Leadership		24	*The strategic leadership* sub-category addresses leadership phenomena at the highest levels of organizations and how executive leaders influence organizational performance. The focal level of analysis involves CEO or other top leader and/or top-management teams (TMT) at the upper echelon levels of the organization
	Strategic/top executive	12	*Strategic/top executive* topics include constraints on executives, top management teams and leadership succession, conditions affecting the need for strategic leadership, and effects of CEO leadership
	Upper echelons theory	9	*Upper Echelons* theory explores how top executives' thoughts, intellectual constructs and values influence how they come to understand their environments; and how this understanding then influences strategic decisions and organizational performance
	Public leadership	3	The *public leadership* focus includes research on public leadership, e.g., president, professional politicians, as they direct large bureaucracies, determine strategy, and are commonly viewed as reasons for success or failure of public initiatives in parallel with their corporate counterparts
Team Leadership		15	*The team leadership* sub-category includes research where teams were the primary focus, or the articles attempted to apply one or more leadership theories to team settings in a novel fashion. The focal level of analysis involves teams and groups at the mid- and lower-level echelons of the organization
	Leadership in team and decision groups	15	Topics encompassed by *leadership in team and decision groups theory* include the nature of leadership in different types of teams, determinants of team performance, procedures for facilitating team learning, guidelines for team building, and leadership function in decision making in groups

Sub-category	Theory	% Frequency	Description
Contextual theories of leadership		15	***The contextual leadership theories*** sub-category addresses leadership in specific context arenas. Social network and integrative perspectives of leadership were also included
	Contextual theories of leadership	6	***Contextual leadership*** theories explore the mediating effect of context such as the national context; function context—e.g., military, health or education setting; and discrete organizational context, and how leadership practices often are constrained by contextual variables (i.e., period of time in organizational processes) and singular events or circumstances
	Social network theories of leadership	4	The ***social network*** theories of leadership explore the contribution of multiple actors and bidirectional influence (top-down and bottom-up) that unfolds along different time scales (from minutes to years). Social network theory emphasizes inter-personal networks as both cognitive structures in the minds of organizational members and opportunity structures that facilitate and constrain leadership understanding and successful action
Complexity and systems leadership theories			***The complexity and systems*** sub-category encompass catastrophe or complexity theory, with the concept of complex adaptive systems (CAS) and encompassed how complexity theory was useful in describing how leaders can be successful in turbulent environments
	Complexity theories of leadership	3	***Complexity theories of leadership*** are based upon the application of complexity theory to the study of organizational behavior and the practice of leadership. In essence, complexity theory is about (1) the interaction dynamics amongst multiple, networked agents, and (2) how emergent events—such as creativity, learning, or adaptability—arise from these interactions. Leadership as mediated and practised by the influence of these factors is the substance of complexity leadership

Sub-category	Theory	% Frequency	Description
Leader Emergence and Development		14	*The leader emergence and development* sub-category is focused on research that prescribed or described pathways or processes by which leaders came to possess leadership capacity, follower recognition of leadership status, and a systems perspective of leadership. Specific topics include leadership training programs, designing effective training, specific techniques of leadership training, learning from experience, developmental activities, self-help activities, facilitating conditions for leadership development, development and identification of leaders, and leadership assessment, appraisal and selection
	Leadership development	9	**Leadership development** theories explore the processes that lead to the expansion of a person's capacity to be effective in leadership roles and processes. It takes two forms: individual leader development; and leadership development, which is the expansion of a one's ability to be effective in leadership roles and processes
	Leadership emergence	5	*Leader emergence* theory concerns itself with how a group member emerges and maintains a leadership position within a group or organization; not necessarily as a function of formal position. The individual acquires emergent leadership through the support and acceptance of other people in the organization and it is the "emergent leader" who is most respected and most followed in any leadership setting
Ethical/Moral Leadership Theories		11	*This ethical/moral* sub-category encompasses leadership theories that have in common a core focus on altruistic behaviour as a foundation for effective leadership
	Authentic leadership theory	4	*Authentic leadership* theory describes leaders who are self-aware, process positive and negative ego-relevant information in a balanced fashion, achieve relational transparency with close others, and are guided in their actions by an internalized moral perspective. The theory emphasizes building the leader's legitimacy through honest relationships with followers which value their input and are built on an ethical foundation

Sub-category	Theory	% Frequency	Description
	Ethical leadership theory	3	***Theories of ethical leadership*** investigate leader moral priorities, including how an ethical orientation toward leadership is developed; how an ethical approach to leadership is important; the consequences of ethical leadership and how it can be sustained.
Leading for Creativity, Innovation and Change		9	The ***leading for creativity, innovation and change*** sub-category investigated creative leadership processes from a variety of perspectives, covering topics like innovation and organizational learning. Research in this thematic sub-category also dealt with leader's roles in organizational change, or larger social changes in society or government, e.g., developing a vision, implementing changes, and influencing organizational culture. These changes were spurred by direct or indirect actions of leaders
	Leading for creativity and innovation	5	***Leading for creativity and innovation*** theories emphasize the use of innovation theory and creativity processes in the practice of leadership. Tangential theories are authentic, complexity, abusive, transformational, organizational change, shared and team leadership
	Leading organizational change	3	***Leading for organizational change*** theories focus on how leaders can unleash the potential of systems and people to adjust and adapt in ways that successfully address the needs of a shifting environment. Topic areas include leadership and ambidexterity, dynamic capabilities, innovation, and paradox and tension. They are also tangential to theories on complexity, leadership and networks, and collective leadership
Identity-Based Leadership Theories		8	***The identity-based*** sub-category of theories includes self-concept and social identity approaches to leadership, i.e., studies adopting the work on leader categorization theory and studies adopting other social identity and self-concept frameworks

Sub-category	Theory	% Frequency	Description
	Social identity theory of leadership	4	***Social identity theory*** describes the emergence of a leader as being based on a group member's resemblance to a prototypical leader as determined by other group members. Leadership is perceived as a group process generated by social categorization and prototype-based depersonalization processes associated with social identity
	Identity and identification process theories of leadership	4	***Identity and identification process*** theories of leadership posit that leaders are perceived in an organizational setting as leaders through a process of mutual influence in which social interaction among individuals as well as contextual factors cause leader and follower identities to shift over time and across situations. Leader identities are constructed through individuals projecting an image as a leader and others mirroring back and reinforcing that image as legitimate
Other		13	A potpourri of ***other individual theories*** is found in the research literature. Two that are profiled here are emotions and leadership; and destructive/abusive/toxic leadership
	Emotions and leadership	8	***The emotions and leadership*** construct encompass leaders' and followers' affect, and a variety of influences that emotions, positive and negative, have at all levels of leadership both on the leader and follower
	Destructive/ abusive/toxic leadership	3	***Destructive/abusive/toxic theories*** encompass cases where leaders misbehaved, acted in ways contrary to the well-being of followers and/or the organization, and the setting where they were leaders, including abusive leadership, toxic leadership, and followers' susceptibility and destructive followership as well

References

1. Forsyth PY. Pericles and Augustus: Ancient Leadership. [Internet]. 2019 [cited 2019 18 Sept]. https://uwlabyrinth.uwaterloo.ca/labyrinth_archives/pericles.html.
2. Creel H. Chinese thought from Confucius to Mao Tse-Tung. New York: Mentor Books; 1960.
3. O'Rourke J. Machiavelli's *The Prince*: still relevant after all these years [Internet]. BU Today; 2013 Jan 6 [cited 2013 Aug]. http://www.bu.edu/today/2013/machiavelli-the-prince-still-relevant-after-all-these-years/.
4. Corrigan P. Shakespeare on management: leadership lessons for today's managers. London: Kogan Page; 1999.
5. Greene R. The 48 laws of power. New York: Penguin Books; 2018.
6. Heraclitus. [Internet]. Wikiquote. 2019 [cited 2019 Sept 9]. https://en.wikiquote.org/wiki/Heraclitus.
7. Tolstoy L. War and peace. Oxford: Oxford University Press; 2010.
8. Dinh J, Lord R, Gardner W, Meuser J, Liden R, Hu J. Leadership theory and research in the new millennium: current theoretical trends and changing perspectives. Leadersh Q. 2014;25(1):36–62.
9. Simpson D, Jackson M. Teacher as philosopher. Agincourt, ON: Methuen; 1984.
10. Dickson S. Ethnographic perspectives on leadership [unpublished working paper]. 10 Sept 2011.
11. Joseph R, Joseph C. Working effectively with aboriginal peoples. North Vancouver: Indigenous Corporate Training Inc; 2007.
12. Nyce A. Nisga'a Cultural Advisor, panel text. Toronto: Royal Ontario Museum, Gallery of First Nations Art; 2019.
13. Aboriginal and Torres Strait Islander leadership [Internet]. Indigenous Governance Toolkit. [Internet] c2019. [cited 2019 Dec 21]. https://toolkit.aigi.com.au/.
14. Lewis RD. When cultures collide: leading across cultures; a major new edition of the global guide. Brealey: Boston, MA; 2015.
15. Oc B. Contextual leadership: a systematic review of how contextual factors shape leadership and its outcomes. Leadersh Q. 2018;29(1):218–35. https://doi.org/10.1016/j.leaqua.2017.12.004.
16. Dickson G. Leadership theory as a driver of executive leadership practice in healthcare. In: Raz M, Loh E, editors. Cases for health executives: the principles of practice. Melbourne: Taylor and Francis Group; 2019–2020 (Forthcoming).
17. Tse H, Troth A, Ashkanasy N, Collins A. Affect and leader-member exchange in the new millennium: a state-of-art review and guiding framework. Leadersh Q. 2018;29(1):135–49. https://doi.org/10.1016/j.leaqua.2017.10.002.
18. Dickson G, Tholl B, Baker, GR, Blais R, Clavel, N, Gorley C, et al. Partnerships for health system improvement, leadership and health system redesign: cross-case analysis. Ottawa: Royal Roads University, Canadian Health Leadership Network, Canadian Institutes of Health Research, Michael Smith Foundation for Health Research [Internet]; 2014 [cited 2019 Aug 22]. http://tinyurl.com/qh6ogzu.
19. Friedman T. The world is flat: a brief history of the twenty-first century. New York: Picador; 2007.
20. Xinxuanet. New study reveals how information spreads on social media. Xinhua [Internet]. Sept 2017 [cited 1 August 2019]. http://www.xinhuanet.com//english/2017-09/25/c_136634636.htm.
21. Organization for Economic Cooperation and Development. Health spending statistics. OECD [Internet]. 2019 [cited 2019 Sept 9]. https://data.oecd.org/healthres/health-spending.htm.
22. Shkud M, Velrop B. Hack: project 10X: a game-changing approach to growing 21st Century 'leadership everywhere'. M-Prize [Internet]. 2019 [cited 2019 Sept 9]. http://www.mixprize.org/hack/project-10x-growing-dna-21st-century-leadership-organizations?challenge=14226.
23. Schein EH. Organizational culture and leadership. 2nd ed. San Francisco: Jossey-Bass; 1992.
24. Buckingham M, Coffman C. First, break all the rules. New York: The Gallup Organization, Simon and Schuster; 1999.

25. Harms PD, Wood D, Landay J, Lester PB, Lester GV. Autocratic leaders and authoritarian followers revisited: a review and agenda for the future. Leadersh Q. 2018;29:105–23.
26. Deloitte. The future belongs to the bold. Toronto: Deloitte Canada [Internet]; 2018 [cited 2019 Aug 1]. https://www.canada175.ca/en/research/the-future-belongs-to-the-bold.
27. Yukl G. Leadership in organizations. 6th ed. New Jersey: Prentice Hall; 2006.
28. Meyer E. The culture map: breaking through the invisible boundaries of global business. New York: Public Affairs; 2014.
29. King ML Jr, Carson C, editors. The autobiography of Martin Luther King, Jr. New York: Grand Central Publishing; 1998.
30. Kuhel B. Power vs. influence: knowing the difference could make or break your company. Boston: Forbes Coaches Council, Council Post [Internet]; 2017 Nov 2 [cited 2019 Aug 1]. https://www.forbes.com/sites/forbescoachescouncil/2017/11/02/power-vs-influence-knowing-the-difference-could-make-or-break-your-company/#2e9e0d9a357c.
31. Ury W. Getting to yes with yourself. New York: HarperCollins; 2015.
32. Marles K. Distributed leadership: building capacity to maximise collaborative practice in a new teaching research aged care service, DBA [thesis]. Freemantle (AUS): University of Notre Dame; 2017.
33. Dinh J, Lord R, Gardner W, Meuser J, Liden R, Hu J. Leadership theory and research in the new millennium: current theoretical trends and changing perspectives. Leadersh Q. 2014;25(1):36–62.

The LEADS in a Caring Environment Capabilities Framework: The Source Code for Health Leadership

3

Graham Dickson and Bill Tholl

> *Leadership is the art of accomplishing more than the science of management says is possible.*
>
> Colin Powell [1]

Leadership isn't management and it's not administration. It's energy, influence, perseverance, resiliency, dedication, strategy and execution—applied in the real world of people to create change. As Colin Powell said, "Leadership is the art of accomplishing more than the science of management says is possible." [1].

The ever-more complex challenges facing modern health systems demand sophisticated leadership. That leadership—as we defined it in Chap. 2—is *the collective capacity of an individual or group to influence people to work together to achieve a common constructive purpose: the health and wellness of the population we serve.* The LEADS in a Caring Environment Capabilities Framework—the focus of this chapter—is the evidence-based translation of that definition into action: what leaders do to respond to these challenges.

G. Dickson (✉)
Royal Roads University, Victoria, BC, Canada
e-mail: graham.dickson@royalroads.ca

B. Tholl
Canadian Health Leadership Network, Ottawa, ON, Canada
e-mail: btholl@chlnet.ca

© Springer Nature Switzerland AG 2020
G. Dickson, B. Tholl (eds.), *Bringing Leadership to Life in Health: LEADS in a Caring Environment*, https://doi.org/10.1007/978-3-030-38536-1_3

LEADS in a Caring Environment

The source code of life is the DNA molecule. Each molecule comprises a common set of nucleotides but combines them in unique ways to produce all the proteins in the human body and create the unique characteristics of each of us. So it is with the LEADS framework in the world of health leadership: its 5 domains, each with 4 capabilities, are the source code of leadership, able to be combined in endless permutations or combinations to respond to the changing circumstances, external pressures and people involved in each situation a leader faces. The framework is outlined below (Fig. 3.1).

Lead self: Self-motivated leaders...

Are self-aware:
- Aware of their assumptions, values, principles, strengths and limitations

Manage themselves:
- They take responsibility for their own performance and health

Develop themselves:
- They actively seek opportunities and challenges for personal learning, character building and growth

Demonstrate character:
- They model qualities such as honesty, integrity, resilience, and confidence

Engage others: Engaging leaders...

Foster development of others
- They support and challenge others to achieve professional and personal goals

Contribute to the creation of healthy organizations
- They create engaging environments where others have meaningful opportunities to contribute and ensure that resources are available to fulfill their expected responsibilities

Fig. 3.1 The LEADS in a Caring Environment capabilities framework [2]

Communicate effectively

- They listen well and encourage open exchange of information and ideas using appropriate communication media

Build teams

- They facilitate environments of collaboration and co-operation to achieve results

Achieve results: *Goal-oriented leaders…*

Set direction

- They inspire vision by identifying, establishing and communicating clear and meaningful expectations and outcomes

Strategically align decisions with vision, values and evidence

- They integrate organizational missions, values and reliable, valid evidence to make decisions

Take action to implement decisions

- They act in a manner consistent with the organizational values to yield effective, efficient public-centred service

Assess and evaluate

- They measure and evaluate outcomes. They hold themselves and others accountable for the results achieved against benchmarks and correct the course as appropriate

Develop coalitions: Collaborative leaders…

Purposefully build partnerships and networks to create results

- They create connections, trust and shared meaning with individuals and groups

Demonstrate a commitment to customers and service

- They facilitate collaboration, cooperation and coalitions among diverse groups and perspectives aimed at learning to improve service

Mobilize knowledge

- They employ methods to gather intelligence, encourage open exchange of information, and use quality evidence to influence action across the system

Fig. 3.1 (continued)

Navigate socio-political environments

- *They are politically astute. They negotiate through conflict and mobilize support.*

Systems Transformation: *Successful leaders...*

Demonstrate systems/critical thinking
- They think analytically and conceptually, questioning and challenging the status quo, to identify issues, solve problems and design and implement effective processes across systems and stakeholders

Encourage and support innovation

- They create a climate of continuous improvement and creativity aimed at systemic change

Orient themselves strategically to the future

- They scan the environment for ideas, best practices, and emerging trends that will shape the system

Champion and orchestrate change

- They actively contribute to change processes that improve health service delivery.

Fig. 3.1 (continued)

Caring

Our research, reinforced since the release of the first edition, is unequivocal: the essence of effective health leadership is the ability to care for the health and well-being of others. The common thread that unites people who work in health care—administrators, physicians, nurses and the thousands of other health and social service professionals working in the system—is caring about the health and well-being of others. For a health provider, caring means delivering the best service with compassion, respect, and empathy. For the leader, it means creating a physically and psychologically safe environment for your team, caring for yourself, and acting in ways in which caring shines through every day. Caring is the *why* of leadership in health care.

However, caring alone does not make an effective leader. Just like clinicians, who if they care too much for others can end up not enough caring for themselves, a leader can develop what is known as compassion fatigue [3], a combination of burnout and secondary traumatic stress in the workplace. One study showed that compassion fatigue inhibits nurses' ability to foster the caring behaviour necessary for optimum patient outcomes. Look what one leader did to counteract compassion fatigue, for herself and her nurse colleagues:

Putting LEADS to Work: Caring in Action

Nurses and doctors are renowned for their commitment to caring. Caring was what nursing was all about for Dorothy, a nurse leader. It was why she went into nursing; it was why she remained in nursing.

She began to wonder why nurse's caring had been silenced. What were they afraid of? Her dream was to give voice to nurse's story of caring, so she did. She met with colleagues in practice circles. The discussions that happen in the circles facilitate a deeper understanding of a hurt or incident, what happened, and ideally lead to greater satisfaction among the people who participate.

Dorothy used the practice circle to allow nurses to share memories of caring and noncaring among themselves; to re-learn the excitement and commitment to caring that brought them to the profession, and to reduce the stress of over caring.

In the practice circles the nurses experienced the power of storytelling to move them from silence to voice, to illuminate their experiences for shared reflections and allow them to imagine their desired future. Practice circles gave them three kinds of sight: hindsight, insight, and foresight, and in doing so, re-energized their ability to care for patients [4].

Just as balance is required in health, balance is also required in care. That requires an individual whose caring is fully integrated with who they are (being) and how they act (doing). Being encompasses your values, beliefs, attitudes and personality. Doing is the action you take, inspired and enabled by your being, so what you do expresses your character. Combined with your interpersonal skills and strategic abilities, being and doing allow you to influence the actions of others to create meaningful change (see Fig. 3.2).

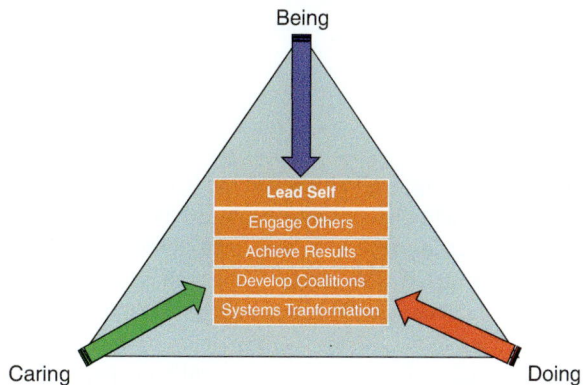

Fig. 3.2 Caring, being and doing interact to generate the LEADS in a Caring Environment capabilities framework

Environment

Originally, the word "environment" in the title of the LEADS framework was used to capture the concept of leadership as an organic system. Now it's often used to denote *context*, which is increasingly used in much of the recent leadership literature to describe the external factors around leadership [5]. We use the two terms interchangeably, to recognize that both the context in which leadership takes place and leadership itself are organic—that is, the ever-fluid human environment of health care is influenced by individual leadership actions and vice-versa.

Jean-Louis Denis and colleagues see the health system in Canada as a series of ever-larger systems, from micro (patient-provider) to mega (systems-citizen), with primary care practices, hospitals and regional health authorities nested within each other [6]. Whether leadership is micro—such as on one nursing station—or macro, at the level of a health authority or province—it interacts with factors in the broader environment that have the potential to change it. Your effectiveness as a leader will come from how you understand and respond to the interdependent dynamics among you, the people you're leading, the environment in which change is happening and whether you can bring others together to work with you collectively on problems.

Peter Senge and colleagues call people who can foster collective leadership "system leaders" (the example they give is Nelson Mandela) and say "At no time in history have we needed such system leaders more." [7] Only through collective leadership, they say, will we be able to solve problems like climate change, youth unemployment, or destruction of eco-systems: problems that all of us face together. System leaders have three core abilities:

- Seeing the larger system of which the problem is a part;
- Fostering reflection and creating generative conversations;
- Shifting the collective focus from reacting to problems to co-creating the future.

Following the LEADS framework should help you to become a system leader, able to work collectively to solve big problems.

Capabilities

Henry Mintzberg, a Canadian guru in leadership and management, advocates moving away from traditional *business* language such as management functions and competencies and referring instead to leadership mindsets or capabilities [8]. We decided early in our work on LEADS to refer to the requirements for exceptional health system leadership as capabilities. We had both practical and cultural reasons for that choice.

First, we think the term competency is most appropriately used in training to refer to a basic skill set—the skills and knowledge individuals need to do their jobs in a predictable environment. In that sense, competencies can be expected of managers whose job it is to address questions such as: *What is it we want to do?* and *How do we do it well?*

Leadership capabilities, on the other hand, lift you beyond a basic skill set, allowing you to build on your training by incorporating your unique knowledge, vision and values into your interaction with colleagues and the environment. Managers tell people what to do in a predictable environment; leaders set a direction and engage people so they are willing to head somewhere new. Competencies are also less likely to continue developing throughout a lifelong journey. Over the years, you may find yourself able to lead well in one situation but not in another; exploring the reasons for that is part of continuously building your capability toolkit and part of lifelong development and growth. To help you with that process, each of the five LEADS domain chapters has a self-assessment exercise at the end that poses questions tailored for five contexts for the practice of leadership—informal leader; front-line supervisor, mid-manager, senior leader and executive leader.

Framework

We use the word framework in connection with LEADS to make it clear the domains and their capabilities outline the parameters of leadership, but don't include all the details that make up leadership. The LEADS framework is designed to be tailored by individual leaders according to their own individual strengths, weaknesses and character.

Another way to look at it is that the five LEADS domains are like the rooms in a house—a kitchen, living room, bathroom and two bedrooms. Each room has features common to all houses—a counter in the kitchen, a shower in the bathroom, closets—which are the capabilities. But rooms are different in different houses and even in the same house they change over time, with redecorating and renovation. You, the leader, are the householder, choosing colours, furniture, art. In the same way, your leadership reflects what you choose to emphasize among the domains and capabilities.

The Validity of LEADS: Can You Depend on It?

How confident can you be that the LEADS framework represents an accurate and valid treatment of health leadership in Canada, and health sectors in general? You might be excused at this point for saying to yourself "Well, some of this sounds good—some of it seems sensible—to what extent can it be validated by research? And even if validated, what traction does it have in the real world of health leadership?"

In the research world, a good study exhibits two forms of validity. The first is *construct validity*: do the findings and results of the research reflect the data and is the logic of interpretation sound and reliable? Researchers go to great pains when they are publishing to show the steps taken to create construct validity. Because this is not a peer-reviewed journal, we will give just an overview on the rigour of our research, and the processes of interpretation that ultimately led us to LEADS.

The second form of validity is called *face validity*, where the findings of the research resonate with people who are the users of the research. The findings make sense to them, considering their own experiences of leadership. The LEADS framework appears to satisfy a growing community of practice of health leaders in both aspects of validity.

Construct Validity of LEADS

Behind the apparent simplicity of the LEADS framework lies a 12-year process of research, dialogue, discussion and use of LEADS. The research was initially carried out by two research teams from Royal Roads University working with health care decision makers across Canada. More recently the LEADS Collaborative, a team of academics and practitioners who are dedicated to ensuring the evergreening of LEADS, has taken the lead. There are more details on research in Chap. 11; what follows is a short summary.

The work on LEADS has been done in three phases. The first phase (2006—2009) was what's called "participatory action research," where research is conducted in cycles of experimentation and reflection by the research team on important questions[1] [9]. This phase was done in three cycles. The second phase (2010–2014) consisted of early efforts to employ LEADS, and a 4-year action research project involving six case studies [10]. The third phase—between 2014 and 2019—comprised an evaluation of the impact of LEADS and a review of the literature published since the original research. That recent research is the focus of this second edition.

Three studies done between 2014 and 2018 confirmed the construct validity for the LEADS framework. The first, completed in 2014, was a Partnerships in Health Systems Improvement research project, funded by the Canadian Institutes for Health Research and the Michael Smith Health Research Foundation in BC. The purpose of the project was to observe leadership in action during ongoing change: six sites, five provincial and one national, were chosen to do the action research. The final report found "Five out of the six case studies…showed LEADS as a useful expression of the leadership qualities required to guide leadership talent management" [11].

Two additional studies found LEADS had robust construct validity [11, 12]. In 2018, a systematic review of the literature was commissioned by the Canadian Health Leadership Network and the Canadian College of Health Leaders. The

---

[1]Traditionally, participatory action research is conducted by a team of both academic researchers and decision makers, who are trying, together, to use inquiry-based methods to generate change in the context of the real world and study it at the same time. It is called the action research phase because most of the activities were formally undertaken using a participatory action research approach. Consequently, the research was conducted in cycles, each consisting of ongoing steps of research; sharing those findings with decision makers, refining the research, and bringing it back to researchers, until the product (ultimately LEADS) was consistent with the 'construct' of the research process.

analysis found that "across all groups of articles anchored in different discipline domains, the articulation of health leadership research aligns with LEADS...the results show that there does not appear to be any domain- or capability-specific revisions needed to maintain the conceptual currency of LEADS at the time of writing." [13] A 2015 study done by the McMaster Health Forum outlined evidence supporting many of the capabilities of LEADS [14].

Face Validity of LEADS

There are two tests of its face validity. First, its initial appeal: is LEADS intuitive enough, accessible enough and accurate enough in its portrayal of leadership to be accepted at all levels of the health system—from executive offices to people on the front lines of care? Second, is LEADS useful and effective for developing leadership, managing talent and planning succession?

LEADS had strong initial appeal. Between 2006 and 2008, the Health Care Leaders' Association of British Columbia, a voluntary professional association of individuals and the province's six health authorities[2] formally endorsed LEADS as a foundation for their leadership endeavours. In November 2009, the Canadian Health Leadership Network[3] (CHLNet) entered a formal agreement with Leaders for Life, a BC legacy organization responsible for giving birth to LEADS, which has subsequently given way to LEADS Canada, to jointly increase awareness of the *LEADS in a Caring Environment* framework and the availability of LEADS-friendly leadership tools across Canada [15]. CHLNet—which has more than 40 regional, provincial and national members—has used LEADS as the foundation for its strategic directions from its inception in 2009 to today. In 2010, the Canadian College of Health Service Executives (now the Canadian College of Health Leaders), endorsed the framework as the foundation of leadership development for its members, and for a certification program for its continuing professional development programs.

The second phase of face validation, from 2009 to the publication of this book, could be called practical research. Over that decade, the LEADS framework was

---

[2]Vancouver Island Health Authority (VIHA; now Island Health); Provincial Health Services Authority (PHSA); Interior Health Authority (IHA); Northern Health Authority (NHA); Vancouver Coastal Health Authority (VCHA); and Fraser Health Authority (FHA) are the six regions in British Columbia, that offer full programs of health services to British Columbians. Note: the PHSA is a quaternary service delivery entity that offers provincial programs in cancer, transplants, etc. in partnership with the other five regional health authorities.

[3]The Canadian Health Leadership Network (CHLNet) is a not-for-profit, **value network** comprised of over 40 health organizations across the country. The network facilitates or brokers joint work among and between its Network Partners; using the LEADS framework as a foundation for much of that work. This joint work cuts across the health disciplines and across the lifecycle of leaders. CHLNet believes that leadership is a life-long pursuit and is Canada-wide. It is through this joint work that CHLNet produces a unique value, adding to the growing number of individual leadership initiatives across Canada.

tested through its use by hundreds of people and organizations, and we give some examples of its impact on them throughout this book.

LEADS has shown itself to be flexible enough to be useful in a broad range of organizations and settings, according to an impact assessment of six organizations commissioned by the Canadian College of Health Leaders in 2016.[4] The assessment found no single best way to implement LEADS. Instead, each organization developed an approach that worked for their context, resources, and strategic aims. LEADS continues to work for the five health organizations, despite ongoing change [16].

LEADS also appeals to both genders—throughout this book you'll see stories from many female leaders who view LEADS as emancipating and empowering, giving them the licence to lead.

LEADS has been embraced by people from many different cultures, including Dr. Arun Garg. Dr. Garg is the founder of the Canada India Network Society, a practising physician for over 40 years, a clinical professor at the University of British Columbia and an adjunct clinical service professor at Simon Fraser University. The following is a condensed version of a piece he wrote about the similarities between LEADS and yoga.

> Even though I was born in the birthplace of yoga, I never understood or related to it. It was an exercise program, difficult postures and twisting of body, which were beyond my comprehension.
>
> This all changed after my meeting with Swami Baba Ram Dev, first in 2008 during his short visit to Vancouver, followed by a visit to India and a personal meeting with him. He told me yoga is a path of action, affirmation and achievement. Rereading the Bhagwat Gita showed me that the narrative is based on yoga philosophy and all our actions are part of yoga fabric.
>
> At the same time, I started to work with the LEADS framework, which stands for: Lead self, Engage others, Achieve results, Develop coalitions and Systems transformation. The program provides a strong basis of leadership through these five areas, which to me resonated with five yogas of raja, karma, bhakti, jnana and gyan.
>
> Raja yoga of Patanjali teaching is the foundation, like a foundation of a home. Its eight limbs form the basis of living, the rules of the game and basis of yoga philosophy and are similar to the five domains of LEADS.
>
> Bhakti yoga and Jnana yoga reflect the LEADS domain of Lead self. Bhakti, the first pillar, relates to consciousness and doing things with passion and commitment. Jnana is the third pillar, and connects meditation, mindfulness and concentration.
>
> Just Baharat speaks to the power of relationships, and the leader should provide opportunity to all to dream and achieve, which echoes engaging others. Another teacher, Swami Patel says "Little pools of water tend to become stagnant and useless. But if they are joined together to form a big lake the atmosphere is cooled and there is universal benefit," which links to Develop coalitions.
>
> Karma yoga, the second pillar of yoga, is following your dreams to action—Achieve results. Gyan yoga is the roof under which all the above live, the overarching guide of building real knowledge and links to Systems transformation.
>
> I marvel at the insightfulness of ancient sages and rishis to express these thoughts so clearly. These are as real today as they were thousands of years ago.

---

[4]The six organizations were: Island Health, Alberta Health Services. Saskatoon Health Region, Sunrise Regional Health Authority, Canadian Agency for Drugs and Technology in Health and Health PEI.

The Ongoing Appeal of LEADS

In 2019 the reach of LEADS—both in terms of numbers of organizations using it as well as the scope and breath of its application—vastly exceeds what it was in 2014. In the first edition, we said four primary factors have driven its widespread acceptance and use—common vocabulary, a collaborative approach, an emphasis on inclusiveness and knowledge mobilization practices.

A common vocabulary is a powerful tool to unite, rather than divide. As Dr. T. Shannon said:

"[If]/when medical leaders are to lead the way forward in this century towards the transformation and improvement of healthcare across the globe then we must work between us towards a simple yet clear vocabulary that we can share with our clinical, management and technical colleagues at every meeting and every report." [17]

LEADS can stake a claim to be that shared vocabulary. As you will see in Chap. 11, LEADS has been adopted as the foundation for leadership learning and practice in almost 70% of Canada's health organizations [18]. It provides the foundation for distributed leadership because people who must practise leadership interdependently can now do so with a shared understanding of how to conduct their work. It limits talking at cross-purposes and mitigates misunderstandings. In addition, a clear and shared vocabulary for leadership helps leaders see themselves as united in a common endeavour: to knit together a system that is increasingly fragmented, yet under pressure to work as a system.

In keeping with the need to overcome system fragmentation, we have focused on collaborative approaches from the beginning. LEADS is a philosophy of distributed leadership that promotes cooperation and collaboration. LEADS categorically states that all of us—regardless of profession, organization, or enterprise—are dedicated to achieving the same results: the health and wellness of the people we serve. We believed Canada needed all CEOs, organizational development professionals, universities and others invested in better leadership to be encouraged—and empowered—to work together to increase collaborative leadership in health.[5]

The third factor promoting acceptance of LEADS is its inclusiveness, the belief that anyone can increase their innate ability to lead, an idea that has gained broader acceptance since the first edition. Evidence shows that well designed and delivered leadership development programs (see Chap. 4) can provide a significant return on investment to organizations [19]. The goal of LEADS is to build leadership capacity throughout the health system, horizontally as well as vertically across organizations. When leadership qualities are distributed throughout organizations

---

[5] In Chap. 11 we discuss the Canadian Health Leadership Network's *Leadership Development Impact Toolkit,* which has been designed for member partners to use to assess the impact of leadership development. This is a consequence of many studies that show that leadership development can make a significant difference, both in terms of individual development as well as organizational development.

and systems, it will be much easier to rally the innovation and flexibility required to meet the challenges of twenty-first century healthcare.

A fourth factor in LEADS' broad appeal is the knowledge mobilization strategies being developed to make research on leadership more accessible and usable. The complex research that went into creating LEADS and the subsequent research that validates it are of little value without products and tools ready for every-day use. This concept underpins the work of LEADS Canada, and the LEADS Exchange Days [20] that are held each year as part of the National Health Leadership Conference put on by the Canadian College of Healthcare Leaders and Healthcare*CAN*.[6]

We think knowledge mobilization has helped make LEADS the predominant approach to building leadership capacity across Canada. For example, let's look at how LEADS is being put to work in Fraser Health, the largest of five regional health authorities in British Columbia and one of the original adopters of LEADS. Fraser Health has worked hard at mobilizing knowledge to make LEADS relevant and practical.

The senior administration at the Fraser Health Authority has been engaged with LEADS from the outset, building it into many different facets of personal and organizational leadership and human-resource development, including by:

- *Integrating LEADS capabilities with management competencies to develop a "leadership and management responsibilities profile" that guides development of new managers in Fraser Health.*
- *Creating personal learning plans that require leaders to assess themselves based on the responsibilities in the leadership and management profile and to keep journals reflecting on their LEADS capabilities.*
- *Using LEADS-based questions and assessments to identify high-quality leaders in its selection and succession processes.*

In keeping with two Systems transformation capabilities—encourage and support innovation and champion and orchestrate change—Fraser Health launched a Centre for Excellence in Health Care Leadership in the spring of 2019. The centre's goal is to provide access to the latest research and trends in leadership and organizational development and help leaders learn and work together.

One of the centre's first actions was to review the value of the LEADS framework in Fraser Health, and whether it was consistent with the leadership qualities found in the survey. Its conclusion was LEADS should continue to be the foundation of Fraser Health's leadership, organizational and human-resource development work.

Moving forward, Fraser wants leaders who are clear, courageous and caring. These qualities sit on top of the LEADS framework, providing clarity about three priorities that all leaders in Fraser should strive to achieve. They are the fundamental principles of leadership important to Fraser Health.

Fraser Health is reaching out to others who share its values and commitment to leadership, in the hope other organizations will join it in the work of the Centre for Excellence in Health Care Leadership (Personal communication, Yabome Gilpin-Jackson and Gabriele Cuff, 2019 Jul 31).

---

[6] Healthcare*CAN* is the national voice of healthcare organizations and hospitals across Canada. Its goal is to improve the health of Canadians through an evidence-based and innovative healthcare system.

LEADS and Other National Frameworks

Further validation of LEADS' effectiveness (and increasing interest in the professionalization of leadership) can be found in the similarity between it and other health leadership frameworks, including Health LEADS Australia and the Health Education and Training Institute of New South Wales Leadership Framework, the United Kingdom's National Health System Healthcare Leadership Model, and the UK's Faculty of Medical Leadership and Management's Standards. LEADS-based programming has also been used in Belgium and India.

The United Kingdom (England)

The National Health Service (NHS) Healthcare Leadership Model, which is designed to help NHS employees become better leaders in their day-to-day roles, has been revised since we first wrote about it. This new framework, like LEADS, encourages distributed leadership: "The Healthcare Leadership Model is useful for everyone because it describes the things you can see leaders doing at work and demonstrates how you can develop as a leader—even if you're not in a formal leadership role." [21] The NHS Leadership Academy developed the evidence-based model, based on what it learned from its previous framework and on "what our patients and communities are now asking from us as leaders." [22] There are nine elements to the framework:

- Inspiring a shared purpose
- Leading with care
- Evaluating information
- Connecting our service
- Sharing the vision
- Engaging the team
- Holding to account
- Developing capacity
- Influencing for results

There are significant overlaps between dimensions of the NHS framework and LEADS. Several of the NHS dimensions can be seen as interchangeable with LEADS domains—Leading with care, Influencing for results and Engaging the team match three of the Engage others capabilities: *Contributes to the creation of a healthy organization, Communicate effectively* and *Build teams*. The NHS dimensions of Inspiring a shared purpose, Sharing the vision, Evaluating information and Holding to account are like the four capabilities of Achieve results, and so on.

There are also differences of emphasis between the two frameworks. LEADS focuses more on system-wide collaborative leadership, while the NHS framework's scope is limited to interpersonal or organizational use. As well, while the NHS

LEADS Standards	UK Leadership and Management Standards for Medical Professionals
Lead Self • Are self aware • Manages self • Demonstrates character • Develops self	**Self** • Self-awareness and self-development • Personal resilience, drive and energy
Engage Others • Foster development of others • Contribute to the creation of healthy organization • Communicate effectively • Build teams	**Team Player/ Team Leader** • Effective teamwork • Cross-team collaborations
Achieve Results • Set direction • Align vision, mission, vision values and evidence to make decisions • Take action to implement decisions • Assess and evaluate	**Corporate Responsibility** • Corporate team player • Corporate culture, improvement and innovation
Develop Coalitions and Systems Transformation	**Systems Leadership**

Fig. 3.3 Comparison of LEADS to the Faculty of Medical Leadership and Management's Leadership and Management Standards for Medical Professionals

model talks about elements of self-leadership, it does not have a specific dimension for leading self, as LEADS does [23].

Since our first edition, the UK's Faculty of Medical Leadership and Management has created standards for medical professionals. These standards define what effective medical leaders do and how they do it (Fig. 3.3).

Australia

In 2010, Health Workforce Australia (since dissolved) was a national coordinating body dedicated to system reform. In 2011 it released the *National Health Workforce Innovation and Reform Strategic Framework for Action, 2011–2015,* calling for "a leadership framework that defines the capabilities needed for leaders in all areas of health." Subsequently a draft document called *Health LEADS Australia* was released for public consultation. The framework (Fig. 3.4) was formally endorsed in June 2013 [24].

The Health Leadership Australia framework is closely related to the Canadian Leads in a Caring Environment framework [25]. Four of its five domains are almost identical; the one that differs is the LEADS Canada domain of Develop coalitions. In the Australian model, that concept is captured in Engages others, while the D in Australia is Drives innovation—which reflects the high priority innovating for reform and improvement had in Australia at the time of the framework's release.

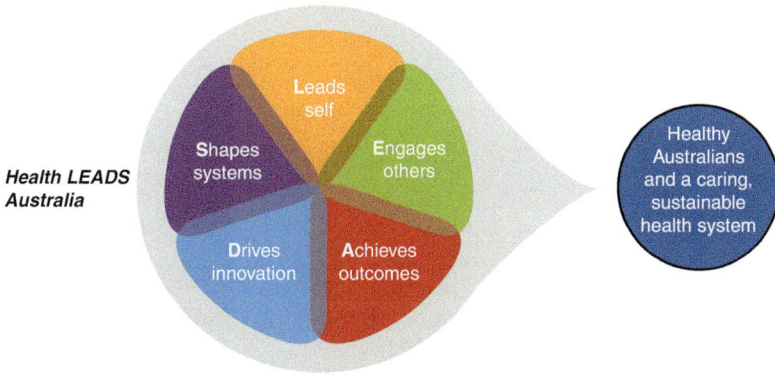

Fig. 3.4 Health LEADS Australia

Fig. 3.5 Health Education and Training Institute: NSW Leadership Framework

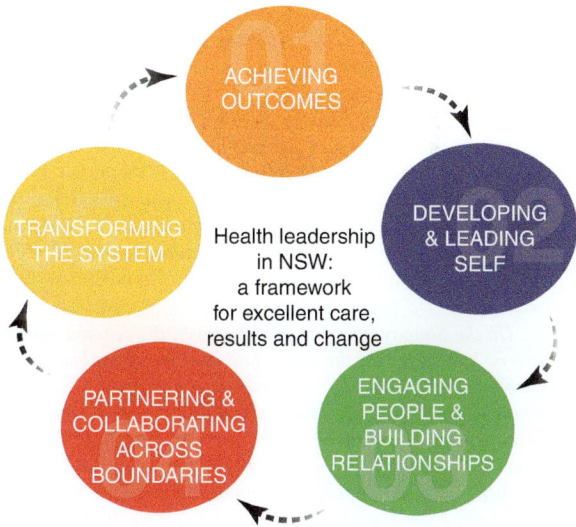

Once Health Workforce Australia was closed in 2014, responsibility for Health Leads Australia was taken over by the Ministry of Health. As a result, the framework has "not yet been fully developed as envisioned…and has only partially fulfilled the purpose" [25] of providing a consistent national approach to develop health care leadership. However, there has been some development by some organizations across Australia. These efforts are described in Chaps. 11 and 12.

The state of New South Wales in Australia endorsed a version of the Canadian LEADS framework in 2013. The Health Education and Training Institute leadership framework for New South Wales Health (Fig. 3.5) lists the five domains in a different order and packaged slightly differently but have very similar content to Canada's LEADS [26].

Summary

We opened this chapter by calling the five domains of LEADS, each with its four capabilities, the source code for health care leadership and a framework for individual, interpersonal, and strategic leadership talent management. Let's close with a story of truly inspiring leadership that underscores how LEADS is being put to work.

Suann Laurent was the chief operating officer of the Saskatchewan Health Authority on April 6, 2018, when the bus carrying the Humboldt Broncos hockey team was in a terrible crash, which killed 16 people and injured 13 others—players, coaches and team personnel. Suann had to respond to the unthinkable, immediately.

Suann's initial reaction—as a senior Saskatchewan health leader—was to focus on her organization's vision: Put the patient and family first. "We had faced nothing remotely like this. Regardless, I knew we had to show up for the victims and for the families. Results for them—not for us—were foremost in our minds throughout the many days of the crisis. They still are today."

In a riveting talk at the National Health Leadership Conference in St. John's Newfoundland a few months after the crash, Suann explained how she has for many years used the LEADS framework as a guide to her leadership. "I use the LEADS framework all the time…it is an inventory for me of the key factors I need to consider in order to show up for others." It kicked in as she prepared to deal with the Humboldt crash.

She and her colleagues, for example, kept the victims' and families' welfare foremost in their minds as they made decisions. Knowing that relatives of the injured couldn't leave the hospital to attend community vigils and memorial services, Suann and her team arranged to have the services streamed into the hospital. "We knew that the relatives of the players still in the hospital wanted to show solidarity with those who had suffered even more than they were, and that the sense of community was central to them. We had to do this." [Achieve results].

On the Sunday after the Friday crash, the coroner informed Suann and her team that two of the victims of the crash had been misidentified: a player who had died had been reported as injured while a player reported dead was, in fact, in the hospital. "We—the whole team—myself, other representatives from the health authority, RCMP, government officials and the coroner—came together quickly," she said. "While we were all very shaken, we agreed we needed to put the families and victims first, so we immediately decided that there would be no finger pointing. Our hearts told us to reach out to the families of those two poor boys. And that's what we did immediately."

Throughout, regular meetings were held with stakeholders including the school system, community representatives, the health authority, the RCMP, government officials and the coroner [Develop coalitions]. Suann credits these ongoing sessions with ensuring the focus was always on the welfare of the victims and families and on helping the community to heal, and that decisions were always made in their best interests.

Another key element of her response was to be present with those delivering the care, who had seen and responded to terrible things [Engage others]. "We couldn't have asked for more from them than they gave. They were caring and professional. Indeed, all we had to do was trust them to do their job. Yet, showing up for them was vital. They needed to see us, to know that we had their back in such an emotionally draining time. After all we weren't on the front line, they were."

Suann had moments of soul searching as she strove to manage herself during conversations with grieving parents, distraught citizens and overwhelmed caregivers—all the while building her own resilience. She did that by debriefing with colleagues, close friends and family. She was also careful to monitor her own mental and physical state. "After the first three days—Tuesday morning—I realized I was out of gas and was going to do others more harm than good. I gave myself permission to go home and sleep, refill the tank. That is something I had never done before at work." [Lead self].

Suann also described what we call an "after-action review" during the crisis: regular meetings of stakeholders to discuss what happened the day before, what they would face that day and how to handle tomorrow. Longer term, the Saskatchewan Health Authority organized a review to determine what went well during the overall response to the crash and what might be done better in the future if there is ever another such event.

Suann concluded her talk by saying "If you use the framework, it helps you lead with integrity. But to do so you need to consider all of the domains as part of a whole. Some people see LEADS as a bunch of pieces; but to me, it is the whole of leadership in health-care; and if you use it that way, it brings integrity to your leadership."

References

1. Wise wisdom on demand. 2013. http://www.iwise.com/TPU7r. Accessed 11 Jul 2013.
2. Leads Collaborative. LEADS in a caring environment [brochure]. CHLNet: Ottawa; 2013.
3. Kelly L, Runge J, Spencer C. Predictors of compassion fatigue and compassion satisfaction in acute care nurses. J Nurs Scholarsh. 2015;47(6):522–8.
4. Dougherty K. Caring leadership: voices of nurses. In: Picard M, Dickson G, editors. Royal Roads University leadership programs. Victoria (BC): Royal Roads University Leadership Programs; 2002.
5. Oc B. Contextual leadership: a systematic review of how contextual factors shape leadership and its outcomes. Leadersh Q. 2018;29(1):218–235. doi:https://doi.org/10.1016/j.leaqua.2017.12.004; and Dickson G. Leadership theory as a driver of executive leadership practice in healthcare. In Raz M and Loh E. editors. Cases for health executives: the principles of practice. Taylor and Francis Group (AUS). Forthcoming 2019.
6. Denis J-L, Lamothe L, Langley A. The dynamics of collective leadership and strategic change in pluralistic organizations. Acad Manag J. 2001;44(4):809–37.
7. Senge P, Hamilton H, Kania J. The dawn of system leadership. Stanf Soc Innov Rev. 2015;13(1):26–33.
8. Mintzberg H. Managers, not MBAs: a hard look at the soft practice of managing and management development. San Francisco: Barrett-Koehler; 2004.
9. Stringer E. Action research. 3rd ed. Thousand Oaks (CA): Sage Publications; 2007.
10. Dickson G, Tholl B, Baker, GR, Blais R, Clavel, N, Gorley C. et al. Partnerships for health system improvement, leadership and health system redesign: Cross-case analysis. Ottawa: Royal Roads University, Canadian Health Leadership Network, Canadian Institutes of Health Research, Michael Smith Foundation for Health Research; 2014. http://tinyurl.com/qh6ogzu. Accessed 22 Aug 2019.
11. Moat KA, Lavis JN. Dialogue summary: fostering leadership for health-system redesign in Canada, Hamilton: McMaster Health Forum; 2014. https://www.mcmasterforum.org/docs/default-source/Product-Documents/issue-briefs/fostering-leadership-health-system-redesign-canada-ib.pdf?sfvrsn=2. Accessed 21 Nov 2015.
12. Marchildon G, Fletcher A. Prioritizing health leadership capabilities in Canada: testing LEADS in a Caring Environment. Health Manage Forum. 2016;29(1):19–22.
13. Cikaliuk M. Pre-phase preliminary intelligence gathering report: LEADS in a Caring Environment capabilities framework. [unpublished research report]. Ottawa: Canadian Health Leadership Network and the Canadian College of Health Leaders; 2017.

14. Lavis JN, Moat K, Tapp C, Young C. Evidence brief: improving leadership capacity in primary and community care in Ontario. Hamilton (ON): McMaster Health Forum. 2015. https://www.mcmasterforum.org/docs/default-source/product-documents/evidence-briefs/leadership-capacity-in-ontario-eb.pdf?sfvrsn=2. Accessed 18 Sep 2019.
15. Philippon D. The leadership imperative in publicly funded universal health systems with a particular focus on the development of the Canadian Health Leadership Network (CHLNET). Ottawa: Canadian College of Health Leaders; 2011. http://chlnet.ca/wp-content/uploads/Don-Philippon-Fellowship-report-.pdf. Accessed 13 Jul 2013.
16. Vilches S, Fenwick S, Harris B, Lammi B, Racette R. Changing health organizations with the LEADS leadership framework: report of the 2014-2016 LEADS impact study. Ottawa: Fenwick Leadership Explorations, the Canadian College of Health Leaders, & the Centre for Health Leadership and Research, Royal Roads University; 2016. https://leadscanada.net/document/1788/LEADS_Impact_Report_2017_FINAL.pdf. Accessed 18 Jun 2019.
17. Shannon T. as quoted in Dickson G, Van Aerde J. Enabling physicians to lead: Canada's LEADS framework. Leadersh Health Serv (Bradf Engl). 2018;31(2):183–194.
18. Canadian Health Leadership Network Breakfast Session. Does Canada have the leadership capacity to innovate? Benchmark 2.0. Toronto: National Health Leadership Conference; 2019. http://chlnet.ca/wp-content/uploads/NHLC-CHLNet-Breakfast-Session-2019-V02.pdf. Accessed 20 Aug 2019.
19. Jeyaraman M, Qadar SMZ, Wierzbowski A, Farshidfar F, Lys J, Dickson G, et al. Return on investment in healthcare leadership development programs. Leadersh Health Serv (Bradf Engl). 2018;31(1):77–97. https://doi.org/10.1108/LHS-02-2017-0005.
20. The LEADS community for practice exchange day. Ottawa: LEADS Canada and the Canadian College of Health Leaders. 2019. https://www.leadscanada.net/site/2019day. Accessed 18 Sep 2019.
21. NHS Leadership Academy. Healthcare leadership model; 2019. https://www.leadershipacademy.nhs.uk/resources/healthcare-leadership-model/. Accessed 13 Jan 2019.
22. NHS Leadership Academy. How the healthcare leadership model has been developed. 2018. https://www.leadershipacademy.nhs.uk/resources/healthcare-leadership-model/healthcare-leadership-model-developed/. Accessed 13 Jan 2018. This website also refers the reader to the secondary research, done by John Storey and Richard Holti, working with the Hay Group, who carried out a review of current literature and research on leadership models and behaviours. You can download Holti and Storey's paper @ https://www.leadershipacademy.nhs.uk/wp-content/uploads/dlm_uploads/2014/10/Towards-a-New-Model-of-Leadership-2013.pdf.
23. NHS Leadership Academy. The nine leadership dimensions; 2018. https://www.leadershipacademy.nhs.uk/resources/healthcare-leadership-model/nine-leadership-dimensions/connecting-our-service/. Accessed 13 Jan 2018.
24. Health Workforce Australia. Health LEADS Australia: The Australian Health Leadership Framework. Adelaide (SA). Health Workforce Australia. 2013.
25. Shannon E, Sebastian A. Developing health leadership with Health Leads Australia. Leadersh Health Serv (Bradf Engl). 2018;31(4):413–25. https://doi.org/10.1108/LHS-02-2017-0002.
26. NSW Health leadership framework. Sydney (NSW): Health Education and Training Institute; 2019. https://www.heti.nsw.gov.au/education-and-training/our-focus-areas/leadership-and-management/nsw-health-leadership-framework. Accessed 31 Jan 2019.

Learning LEADS: Developing Leadership in Individuals and Organizations

4

Graham Dickson and Bill Tholl

"Leadership cannot really be taught. It can only be learned"

Harold S. Geneen

The old adage "leaders are born, not made" is wrong. Leaders are born *and* made. Our premise in developing the LEADS framework and writing both editions of this book was that leadership can be learned and developed. As Malcolm Gladwell points out in his book *Outliers* [1] an individual must be nurtured in an environment that creates the conditions for success. In this chapter, we describe two approaches for using LEADS to develop leadership. The first is an approach where it's up to you, the leader, to create a nurturing environment for yourself. For this approach we focus on self-directed learning and personal leadership development as a life-long pursuit. The second approach shows how people designing leadership programs can use LEADS for organizational growth and development. It's a recognition that leadership development should not be limited to individuals, because research shows leadership training aimed at groups of leaders who are committed to distributed leadership can create workplace cultures that are vibrant, adaptive and productive.

Most leaders develop their craft in the workplace through experience. The point of development programs is to speed up that experience by focusing on the lessons inherent in it. The *LEADS in a Caring Environment* framework describes the capabilities needed to be an effective leader in health care. You'll learn them best by trying them out in the real world. To ensure you learn as much as possible as you do that, we're recommending you use experiential learning. It's an approach that has

G. Dickson (✉)
Royal Roads University, Victoria, BC, Canada
e-mail: graham.dickson@royalroads.ca

B. Tholl
Canadian Health Leadership Network, Ottawa, ON, Canada
e-mail: btholl@chlnet.ca

people work together on real issues, but in a structured way that encourages discussion and reflection so what happens is carefully considered and its impact studied to shape future activity.

Learning from experience is not an easy path. Mark Twain said: "A man who swings a cat by its tail learns something he can learn in no other way." Many of us who've learned leadership on the job feel like that: scratched and bitten, but wiser. The self-directed approaches in this chapter and throughout the book are designed to minimize scratches and bites while creating a safe place for reflection, contemplation and practice.

Because connecting leadership development to real-life problems provides context for new ideas, it has immediate relevance and more power to engage people. If the exercise also emphasizes results the organization wants—such as a healthier workplace or better service for patients and their families—everyone benefits.

Learning Leadership: Why It's Different from Learning Anything Else

Learning leadership differs from learning anything else in several important ways. The first is the tools of the craft. A hockey stick and skates are the tools of hockey, for carpentry it's a hammer and saw. For individual leadership development, your core attributes—values, attitudes, beliefs and talents—are your tools. You can change superficial behaviour to influence others but to truly be effective, your behaviour must express who you are. Kouzes and Posner [2] put it this way: "Leadership is an art—a performing art—and the instrument is the self." You are the instrument and striving to improve as a leader is tuning yourself.

The second reason learning leadership is different is because the context for it is unique for each of us and can be fluid and unpredictable. Leaders must constantly learn (or unlearn: more later) the appropriate response to that context [3]—time, place, events, the specific challenge presented and the needs of followers. Leaders need to be able to read the moment to decide what to do—what works in one context may not work in another. This takes judgement; there is no standard recipe.

Other factors that make learning leadership different:

- Learning leadership means learning followership;
- Learning leadership comes from emotional as well as practical experience;
- Learning leadership includes unlearning; and
- Learning and leadership are indispensable to each other.

Learning Leadership Means Learning Followership

Followership may not be a term you're familiar with, but it is essential to understanding distributed leadership, in which leadership is a function, not a position. Depending on the situation, a formal leader may assume the role of follower; sometimes the role of leader. At any time, a person previously following may have to lead. This idea is at odds with the traditional leader-as-hero scenario, where one person is always the leader and others always follow. It can be a challenge for organizations with typical managerial structures to adapt to this complex leader-follower dance.

Leaders Learn from Emotional Experience as Well as Practical Experience

Emotions are an important part of experience. The whole field of emotional intelligence described in Chaps. 5 and 6 (Lead self and Engage others) underscores the relevance of emotions to the practice of leadership. Leaders need to realize that emotion is part of the context in which they work, including the impact of unchecked emotions and the power passion can give when it's effectively channelled. Leaders need to be conscious of and reflect on the emotion in an experience, and respond to it appropriately.

Learning Moment
The following story shows the power of emotions:

Lana was working at her desk in a ministry of health cubicle and was startled to hear raised voices in the centre of the room. The assistant deputy minister of finance—Frank—was berating his direct report, Valerie. Valerie was an accomplished leader from everything Lana had experienced and knew about her. As Valerie quietly remonstrated with Frank to control himself, he got even louder and ruder, calling her incompetent and unfit for her job. Finally, Frank turned on his heel and stomped off down the hallway, leaving Valerie—and Lana too—feeling distraught and wrongly shamed. A pall fell over the room, with everyone who witnessed the incident feeling demoralized, subdued and ashamed.

Sometimes, however, there is karma in organizational life. A week before the incident, a new government had come to power. A week after, Valerie was promoted to deputy minister—with Frank directly reporting to her.

Reflective Questions
- Have you ever been in a similar situation to Valerie's? Lana's? If so, how did you feel? If not, can you imagine your feelings?
- If you were Valerie, how would you respond to becoming Frank's boss?
- If you were Lana, how might this experience influence your attitude to work?

Situations like this one can flare up at any time. The incident itself may be brief, but the fallout can be far reaching and long lasting. Shaming others—humiliating them in front of colleagues—breeds anger and drives employees away, if not actually to another job, certainly to a different attitude toward work. Knowing the emotional climate of a team or organization—and working to improve it if necessary—is vital to being an effective leader.

It's equally vital, however, for leaders to learn from emotional turmoil. Both Valerie and Frank need to know how to manage their feelings. Frank must learn to control his anger and Valerie needs to resist looking for revenge. Even Lana needs to consider whether what she witnessed will make her fear reprimands so much she is afraid to act. Learning to reflect on feelings and their impact is an important leadership lesson to learn—keeping a journal or talking with a coach or a peer you trust may help you understand lessons from an emotional incident.

Strong emotional outbursts, or emotional issues that bubble up in an organization, should never be ignored or suppressed. The former, as we've said, can have considerable fallout and the latter may be symptoms of underlying ethical or practical issues or significant disagreements that could stall progress or spiral into dysfunction if left unaddressed. Openly exploring emotional issues is fundamental to effective culture change. Because dealing with emotions (at any level) is hard for many people, leadership programs can provide safe places to explore them and effective lessons for managing them.

Learning Includes Unlearning

According to Chris Argyris, a professor at Harvard Business School known for his work on learning organizations, learning is when you add new behaviour you need to be successful in a future endeavour, while unlearning is taking away behaviour that gets in the way of your effectiveness. Both are important for developing successfully, he says [4].

In an article titled "Teaching Smart People to Learn" [5]. Argyris says successful people are not used to failing and therefore have never learned how to learn from it. However, they do have a tendency to let certain approaches become habitual because they have worked over time. If a time comes when a go-to approach doesn't work, they get defensive, blaming other people or circumstances, but unable to admit they might have made mistakes. The trouble is, those ingrained habits are unconscious and the people who count on them can't see when habits are getting in the way of responding effectively to new situations.

Peter Senge [6] calls these habits mental models, defined as "deeply ingrained assumptions, generalizations, or even pictures or images that influence how we understand the world and how we take action. Very often, we are not consciously aware of our mental models, or the effects they have on our behaviour." Those unconscious mental models can lead to what he calls "the delusion of learning from experience," doing the same thing over and over, but not taking the time to plumb the experience for its natural lessons.

Unlearning is also important for organizations, which need to purge organizational culture of beliefs and practices that no longer fit with what the organization wants to achieve. Culture can be seen as shared mental models (held by groups or the entire organization) which create adherence to beliefs and practices that may be getting in the way of progress. Organizational unlearning is required.

Unlearning doesn't, however, always mean eliminating and forgetting a mental model or cultural attribute. In many cases, habitual behaviour needs to be brought into the open and examined, to recognize when it's an appropriate action and when it isn't [7]. Some habits, like teaching, are often, but not always, a good thing to do. Others—like micro-managing, which really means taking power away from people—should be flushed out permanently.

Leadership and Learning are Indispensable to Each Other

A recent review of the literature found most theories of leadership include the need for leaders to be constantly and systematically learning their craft.[1] Or, as John F. Kennedy was intending to say in a speech on the day he was assassinated, *"Leadership and learning are indispensable to each other."*

Effective leaders understand that and they recognize their jobs and organizations are always evolving and they must change with them. Some knowledge and skills will serve you throughout your career, but often what's required to lead effectively is dictated by the role you occupy. Clinical skills won't suffice when you become a manager and to move up to CEO you must develop many new capabilities.

Recent research says resilient organizations are those that pursue learning and development. Leadership development programs for organizations should teach that leadership includes embedding ongoing training and development in the organization's culture and processes. According to the Oxford Review, that's called "absorptive capacity," which it defines as:

> …an organization's ability to identify, assimilate, transform, and use external knowledge, research and practice. In other words, absorptive capacity is the measure of the rate at which an organization can learn and use scientific, technological or other knowledge that exists outside of the organization itself. It is a measure of an organization's ability to learn [8].

The theme of learning—as an individual, organization, or system—is foundational to good leadership.

Learning Individual Leadership: The Hero's Journey

According to cultural anthropologist Joseph Campbell, in times of darkness and confusion we often look to heroes to give us courage and hope. He defines a hero as "the champion not of things become but of things becoming….The dragon to be slain by him is precisely the monster of the status quo. The hero's task always has

[1] For another publication we completed a review of the literature on key principles of leadership theories that apply to modern health executives. In the analysis of the traditional and emerging theories of leadership it was clear that today—partly because of the exponentially changing circumstances surrounding leaders—formal and informal learning are vital to their ability to get and keep senior leadership jobs.

Fig. 4.1 The hero's journey of experiential learning

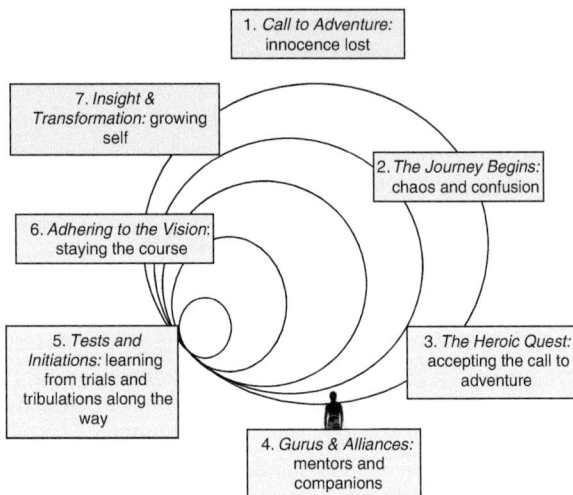

1. *Call to Adventure:* innocence lost
2. *The Journey Begins:* chaos and confusion
3. *The Heroic Quest:* accepting the call to adventure
4. *Gurus & Alliances:* mentors and companions
5. *Tests and Initiations:* learning from trials and tribulations along the way
6. *Adhering to the Vision:* staying the course
7. *Insight & Transformation:* growing self

been and always will be to bring new life to a dying culture." [9]. Like leadership, the ability to act heroically can reside in each of us.

Jim Kouzes and Barry Posner echo that idea, describing leadership as the ability of an ordinary person to rise to the challenge of situation and circumstance and do extraordinary things in response [2]. Sometimes leadership is charismatic and sometimes quiet and unassuming, but the result is the same: followers are empowered to act, rather than remain victims of circumstance.

In his book *The Hero of a Thousand Faces*, Campbell describes the hero's journey[2] [9]. The title reflects the numerous examples, in many cultures, of how an ordinary person can be transformed into a leader by experience. In Herman Hesse's *Siddhartha*, the central character goes on a journey to attain spiritual enlightenment. In Homer's Iliad, Ulysses is transformed by his experiences. Even Dorothy in the *Wizard of Oz* undertakes a hero's journey. There are also many true examples: Nelson Mandela's transition from insurrectionist to president personifies the hero's journey.

Figure 4.1 shows the journey as a series of experiences that ultimately lead to personal growth and transformation: [10].

1. *The call to adventure: innocence lost.* Experiential learning, like a hero's journey, begins with the leader in a state of unconscious innocence—chugging along comfortably in his or her role. But something happens that disturbs that world, and forces the leader onto a journey (desired or not).

---

[2] Some critics have interpreted the use of the term hero in the title as implying only special individuals can lead and that the concept seems to support the "great man" theory of leadership. We interpret the title as the exact opposite—there are thousands of heroes; because the ability to be heroic resides in all of us. The way to realize that potential is to recognize the power of experiential learning, as represented by the hero's journey, and to make it the discipline we employ to grow our leadership capability.

2. *The journey begins: chaos and confusion.* What happened? What do I do now? Do I just hunker down and wait out the change? Why can't we just go back to the old way? Sometimes the individual resists the call, at least initially. Finding a way out of chaos and confusion seems daunting—and the way forward is anything but clear.

3. *The heroic quest: accepting the call to adventure.* This is crucial. The leader must choose between remaining awash in confusion or acting. This is not to say the leader knows what to do and how to do it; but she is willing to begin a journey to a more desirable future state. This is the essence of leadership; and in the case of experiential learning, the step at which the leader chooses to learn or unlearn, as the case may be.

4. *Gurus and alliances: mentors and companions.* In almost all hero's journey myths, the protagonist cannot learn or lead alone. Along the journey, others provide guidance, insight, and friendship (such as the Tin Man, the Lion, and the Scarecrow from the Wizard of Oz). In leadership, your companion may be someone you work with or an expert who can mentor you.

5. *Tests and initiations: learning from trials and tribulations along the way.* Not everyone will share your vision and goal. People may resist, not understand, or lack energy for change. There may be active opposition or obstacles such as policy, practice or culture that are antithetical to the vision. But difficulties are often the learning moments with the greatest potential for insight.

6. *Adhering to the vision: staying the course.* Many leaders abandon their vision, perhaps tired out by effort—but leaders must be resilient. An old Chinese proverb says "A leader is someone who is knocked down seven times and gets up eight." So it is with learning leadership: it's a lifelong endeavour. Many of us abandon learning too early in our career. Learners and leaders must stay the course to realize their learning potential.

7. *Insight and transformation: increasing capacity.* The ultimate benefit of going on a leadership journey is achieving your goal. For an experiential learner, that goal is insight and knowledge of practices that will make you the leader you want to be. The journey will take you there, if you retain the wisdom you have gained, integrate it into your practice, and share it with those around you.

We're using the hero's journey as a metaphor for experiential learning, to show the adventure and risk in setting out on a learning journey. Adventure has no certain outcome; if it did, it would be a plan. T.S. Eliot, in his poem *The Waste Land* [11], suggests the hero's journey is the stuff of life, and as long as one is open to opportunity, never over:

> *We shall not cease from exploration*
> *And the end of all our exploring*
> *Will be to arrive where we started*
> *And know the place for the first time.*

Let's explore the hero's journey further with Brenda's story. Brenda Andreas, a seasoned patient advocate, shares first-hand how her experience with the Canadian health system led her through a process to become a surveyor with Accreditation Canada, and a patient advisor to the Saskatchewan Health Authority. The stages of her journey are noted in square brackets.

> *In 2010 I suffered a traumatic loss in my family. Six loved ones, including my parents, died of cancer* [innocence lost]. *I was devastated. In reflecting on my experience, I began to perseverate on many incidents that did not go well. We as a family did not get the care and the support that we needed from our hospital. I felt hurt and angry* [chaos and confusion].
>
> *I took this pain to the media. My mother, living through her pain and who, as a nurse, had given 50 years of her life to our then 40-bed rural hospital remonstrated with me: "Bunna Jean, you have embarrassed me." "But Mom, look what they have done to our family!" I cried. "It doesn't matter, sweetie—they, and I—have done my best. Don't belittle that."*
>
> *I was deeply chagrined. I replied, "Mom, I will never speak ill of the health care system again. I am going to get involved and try to fix it* [heroic quest]. *As my tears flowed and my heart pounded, I was given the opportunity by the former CEO of the local health region to tell my story to the board* [gurus and allies] *and so began my journey as a patient and family advisor.*
>
> *I started from a place of deep pain and, over time* [trials and tribulations], *moved to a place where I felt like I was being heard, where I could make a difference and I started to feel safe* [insight and transformation]. *The place where I am at now is one of belief and confidence as I engage and collaborate equally in the determination of my health care, and that of my village.*

Brenda has made the journey from citizen to health care leader. In 2017, Brenda applied for a position as a patient partner surveyor with Accreditation Canada. The three-day training experience was quite demanding; in her words, "not unlike boot camp." But this opportunity greatly deepened her knowledge. Along the way she has learned that lived experience "is what patients and family bring to their health care journey. Expertise is what providers bring to the patient journey. Imagine a world where experience and expertise go hand in hand, equal partners on the patient journey." Brenda is a co-author of Chap. 13 on LEADS and People-Centred Care.

We encourage the readers of this book to see their leadership learning journey as an opportunity, adventure and exploration that will ultimately bring personal fulfillment as a leader.

The Hero's Journey and Experiential Learning

Experiential learning is a way to operationalize leadership learning with the work environment as the classroom; it works for either individual or organizational learning. Experiential learning helps to:

- Make sense of the chaos and confusion of changing experiences;
- Reduce unknown elements of change to a manageable level;

Fig. 4.2 Marilyn Taylor's model of experiential learning [13]

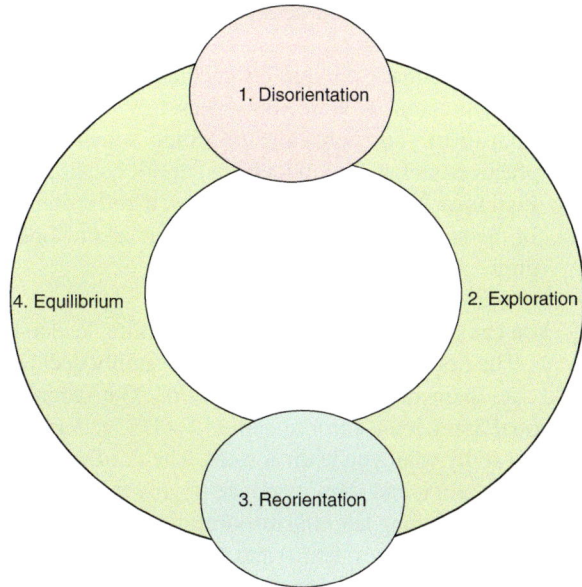

- Develop ways to determine responses to changing internal and external environments; and
- Define where we are in a change and our view of its context [12].

Marilyn Taylor has characterized experiential learning as a continuous process of disorientation, exploration, reorientation and equilibrium. It's a cycle that can repeat itself, each time moving to a next level of excellence. The cycle is pictured in Fig. 4.2.

The Ten Commandments of Individual Leadership Learning

We integrated the experiential learning cycle and the hero's journey to create these top-ten guidelines for learning leadership in the workplace:

1. Look for the leadership opportunity in any situation.
2. If that situation feels chaotic, confusing, or perplexing to you—and you are uncomfortable with the result—it represents an opportunity to learn (or unlearn).
3. Reflect on the situation to make sense of it: what do the people I am trying to lead need from me that they are not getting?
4. Enlist others you trust (it could be colleagues, mentors or writers) to support and guide you as you learn.
5. Use what you've learned this time to set a goal for personal improvement—what aspect of your behaviour do you need to change?

6. Practise your desired behaviour in the workplace. Look for situations where you can test yourself.
7. Gather feedback on your effort, then reflect on what you heard. What insights have you gained? Were you successful? Why? Why not?
8. Transform your behaviour by doing something new, or unlearning habitual practices and mental models that aren't constructive.
9. Find time for ongoing, systematic self-reflection.
10. In the spirit of lifelong learning, start again. Look for opportunities to learn, grow, contribute and feel valued.

You can apply these guidelines for learning leadership in the workplace in three ways. The first is completely informal—simply decide to use them and take care to integrate them in your day-to-day work. The second way is a mixed formal and informal approach—enrol in some LEADS leadership training and use the guidelines to apply what you learn at work. The third way is to participate in formal training, document it and show evidence of growth and success. All three approaches are enhanced by adding learning resources to the mix, including the LEADS framework (as a guide for what to learn) and this book, particularly the learning moments and the many tools and techniques we outline in it.

The following example shows how the concepts and ideas of experiential learning can be operationalized in a leadership program:

> Your two authors were recently coach-mentors at a leadership program offered by the University of Alberta's School of Public Health. Called the Fellowship for Health Systems Improvement, the program involved five weekend retreats, a peer-learning project and, to encourage participants to be disciplined, self-directed learning.
>
> The foundation for the personal learning component was the LEADS framework. Using LEADS as a guide, each participant undertook a self-assessment, and through self-reflection and talks with a mentor, chose a stretch goal that would benefit them as they progressed through the program on their own.
>
> There were five key elements to the self-directed learning process:
>
> - A pre-program webinar, to introduce the discipline of individual experiential learning.
> - Five coaching/mentoring sessions, one after each retreat, with the two authors doing the coaching and mentoring.
> - A peer mentor/coach: either someone the participant worked with or another program participant, who would meet regularly with the individual learner to discuss what they were learning.
> - A collection of eight self-directed-learning tools including a personal vision tool, personal learning plan and a feedback tool. These were to be used at work to maximize learning opportunities.
> - A series of recommended learning resources including websites, You Tube videos, articles or books, depending on the individual's learning goals.
>
> Coaching/mentoring discussions focused on contextualizing what the participant was learning—both in the workplace and from the peer-learning project. What the learners experienced in those two areas helped them choose their learning goals (using LEADS as the guide) and their choice of learning methods.

The Fellowship for Health Systems Improvement program will be offered to a fifth cohort and given the success of this LEADS-based experiential learning process, the coaching/mentoring sessions are now a permanent part of the program and being modelled by other leadership development programs.

A Disciplined Approach to Learning Organizational Leadership

Recent literature in the field of leadership development suggest the same tactics that work for individual leadership development can be deployed for organizations. Distributed, shared and collaborative leadership theories emphasize the need for all members of an organization to have the initiative and skills needed to enable others to work together, but also the ability to recognize when they have the capacity to lead and when they should follow.

However, too often hierarchical organizations discourage leadership in people who don't fit a classic concept of leader. One unpublished study that looked at this issue in Saskatchewan found that "In a hierarchical health system structured by rules and protocols to ensure accountability, front-line leaders have been habituated to manage rather than "empowered to lead." [14] Too often, people selected for programs that will develop their leadership capacity return to an organization where the culture dictates followership. It's why so many individuals rightly claim their organization prevents them from exercising their new leadership skills.

No surprise then, that initiatives to increase leadership capacity are more successful when the goal is not just to make existing leaders more capable, but also to shift organizational culture to distributed leadership [15, 16]. Organizations that commit to distributed leadership can use collective learning to bring about organizational change at the same time.

Similarly, both individual and collective leadership can shift the culture of an organization. The first step is to recognize the organization can't keep on doing the same old thing and then launch a learning process in which the challenge is presented as a quest to be undertaken. Using LEADS as the foundation for learning leadership, development programs can employ an array of practices known to be effective in developing organizational leadership.

Learning Moment
1. Review the stages of the hero's journey and the Taylor model.
2. Can you identify the specific tactics used in the *Fellowship for Health Systems Improvement* example to put various stages of the journey into practice? Can you do it for Taylor's model?

The following vignette, courtesy of Dr. Susan Drouin, is an example of how individual and collective leadership development was used at the McGill University Health Centre in Montreal, Quebec.

The McGill University Health Centre was created by the 1997 merger of five of the university's affiliated health providers. When it came time to move three of the hospitals (the Royal Victoria Hospital, the Montreal Children's Hospital and the Montreal Chest Institute) to a new building in April 2015, the health centre collaborated with the university's School of Continuing Studies to prepare its management staff for the move. The program's purpose was to redesign the organization and create a new organizational culture to suit the move to shared space. It used LEADS as a foundation for its curriculum.

Dr. Susan Drouin, an associate director of McGill's Ingram School of Nursing, evaluated the program. Her study found the program met its goals on increasing leadership capabilities, improving attitudes toward resolving challenges, creating networks and better equipping participants to handle the upcoming transition [17].

Leading Practices for Developing Leadership in Organizations

Recent literature in leadership development and your authors' years of experience with designing and delivering leadership programs suggest a number of design features that should be strongly considered in designing programs for organizations[3] [16, 18–20].

Jaason Geerts provides a detailed analysis of design elements, tactics, ways of measuring and learning transfer strategies that must be chosen artfully to maximize the principles of experiential learning [21]. Programs that choose and use a selection of these approaches effectively—that is, consistent with the principles of experiential learning and the hero's journey—can increase their organization's leadership capacity and in the process accomplish organizational goals such as changing the culture and improving organizational outcomes [22].

However, as Geerts also points out, to take advantage of such programs an organization must have a clear leadership doctrine that states why better leadership is important, and how it will improve organizational wellness and productivity. There needs to be a vision and ethos for leadership development that is shared, endorsed, and supported across the organization.

Effective Features for Maximum Leadership Program Impact

As you design your leadership program, the factors listed below will contribute to maximum impact. You should:

- Use adult learning techniques. Adults learn best through discussion, self-discovery, reflection, team learning and question-based approaches. Lecturing and lengthy presentations don't work.
- Provide ample dedicated time for learning. Allow sufficient time for learning and mix active learning and more formal learning events to encourage reflection and

---

[3] One of the virtues of a capability framework like LEADS is that it provides a lifelong learning pathway of graduated growth and development so that one workshop, one on-line course, can all become parts of a whole, built into a long-term developmental plan.

practice in the workplace. Connect learning programs with activities that give people the chance to transfer their skills to the workplace.

- Learn about the learners. People have different capacities to lead and have an array of experience in leadership before entering courses or programs. Knowing how each person's background and makeup prepares them to learn is extremely helpful to creating a successful program.
- Emphasize strengths. Design your program to allow participants and their organization to develop strengths they already possess. Only work on areas for improvement when a threshold level is necessary for success and the individual or organization does not meet it.
- Offer many ways to learn. Try group work, coaching or mentoring, self-reflection tools such as 360 assessments or journaling. Create opportunities for personal and organizational growth and maximize transfer to the workplace.
- Integrate multiple teaching models. Today's technology allows you to blend face-to-face sessions with online discussion, webinars, coaching, self-directed learning tools and more. You can reach more people more efficiently, while keeping them on the job, where they can apply lessons in real time as they work.
- Work with a diverse group. Make an effort to get a good mix in your program— of age, gender, ethnicity, etc. Participants will benefit from the mind-broadening experience of seeing problems from different perspectives and develop an appreciation for the power of diversity.
- Incorporate real and timely organization issues. Strong programs provide participants with challenges that engage their emotions, have inherent conflict, and that are relevant to the real world. Participants should be able to apply what they're learning immediately to their work.
- Design for context. Participants need to be conscious of how their organizational culture will shape their ability to implement what they have learned. This could work well for multidisciplinary teams learning about leadership together.
- Try these online learning approaches:
  - Assign electronic teamwork where participants can discuss and work through leadership challenges.
  - Use online discussions, resources, journaling and individual learning plans as tools for self-awareness and self-development.
  - Provide just-in-time material to provide learners with up-to-date leadership resources.
  - Give access to online libraries and video streaming and simulations.

Covenant Health is the largest Catholic health care provider in Canada. It has a comprehensive leadership development program, called *Leadership Pathways,* aimed at developing individual and organizational leadership capacity over time. The program is LEADS-based in both philosophy and content and employs many of the learning strategies outlined above. Here's Covenant's story, courtesy of Kyla Coole (Personal email, 2019 Jul 9):

Covenant's mission is to "...provide quality health care to all Albertans. Our mission calls us to serve with compassion, uphold the sanctity of life at all stages and serve the whole person body, mind and spirit....While providing a full spectrum of care from birth to end-of-life, our unique focus is on four of the most vulnerable populations: seniors, mental health and addiction, palliative end-of-life and rural care."

Leadership Pathways is Covenant Health's leadership development program designed to support its mission, vision, values, strategic plan and leadership charter. It consists of seven levels of development (see Fig. 4.3).

Supported by LEADS in a Caring Environment, certified LEADS facilitators at Covenant have designed seven pathways to leadership for everyone from front-line employees to board members. These pathways are flexible and provide learning experiences based on the five domains of LEADS.

Following course and activity work, integrating and using the lessons is strengthened with a variety of learning resources, tools and experiences, including:

- *Comprehensive courses on Covenant Health's required capabilities*
- *Experiential learning in team, focused on organizational challenges*
- *Discussions*
- *Tools and techniques*
- *Online discussions on Covenant Health's web-based workspace for leadership development*
- *Assessment of learners' progress measured against Covenant's leadership development inventory*

All participants in Leadership Pathways are expected to strengthen their ability to model LEADS capabilities in Covenant Health. The program is optional and allows participants to work at their own pace.

Covenant Health's Leadership Pathways is offered to every employee. To get the most out of the program, Covenant encourages all employees to discuss participation with their managers so they can incorporate their personal goals in their individual learning plan.

The Covenant story shows how individual and organizational leadership development programs can be integrated in a comprehensive process of lifelong learning (Fig. 4.3).

In his book, *Constructivist Leadership*, Richard Kelly takes some of these ideas further, exploring what leadership development should look like in an era of digital transformation and empowered consumerism. He says "The knowledge/skills/competency-based model to developing leaders, which has dominated business leadership development for four decades, is not fit for purpose... New methodologies are needed." [23]. His suggestions support many of the notions in this book, including that leadership developers embrace virtual, augmented and mixed learning approaches. He also says approaches similar to what we've described earlier can be combined in "networked learning:" voluntary participation in leadership development using networks that provide access to resources for learning.

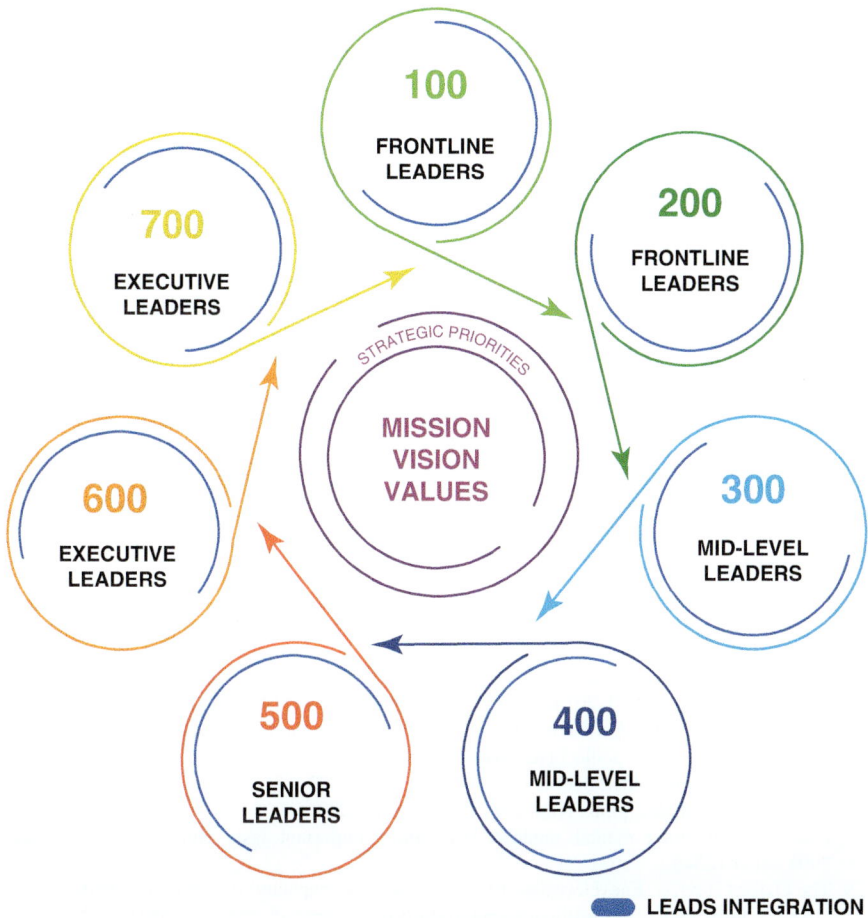

Fig. 4.3 Seven levels of leadership programming at Covenant Health

Summary

In this chapter we've discussed the significant evidence that leadership can be learned and developed, like music or athletic ability, through acquiring skills and knowledge and practising. We've learned that leadership and followership are symbiotic; and all leaders will do both over time. Learning can happen at both the individual and organizational levels. When the two are combined, the potential for developing distributed leadership is enhanced. We have identified some key factors, based on the metaphor of the hero's journey, which can facilitate both individual and organizational leadership development. Regardless of the approach taken, the discipline needed for success will depend on the will and commitment of people who want to increase their leadership capacity.

As this chapter underscores, what is most important is that you, the leader, need to see leadership development as a life-long learning process. Malcolm Gladwell, in his book *Outliers,* suggests in order to be truly proficient a person must practise a specific task for a total of around 10,000 hours [1]. The more deliberate you are in shaping that process (using the experiential tactics outlined in this chapter, for both individual and organizational leadership development), the quicker you will progress in your development journey. As we have shown in the Covenant Health example, your organization can (and should) provide support for learning.

We now invite you to embrace the opportunities to learn that the workplace provides for you and to use LEADS as a guide.

And that takes us to the first of the LEADS capabilities: Lead self.

References

1. Gladwell M. Outliers the story of success. New York: Little, Brown and Company; 2008.
2. Kouzes J, Posner B. The leadership challenge. 4th ed. San Francisco: Jossey Bass; 2007.
3. Oc B. Contextual leadership: a systematic review of how contextual factors shape leadership and its outcomes. Leadersh Q. 2018;29(1):218–35. https://doi.org/10.1016/j.leaqua.2017.12.004.
4. Argyris C, Schön D. Organizational learning II: theory, method and practice. Reading, Mass: Addison Wesley. Asia Pacific J Hum Res. 1998;36:107–9.
5. Argyris C. Teaching smart people how to learn. Sol J. 2002;4(2):4–15.
6. Senge P. The fifth discipline. New York: Doubleday; 2002.
7. Pfeffer J. Changing mental models: HR's most important task. Hum Resour Manage. 2005;44(2):123–8.
8. The Oxford Review. Encyclopedia of terms. Absorptive capacity: definition and explanation. 2018. https://www.oxford-review.com/oxford-review-encyclopaedia-terms/encyclopaedia-absorptive-capacity/. Accessed 20 Dec 2018.
9. Campbell J. The hero of a thousand faces. New York: Pantheon Books; 1949.
10. Brown J, Moffat C. The hero's journey: how educators can transform schools and improve learning. Alexandria, VA: Association for Supervision & Curriculum Development; 1999.
11. Eliot TS. The waste land. Poetry Foundation; 2019. https://www.poetryfoundation.org/poems/47311/the-waste-land. Accessed 18 Sep 2019.
12. MacKeracher D. Making sense of adult learning. 2nd ed. Toronto: University of Toronto Press; 2004.
13. Jarche H. Disorientation in learning; 2007. http://www.jarche.com/2007/06/disorientation-in-learning. Accessed 20 Jul 2013.
14. Marchildon G, Philippon D, Fletcher A. Prairie Node Case Study Final Report. [unpublished working paper]. Partnerships in Health Systems Redesign; Canadian Institutes of Health Research and the Michael Smith Research Foundation, 2013.
15. Ekington R, Pearse NJ, Moss J, Van der Steege M, Martin S. Global leaders' perceptions of elements required for effective leadership development in the twenty-first century. Leadership Org Dev J. 2017;38(8):1038–56. https://doi.org/10.1108/LODJ-06-2016-0145.
16. Johnstal SP. Successful strategies for transfer of learned leadership. Performance Improvement. 2013;52(7):5–12.

17. Drouin S. Developing organizational leadership capacities in preparation for a major transition in healthcare. PhD [Dissertation]. Victoria (BC): Royal Roads University; 2015.
18. Petrie N. Vertical leadership development—part 1. developing leaders for a complex world. Greensborough, PA: Centre for Creative Leadership (Parts 1 & 2); 2014. p. 1–14.
19. Konings KD, de Jong N, Lohrmann C, Sumskas L, Smith T, O'Connor SJ, et al. Is blended learning and problem-based learning course design suited to develop future public health leaders? an explorative European study. Public Health Rev. 2018;39:13. https://doi.org/10.1186/s40985-018-0090-y.
20. Dugan JP, Humbles AD. A paradigm shift in leadership education: Integrating critical perspectives into leadership development. New Dire Stud Leadersh. 2018;159:9–26. https://doi.org/10.1002/yd.20294.
21. Geerts J. Optimal leadership development for professionals. PhD [dissertation]. London: University of Cambridge; 2017.
22. Jeyaraman M, Qadar SMZ, Wierzbowski A, Farshidfar F, Lys J, Dickson G, et al. Return on investment in healthcare leadership development programs. Leadersh Health Serv (Bradf Engl). 2017;31(1):77–97. https://doi.org/10.1108/LHS-02-2017-0005.
23. Kelly R. Constructing leadership 4.0. Swarm leadership and the fourth industrial revolution. Palgrave-MacMillan: Swam (SUI); 2019.

The LEADS in a Caring Environment Framework: Lead Self

5

Graham Dickson and Bill Tholl

Tzu-kung asked, "What is kingcraft?"
The Master said: "Food enough, troops enough, and a trusting people."
Tzu-kung said: "Were there no help for it, which could best be spared of the three?"
"Troops," said the Master.
"And were there no help for it, which could better be spared of the other two?"
"Food," said the Master. "From of old all men die, but without trust a people cannot stand." [1]

Introduction

"Without trust people cannot stand." But what is trust? A word we often use but spend little time reflecting on. Webster's Dictionary defines trust as "believing in the reliability, truth, ability, or strength of." But of what? A quick response is, believing in the reliability, truth, ability, or strength of another person. But what if the true source of trust is in ourselves?

A colleague once said to one of your authors that "you can only trust others when you trust yourself in their presence." The author puzzled over this comment for a long time: what does it mean? What does trusting yourself in another's presence look like? How does trust revolve around how I see myself, rather than how the other person behaves? Six months passed and the enigma remained. And then it was revealed, as the following story demonstrates.

G. Dickson (✉)
Royal Roads University, Victoria, BC, Canada
e-mail: graham.dickson@royalroads.ca

B. Tholl
Canadian Health Leadership Network, Ottawa, ON, Canada
e-mail: btholl@chlnet.ca

© Springer Nature Switzerland AG 2020
G. Dickson, B. Tholl (eds.), *Bringing Leadership to Life in Health: LEADS in a Caring Environment*, https://doi.org/10.1007/978-3-030-38536-1_5

While preparing to teach the final day of a week-long university program on diversity in leadership to senior governmental employees, the faculty team—of which this author was a member—were told a small group of participants were going to announce to the class the program was not delivering what they needed, they were disenchanted and going home.

The plan had been to lead a large group session before final group presentations, and the team feared the complaint could derail the program and disrupt the presentations. One faculty member said proceeding as planned would potentially mean the disenchanted could sway some in the larger group to also leave, damaging our program's reputation. Two others called for cancelling the session and switching to small seminar groups so the malcontents would lose their audience and the dissension would not spread.

And then the words of my colleague came back to me—"You can only trust others when you trust yourself in their presence."

I realized we were projecting our fears onto the program participants. The real issue was that we were worried we could not handle the discord. We were afraid we might get angry, or not respond productively, leading other program participants to quit and leaving us looking like fools.

In fact, I realized, we weren't trusting ourselves in the presence of others. At that point I understood the way to deal with the situation was to build trust in myself, or in this case, my team: to believe in the reliability, truth and strength of our ability to respond to whatever happened the next day. We discussed what we would say, how we would handle our emotions and what we would do if people left anyway.

Bolstered by our talk we entered into the fray—and quickly realized only one person was disgruntled. We asked her calmly about her concerns and gave her the opportunity to speak in front of the group. That meant it wasn't us who had to respond: the other participants stepped up to support her in her discomfort and suggest how her concerns could be alleviated. In the end, it was a bonding event, not a divisive one and a great lesson in not projecting one's fears on other people.

The leadership lesson: Deal with your own fears. Prepare for the worst and accept your responsibility to respond to it. And trust—there's that word again—most human beings are motivated to act for the right reasons.

Learning Moment

Take a moment to reflect on the past six months at work.

- Have there been moments where you have not trusted yourself in a challenging situation, or in dealing with another person?
- Reflect on one of those moments. If you had looked internally at the time, to understand yourself and your reactions better, how might the situation or your reaction to it have changed?
- What might you do differently in the future if a similar situation arises?

This anecdote lays the foundation for the Lead Self domain of the LEADS framework.

In a nutshell, the principle underlying the first of five LEADS domains, Lead self, is that we can't lead others without first leading ourselves—we are all CEOs of self.

Recent research provides a strong foundation for our understanding of Lead self. Some of the theories that emphasize the internal focus of leadership variously label it as "authentic," "servant," "neo-charismatic," "spiritual" or "toxic/destructive." [2] These theories echo Chap. 2's definition of leadership and suggest elements of character, virtue and service (or the lack of them) are part of a leader's actions at home and at work. Practicing moral leadership, which is what these theories describe, is directly linked to feelings of well-being among workers and vice-versa—toxic/dark leadership helps create unhealthy workplaces [3].

To develop your own leadership skills, the Lead self domain asks you first to look internally, to discover your sense of duty, consideration and respect for others and then hone it, until you understand the core purpose of leadership is to enhance the health and wellness of people. The next step is to demonstrate that purpose in everything you do (putting the *caring* into the LEADS framework). Good intentions are not enough: you must act, or your capacity to lead will be diminished.

Lead self is the foundation of all the domains. You cannot have productive relationships dedicated to people's health and wellness (Engage others) without looking inward for your purpose; nor can you ask your organization to deliver caring health services (Achieve results) if the motivation to care does not permeate every decision you make and all activities you direct. You can't Develop coalitions to improve patient care if the motive for those coalitions is not to improve service. Finally, you will not succeed in Systems transformation if you have not transformed your own ways of thinking and acting.

To help you bring the Lead self domain to life, we outline four capabilities necessary for people to lead themselves. Leaders need to (1) be self-aware; (2) manage themselves; (3) develop themselves; and (4) demonstrate character. We'll explore each of these capabilities now.

Are-Self-Aware

To know oneself is the first step toward making flow a part of one's entire life. But just as there is no free lunch in the material economy, nothing comes free in the psychic one. If one is not willing to invest psychic energy in the internal reality of consciousness, and instead squanders it in chasing external rewards, one loses mastery of one's life, and ends up becoming a puppet of circumstances.

Mihaly Csikszentmihalyi [4]

What is the self? It's commonly understood as a person's essential being. What we believe, what we stand for: our souls. And as Csikszentmihalyi says, we should make an effort to know our internal reality for what it is. But the self is also changeable and self-awareness—knowing how your thoughts, actions and practices reflect the essence of you—requires ongoing work. In the absence of self-awareness, your actions may be more convenient than principled, just a response to the demands of the moment.

Brain research by Baron and colleagues has shown that one of the hallmarks of self-awareness is the ability to reflect on one's own thoughts, feelings and actions

[5]. Brain imaging studies show when people reflect on their own experiences, they activate the brain circuitry used when empathizing with someone else. As an expression of that research, and to counter the predilection of knee-jerk responses to the demands, Baron and colleagues propose *mindfulness* as the foundation of leadership flexibility.

Mindfulness is a form of self-awareness with two components. The first is to focus attention on one's immediate mental experiences. The second is the willingness to explore those current mental experiences in a non-judgmental manner, through a combination of openness, curiosity, and receptivity. Mindfulness is associated with authentic leadership. Louis Baron's study in 2016 showed action learning in a leadership development program can increase mindfulness, which in turn is associated with improvements in authentic leadership [6].

Ellen Langer is a professor of psychology at Harvard. After four decades of research on mindfulness, she argues mindfulness training makes it easier to pay attention, particularly in a complex environment such as health care. "You remember more of what you've done. You're more creative. You're able to take advantage of opportunities when they present themselves. You avert the danger not yet arisen. You like people better, and people like you better, because you're less evaluative. You're more charismatic." [7] Some studies have found that mindfulness education also increases empathy [8].

Components of Self-Awareness

Psychologist Carl Jung said: "Your visions will become clear only when you can look into your own heart. Who looks outside, dreams; who looks inside, awakes." [9] The LEADS framework describes the components of self-awareness as your own deep-seated motives, emotions, beliefs and assumptions. Without self-awareness, how can you know if your leadership is caring? Or inclusive? If you aren't aware of your inner biases around, say, mental health or diversity issues, how can you know their impact on your ability to lead? If you can recognize your own biases, you can challenge and alter them, so caring and inclusiveness can become part of your authentic self, and you can act accordingly.

None of this is to say a leader must be perfect. Everyone has flaws, but most can still lead if they admit to them—the issue is whether they are willing to challenge and change them. What most people find impossible to accept in a leader is deception. Leaders who dissemble, who cover up motives or are hypocritical, are clearly not people who care, either about their employees or the people their organizations are supposed to serve. They just want power.

When dishonesty is all about self-aggrandizement, getting power for its own sake, we don't tend to forgive. We don't like fakes and we're even more uncomfortable with people who start to believe the image they've created for themselves.

Learning Moment
Take a moment to reflect on a political leader in your country.

- Do you know who he is—the real person? Is she authentic—true to herself—or pretending to be something she is not?
- When you see authenticity, are you more likely to support someone? Why or why not?
- Why should others follow you? What do you say or do that shows people who you truly are?

Authentic leaders choose appropriate times to admit their vulnerabilities, are aware of who they are and accept it, flaws and all [10].

Self-delusion is the opposite of self-awareness. Whether it's rationalizing decisions, refusing to acknowledge your true nature or being unaware of what you truly believe, self-delusion lets you justify actions that are easy and self-gratifying, rather than doing the difficult thing for the common good [11]. Self-delusion is easy because it allows you to retreat into your own world view, and not attempt to understand the world view of others [12]. Research has shown all humans are prone to self-delusion—it's almost necessary for survival—but it's a matter of degree. Self-awareness lets us expose internal frauds that get in the way of our purpose.

In health care, separate, unchallenged world views can create disconnects between groups. Physicians, for example, may persuade themselves they alone are patient advocates and champions of quality—often to the point of thinking that physicians who move into administration have gone over to the "dark side." [13, 14] In turn, administrators may think themselves the guardians of value for money while physicians ignore the need to manage finances. These contrary world views can cause rifts between physicians and administrators and undermine the chances of them working together for health reform [15].

To use self-awareness to combat self-delusion, we need to start by acknowledging our potential for self-delusion, then, through self-reflection, expose what our world views, mental models and biases are, before rigorously challenging each of them to root out delusional notions [16]. Self-reflection can be developed in several ways [17]. It can be done through workshops and exercises devoted to building self-awareness, by asking others for feedback, by working with counsellors or mentors, by keeping a journal and through psychometric development assessments (a scientific approach to measuring individuals' mental capabilities and behavioural style). On your own you can seek out books and movies that explore power and self-delusion; there is no shortage of examples of this Achilles heel of leadership.

Learning Moment
Take the opportunity to have a conversation with a trusted colleague or friend.

Directions: Part 1
1. One of you is A, the other B. A interviews B, then B interviews A. Each interview is approximately seven minutes.
2. Each interviewer starts by asking *"Why do you want to be a leader in health care?"* and the interviewee answers.
3. Next, the interviewer asks, "Why is that important?" following up by asking the interviewee to reflect, introspectively, on the rationale for the original answer, and explain it.
4. The interviewer repeats "Why is that important?" three more times, pressing the interviewee to reflect and explain the rationale.
5. Repeat with roles switched.

Directions: Part 2—Consider these questions
1. What do your answers tell you are your true beliefs when it comes to your reasons to lead in health care? Are these beliefs consistent with concept of people-centred care?
2. Reflect on the past six months. Would others in your workplace see you acting in a manner consistent with your beliefs? Why or why not?

This "five whys" exercise is designed to help you uncover your internal stories, test them, and decide whether you want to adjust your world view. But internal adjustment is not enough. You must also consider whether your actions reflect your changed world view and if not, reshape them for the good of the group.

Manage Themselves

The second capability in the Lead self domain is that leaders manage themselves, taking responsibility for their own performance and health.

Self-management is introspection in action, where *manage* means applying mental discipline and rigour to the mindset and behaviour of the *self*. It means internal discipline (the psychic energy mentioned in the *Csikszentmihalyi* quote) is brought to bear on the mental landscape that shapes your practise of leadership, which if not managed, leads to non-productive behaviour. The capability Manage themselves, in its purest form, is action learning, a combination of mindfulness and action needed to respond productively with the agility that modern health workplaces require.

In this section we explore three key elements of self-management, which are:

- demonstrating emotional intelligence;
- building a productive leadership mindset; and
- balancing the demands of personal responsibility and accountability [18].

Demonstrating Emotional Intelligence

Emotions are a source of much energy. According to Swart and colleagues, in their book *Neuroscience for Leadership* [19], there are eight emotions that fuel our desire, commitment and will to do productive work. Five are survival emotions—fear, anger, disgust, shame and sadness; two are attachment spectrums (love/trust and joy/excitement) and the last is surprise. As the eight combine, in response to external stimulus, they construct feelings, which can either help you reach your leadership goal or get in the way of it. Recognizing the existence and power of these emotions—in ourselves and those we lead—is fundamental to managing ourselves and our relationships with others.

Managing one's emotions for personal satisfaction and efficacy is key to being an effective leader. Modern neuroscience tells us emotions may be innate, but it also tells us the brain has multiple information processing systems that can override emotions and determine how they are expressed. Stephen Pinker says "…minds are packed with combinatorial software that can generate an unlimited set of thoughts and behaviour." [20] This ability, when directed at managing our emotions, is called emotional intelligence.

In the book *The EQ Edge* by Harold Book and Steven Stein, emotional intelligence is defined as "an array of non-cognitive capabilities, competencies and skills that influence one's ability to succeed in coping with environmental demands and pressures." [21] Their research shows emotional intelligence can change over time and can be learned and expanded throughout life. Emotional intelligence can be measured through a test called the E-Q-I 2.0. Developed by Reuven Bar-On, the EQ-i has been validated by the American Psychological Association [22]. Based on 15 constructs of emotional intelligence in five realms, the test has demonstrated in many studies that individuals with higher emotional intelligence scores outperform those in similar contexts with lower emotional intelligence. The 15 components of emotional intelligence are shown in Table 5.1:

The aspects of emotional intelligence in the shaded boxes apply to Lead self. They are subject to triggers but can be controlled with effort. The other dimensions are called social intelligence and are more likely to be a function of interpersonal relationships. They are dealt with in Chap. 6: Engage others.

Table 5.1 Elements of emotional intelligence [19]

Self-perception	*The Interpersonal realm*
• Self-regard	• Empathy
• Self-actualization	• Social responsibility
• Emotional self-awareness	• Interpersonal relationships
The stress-management realm	*Decision making*
• Flexibility	• Problem solving
• Stress tolerance	• Reality testing
• Optimism	• Impulse control
Self-expression	
• Emotional expression	
• Assertiveness	
• Independence	

There are numerous exercises and programs to help you build your emotional intelligence muscle. We use the word muscle, because developing emotional intelligence is not unlike going to the gym to tone up—it must be done consistently and deliberately. We share one of these with you in our learning moment.

Learning Moment

In their book, *Neuroscience and Leadership*, Swart, Chisholm and Brown provide an exercise to make self-management a part of your leadership backpack. They call the exercise an interoception activity: being in touch with the physiological condition of your body. We have adapted it to reflect self-management.

At least once a day for a week or two, make a brief note of how you feel each day—physically and mentally—as you work with your leader. Use language that is as accurate as possible. At the end, ask yourself what you now know about your emotional and physical reactions that you did not know before. This will help you recognize data—coming from you—about the mind-body connection.

This is an activity you can use periodically to remain grounded and to increase your own self-management capacity.

Build a Productive Leadership Mindset

A second dimension of managing self includes consciously adopting a mindset that can balance the complex demands of leadership. Mindset is defined as "a state of psychological preparedness to perceive or respond to an anticipated stimulus or situation." [23] A leadership mindset is a conscious orientation of thought, based on our best knowledge and continuously enriched by experience and reflection. Unless you pay constant attention to your mindset, you might not recognize situations in which your emotions and actions need to be managed, or why.

A leadership mindset requires you to balance the tension between what might be perceived as competing choices. In the heat of the moment we often rush to choose one idea over another, rather than trying keep them in productive balance. One example is balancing friendship with a professional colleague who deserves corrective feedback and the obligation to provide that feedback. Another example is finding ways to minimize the moral distress a caregiver may feel faced with conflict between the welfare of one patient and a required hospital practice. Managing these opposing situations and doing your best to keep them in productive balance requires a certain mindset. Let's look at a few different mindsets that reflect a commitment to managing self.

One leadership mindset is "pursuing the 100-year vision in the immediate moment." A colleague who was proud of his Chinese ancestry told us that to maintain perspective on day-to-day progress, he damped down impatience for short-term success by putting it in a 100-year time frame. This is a kind of mindfulness—the leader has to be in the moment *and* see the moment in the long-term context. Our colleague understood a 100-year vision meant divorcing his self-esteem from immediate gratification and ongoing frustration and attaching it to a long-term purpose. At the same time, however, he had to be present in the moment: fully conscious and committed to what he was doing to achieve the long-term goal.

A second mindset you are encouraged to develop is *embracing chaos to discover order*, described by Beverly Kaye as leaders being comfortable in ambiguity and chaos [24, 25]. Chaos suggests an underlying flow of ideas or forces, which disrupt expected order and open up opportunities. On a psychological level, this means balancing the need to be in control (reflecting fear and anxiety) with seeing opportunity in chaos (reflecting trust and excitement).

One way to embrace chaos is to shift your focus from looking for stability to appreciating the dynamics of change. Change is triggered by a surge of new values, but stability, through long-standing values, perpetuates the status quo. It's important for leaders to explore surface chaos to determine its underlying values. Knowing the tension between new values and status quo values is the key to understanding why we need to change and the difficulties we—and others—will have with it. Value shifts are difficult places to be in, but we, as leaders, will find ourselves there.

An alternative way of embracing chaos is to see it as an opportunity to be creative, to explore, to generate new goals and directions—in other words to envision a better future. For followers, chaos is uncomfortable; it creates (in the words of the hero's journey) confusion and sometimes resistance or fear of being inadequate. Followers don't know how to move forward in chaos; it is a leader's heroic quest that engages their will to act. But if the followers don't share what the leader is questing after, they won't align their journey with those aspirations. In this case the leader's journey could easily be interpreted as self-gratification. The following story illustrates this.

Joan was an executive coach, working with Jack, a physician, who was vice-president of quality in a large health authority. Jack was describing getting pushback from some nurses and doctors over quality improvement policies he wanted implemented. He had no idea where the resistance was coming from.

"I told them we have to be the best of the best, this is about meeting quality benchmarks, it's a question of proving how well we perform on the most important measures there are. If we're not the best, we can't claim to be excellent providers. For some reason I got a really lukewarm response. What's wrong with them? Why don't they see how important quality is?"

Joan thought for moment, then asked "So Jack: why is being the best so important to you?"

Jack responded immediately. "Ever since I was a child I've strived to be the best at whatever I do. In school, I was always top of my class. It was really important to be the best and it's still a real strength of mine."

"And," Joan said, "Why is that important?"

"Well," Jack responded, "You can't get into medical school if you're not the best of the best. I wouldn't have become VP of quality if I weren't the best.

"Jack," Joan responded. "Why is being the best at quality important? Is there a reason beyond simply being the best?"

"Excellence is a goal in its own right," said Jack. "It's part of being a strong leader, it's who I want to be."

"But is that the message you wanted to give your colleagues?" Joan asked, "Isn't performing well at quality important because it's in the best interests of your patients—the goal you all share? Isn't giving patients the best care possible the ultimate quality goal?"

"That goes without saying," said Jack. "That's exactly why I want to be seen to be the best and why it's important people understand that I will not be satisfied with less."

"I get that Jack," Joan said, noting how quickly the conversation veered away from patients to Jack's need for recognition. "Being the best at something, especially quality—is important. But why is it important? Remember, you asked me why your colleagues were lukewarm. Could it be because the message they were hearing is that improving quality matters because you need to be the best? In other words, more to satisfy your needs than the patients? Is that possible?"

"Maybe," said Jack. "But I'm not sure what you mean. Isn't being the best at quality obviously in the patients' interest?"

"Jack," responded Joan. "Reflect on the meeting—what you said, your tone of voice, your motivation. If your message was 'Do this for me because being best is important to me,' rather than 'Do this because excellent quality is good for patients,' you might have a clue why the meeting didn't go well. Please think about that before our next call, and when you're in meetings over the next week or so, be mindful of what message you're trying to deliver, and how best to deliver it so it reflects a shared vision with others, rather than your own needs."

Jack agreed and used some of the self-directed learning tools (introduced in Chap. 4) to explore why he was preoccupied with excellence. He also worked to ensure he grounded his messages in the shared commitment he and his colleagues had to patients and families.

Jack's story shows how the "five whys" mentioned above work, and emphasizes two key aspects of self-management: the value of reflection and mindfulness. Joan and Jack used the dissonance between Jack and his colleagues to discover how to bring order to the situation. The solution is consciously reinforcing the vision of higher quality care that is the bond between Jack and his colleagues. As well, urged by Joan, Jack was reminded of the value of reflection and mindfulness as he examined the experience, motives, and feelings of both himself and his team and then used them to understand how his message could unite people in a common cause.

Productively Balance the Demands of Personal Responsibility and Accountability

As leaders, we have responsibilities and accountabilities. Our primary responsibilities come from leadership itself: *the collective capacity of an individual or group to influence people to work together to achieve a common constructive purpose: the health and wellness of the population we serve.* They are:

- Integrating the work of professionals and staff, so they can act collectively as agents of health and wellness;
- Working with all members of the system to improve health and wellness through people-centred care; and
- Achieving results that improve and promote the health and wellness of the population we serve.

Managing your responsibilities and accountabilities is an important dimension of the Manage self capability. To understand their relationship to self-management, consider Steven Covey's definition of responsibility (or as he phrases it, *response-ability*): the ability to respond, productively, to the duties of your role [26]. For a front-line leader, that means responding productively to patients or families. If you're a finance manager your immediate clients are clear but your relationship to patients/families is not. Your responsibility is to understand the impact of your decisions on them and act accordingly. For patients or patient advocates (leaders in your own roles) your responsibility is to balance your personal demands with understanding the personal health and the safety needs of those being advocated for; and to act accordingly. We cannot be *response-able* if we don't thoughtfully understand and accept what is needed by self and others to achieve our collective goal of health and wellness.

As Jack's story shows, the motives behind our actions and how we express them have an impact we need to be aware of. We also need to be able—as Jack initially was not—to accept accountability.

Finally, the challenge of managing self includes an overriding obligation to take responsibility not only for your performance, but for your health. We can't lead effectively if we are mentally or physically unhealthy. Also, there is deep power in modelling health and wellness for others. Not accepting responsibility on this front undermines our authenticity as leaders.

Develop Themselves

Carol Dweck, a psychology professor at Stanford, has done work on mindsets that is fundamental to the Lead self capability of Develop themselves. Her research, based on evidence the brain is capable of lifelong learning and development, shows leaders can move from a fixed mindset (such as a belief your qualities are unchangeable) to a growth mindset: whereby personal qualities can be cultivated through deliberate effort (as we discussed at length in Chap. 4) [27]. You can change who you are if you're self-aware and follow the approaches described throughout this book.

Our analysis of leadership theories and research reinforces the importance of developing oneself. Modern health leaders have to keep growing and developing. Why? Leadership scholar Kets DeVries and his fellow authors say "In a knowledge-driven society, many learned competencies become obsolete at the speed of light… The challenge of unlearning old things and learning new ones is exacerbated by the fact that executives have less and less discretionary time." [28]

To develop self is to keep learning and since the context and work of leading is creating change, learning is continuous. If we as leaders are not open to changing ourselves, how can we ask others, or the organization, to change? Demonstrating how you manage change is modelling for others what you expect of them. As the noted consultant and scholar Peter Senge has said: "There is an old tradition that you see in many parts of the world that if you're going to be in a position of authority, you should be a *cultivator*. Leaders should be people who are deeply involved in their own realization of becoming a human being." [29]

Margaret Cromack, a former CEO in Canada's health system, was trained as a nurse. She has written "The LEADS framework provided a structure to situate my career path and my personal journey toward the position of chief executive officer." [30] But it's clear some of the capabilities we describe as part of LEADS came naturally to her, as these examples of developing self and managing self show:

> Early in my career, I recognized that the ability to manage myself under any circumstance made a significant difference to the people around me. While rushing to the emergency room, I took the few minutes that we had in the elevator, prior to the run and push with the arrest cart, to collect myself, calm down, breathe deeply, and think about what I needed to do when we arrived. What a difference it made to my being able to contribute to calming the people in the room when we arrived.
>
> Over time, I worked on this skill to manage my reaction to stressful experiences by calming my physiological reaction with deep breathing, listening, and taking time to develop a thoughtful response rather than reacting. It has become a defining character trait of my leadership capability [30].

The article describes challenges and successes on her journey that show the importance of a growth mindset and always developing leadership capacity.

Develop self has three fundamental principles. The first is to know your personality, strengths and limitations—what you do well and what you don't. The second is to take a systematic approach to learning. Make it part of your daily routine (including getting formal feedback on your development). The third is the commitment to applying what you learn. The LEADS framework helps you put all three principles into practice with guidance on what's important to know, tools and activities to help you learn and as a guide for continuous learning by defining the qualities of leadership valued in the workplace.

Personal Mastery: A Discipline for Self-Development

A self-directed approach [31] to developing your leadership is sometimes referred to as personal mastery. Peter Senge defines it as "the discipline of continually clarifying and deepening our personal vision, of focusing our energies, of developing patience, and of *seeing reality objectively.*" [32] It's the last aspect that obliges leaders to evaluate their personal performance so they can set directions for growth. In many of the learning moments in this book we use activities designed to help you see your leadership "objectively." We're putting quotation marks around objectively because we would rewrite Senge's definition to seeing reality *subjectively.* Yes, we should gather evidence and feedback on our performance as a leader, but even 360 evidence is based on someone's subjective interpretation. Objectivity toward leadership—like beauty—is not possible; it can only be approximated.

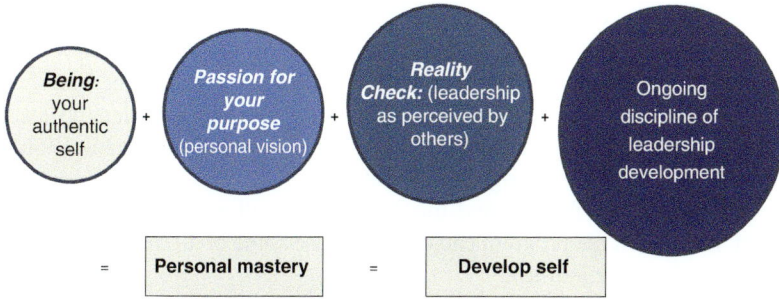

Fig. 5.1 The dynamics of personal Mastery

Astute readers will see that personal mastery is a disciplined approach to their hero's journey, using experience, allies and insight to grow. Personal mastery puts self-management and self-development into practise. Its skills include:

> …self-observation, self-goal-setting, self-reward, rehearsal, self-job redesign, and self-management of internal dialogues and mental imagery….These principles require the leader to gather data through self-reflection, using instruments, directed learning tools, and journaling, and to use that data to set goals and monitor progress through a personal learning program [33].

Personal mastery, as Fig. 5.1 illustrates, begins with examining the challenges you face as a leader in the health system and your role in it. Facing those challenges requires you keep your values, personality, emotional reactions and talents always in mind and ensure they are in the forefront of what you do. Then you move to clarifying your vision and infusing it with passion, so you can bring your leadership energy to bear on workplace issues. As you do that you interact with others and, in keeping with your personal mastery regimen, gather feedback on how your actions resonate with followers—what we call seeing reality subjectively. The final step is establishing directions for growth. Personal mastery is the route to becoming a master of your profession by maximizing the instruments of self, as we described in Chap. 4.

Putting LEADS to Work: Operationalizing Personal Mastery

The University of Alberta's Fellowship in Health Systems Improvement, mentioned in Chap. 4, has built a personal mastery component into the program, using self-directed learning. Each participant chooses a goal for self-improvement, designs their learning method and participates in a coaching/mentoring[1] conversation with

---

[1]The facilitators use a combination of coaching and mentoring techniques in working with their coachee/mentee. When acting as a coach, the facilitator will ask questions and probe to draw out answers from the person rather than provide them. When acting as a mentor, they will provide guidance and expertise that is needed by the mentee.

facilitators who are knowledgeable about LEADS and have experience in health care leadership.

Using LEADS as a guide, each participant does a self-assessment, and through self-reflection and a coaching/mentoring dialogue, chooses a leadership learning goal that represents a benefit to themselves—and their sponsor organizations—to focus on as they progress through the program.

To operationalize reflection and mindfulness, self-directed learning tactics are provided. Leaders in the program can choose to use some or all to bring structure to their personal mastery journey.

A Strengths-Based Approach

Developing leadership requires us to know our strengths and how to use them for maximum effectiveness. "Research is showing that the more leaders use their unique strengths, the higher their performance will be in the workplace…and their levels of happiness, fulfillment, authenticity, goal accomplishment, and optimal functioning will increase." [34]

Focusing on weakness leads to mediocrity, not mastery, but developing strengths leads to exceptional performance.

> Proactive leaders work from their strengths, have a clear purpose and vision, have a plan, and understand that they have choices in any given situation. They achieve greater success by focusing on things they have direct control over, such as their own behaviour and reactions, and spend less time on things they have indirect or no sway over, like other people's behaviour and reactions [17].

Welch and colleagues provide interesting insights from expert coaches on methods to build on your strengths [34]. They suggest you should identify your strengths through the use of validated instruments such as the StrengthFinder [35], reflect on situations and circumstances where your energy is at its highest, and grow your own awareness of how your strengths contributed to that situation. They also recommend spending some time reflecting on how your strengths can be applied in different situations and circumstances and that you engage in dialogue with a trusted peer or coach to explore how to use your strengths more effectively.

However, focusing exclusively on your strengths is not a guarantee of success. In fact, a strength used inappropriately or excessively can be a weakness [36, 37]. For example, your strength may be that you're results oriented, but if you employ it when compassion is needed, it'll be a fail. Also, focusing solely on your strengths could lead to complacency and stagnation, leaving you unready to deal with new situations. You can avoid those pitfalls by taking on new assignments, which can help you develop by demanding different skills.

Learning Moment

There is the charming story of the animal school, in which the hare, the tortoise, and the monkey were being scheduled for their next year's program. The school counsellor looked at the hare's transcript and noted that she was extremely good at hopping but had failed climbing. So she took her out of Hopping 2 and enrolled her in a remedial climbing program.

The tortoise had excelled at swimming, but was deplorable at hopping: so he was scheduled into remedial hopping. The monkey was excellent at climbing, but really poor at swimming…and you can guess how this goes.

Reflect on the following questions:

1. How productive do you think the remedial programs would be? Either in terms of personal motivation, or improved results?
2. How does this story relate to Carol Dweck's concept of fixed and growth mindsets? Is leadership a function of physical wiring or a mental muscle that can be developed?
3. If you were to identify one strength and one weakness you bring to the practice of leadership, what would they be?
   - How might working on the strength enhance your leadership capability?
   - Is it worth working on the weakness, or are there better ways to compensate for that?

Demonstrates Character

"Character is the voice inside which speaks and says, 'This is the real me.'
Effective leaders, and effective people, know this voice very well."

Warren Bennis

This quote from Warren Bennis, founder of the Leadership Institute at the University of Southern California, was echoed in recent research that asked senior leaders from across Canada to identify qualities of leadership. The qualities mentioned most—passion, integrity, focus, resilience, commitment, persistence, courage and credibility—all spoke to character [38]. We noted a similar trend when we were doing the research for LEADS, which led us to this capability, *Demonstrates character*. As one interviewee said about integrity and credibility, "In reality you only have one tool in your toolbox and that is your word. Your word has to mean something."

Does it pay to demonstrate character? An article in the Harvard Business Review said it does. The researchers found CEOs whose employees gave them high marks for character had an average return on assets nearly five times as much that of those with low character [39]. Bernard Bass, the father of transformational leadership, says character does matter in leadership. "This is not to deny that evil people can bring about good things or that good people can lead the way to moral ruin. Rather, leadership provides a moral compass and, over the long term, both personal development and the common good are best served by a moral compass that reads true." [40] In health care, studies have shown transformational leadership has a positive impact on organizational culture, such as employee stress, job satisfaction, and psychological health [41]. Moral character provides followers with a sense of predictability, which may help them cope with uncertainty.

The degree to which one demonstrates character is closely associated with emotional intelligence. For example, when making complex decisions that require moral or ethical considerations, the more primitive emotional centres of your brain (the limbic system) coordinate with the newer part involved in planning and social empathy (the prefrontal cortex). Clinically, people who have underdeveloped character, such as sociopaths, have been shown to have poor connection between those brain centres. So, the ability to act morally, in other words, requires a healthy connection between the feeling and thinking centres of your brain.

Recent research in health care leadership has shown the importance of *resilience*, defined as "the ability to bounce back from adversity, frustration, and misfortune." [42] Resilience comprises many other elements of character including integrity, adaptability, patience and courage. Recent research suggests, similar to emotional intelligence, resilience can be developed like a muscle, in both people and organizations [43]. What can individuals do to increase their resilience? Welcome feedback through LEADS-based 360s such as the LEADS self-assessment at the end of this chapter or through regular bilateral meetings with your coach, mentor, supervisor or board chair. Look for new challenges: opportunities to grow, learn, contribute and feel valued. See adversity as a challenge and willingly take on risks, looking for success but knowing with failure comes an opportunity to learn and "fail forward." Stretch yourself, test your strengths, and admit vulnerabilities, to learn more about potential weaknesses. Build strong, personal, and professional networks.

Building Character, Building Resilience

Character, like any other attribute we are born with, can be developed. To do that, leaders must be conscious of what constitutes character, and want to develop it. One of the most important ways to develop character is to focus on it. Recognize it in yourself, the challenges to it and reflect how you react to those challenges. Journal your reflections or share them in conversations. Listen carefully to what others did in situations they've faced and think how you would want to react in similar circumstances. Gene Klann, in collaboration with the Center for Creative Leadership in the United States, has devised a five-step process called the Five E's of Character

Development. He says you develop your character by focusing on examples, education, environment, experience and evaluation [44].

According to the Mayo Clinic, the most important exercise for improving your personal resilience is to train your attention and awareness. "Becoming more intentional and purposeful will decrease your negative thoughts and draw your attention to what is most meaningful around you." [45] As we said earlier in this chapter, being more intentional and mindful can substantially decrease stress and anxiety while enhancing overall quality of life. Resilient leaders stay focused on their "north star" within the overall context of organizational resilience (more on this in Chap. 7: Achieve results).

Summary

As we've seen, leadership is an ongoing, lifelong process of development. Those pursuing it:

- Are self aware
- Manage themselves
- Develop themselves
- Demonstrate character

Each of the four capabilities of the Lead self domain is aimed at clarifying and focusing you on building internal strength so you can lead others with confidence, purpose and conviction. Remember: you have to trust yourself before you can be trustworthy in the presence of others. The exercises and stories in this chapter highlight how the Lead self capabilities reinforce each other to build trust in yourself that can be conveyed to others. Circling back to where we began this chapter on the importance of trust, the Rt. Hon. David Johnston, formerly Canada's governor general, said in his book called *Trust*: "While it is something that most of us take for granted, trust is a vital quality that grows stronger as it is acknowledged and cultivated (like a garden) attentively." [46]

To help you lead yourself, we'll end this chapter with a self-assessment exercise. Please evaluate yourself, then based on your results identify one capability you think you should work on to improve your leadership.

Learning Moment
Using the following LEADS self-assessment, assess how well you demonstrate the four Lead self capabilities. Choose the appropriate level (relative to your level of responsibility) to make that assessment.

If there was one capability you would like to improve upon, what is it? Why?

Lead Self Self-Assessment (For on-line access to self assessment tool, please visit www.LEADSglobal.ca.)

Informal leader (patient, family member, citizen) responsibilities

In order to use my attributes of self to be a better leader, I

1.	Make a conscious effort to continuously surface my assumptions, values, principles, strengths and limitations; understand them as it relates to my own health; and my expectations of care providers or the healthcare system	1 2 3 4 5 6 7 N
2.	As a respectful consumer of healthcare services or engaged citizen, take responsibility for managing my emotions, mindsets and my personal responsibilities	1 2 3 4 5 6 7 N
3.	Systematically seek out opportunities for learning and developing myself in order to influence others effectively	1 2 3 4 5 6 7 N
4.	Recognize the qualities of character as demanded of me in my advocacy role; and try to exercise them accordingly	1 2 3 4 5 6 7 N

Front-line leader responsibilities

In order to use my attributes of self to be a better leader, I

1.	Make a conscious effort to surface my assumptions, values, principles, strengths and limitations; and understand them in the context of my supervisory role	1 2 3 4 5 6 7 N
2.	Take responsibility for managing my emotions, mindset and role expectations as they relate to my role of supervisor	1 2 3 4 5 6 7 N
3.	Systematically seek out opportunities for learning; and be disciplined in developing myself in the context of my supervisory role	1 2 3 4 5 6 7 N
4.	Recognize the qualities of character demanded of me in my supervisory role, and I am deliberate in demonstrating them	1 2 3 4 5 6 7 N

Mid-manager leader responsibilities

In order to use my attributes of self to be a better leader, I

1.	Make a conscious effort to surface my assumptions, values, principles, strengths and limitations; and understand them in the context of my mid-management role, connecting senior and supervisory leaders	1 2 3 4 5 6 7 N
2.	Take responsibility for managing my emotions, mindset and role expectations as they relate to my role of mid-manager	1 2 3 4 5 6 7 N
3.	Systematically employ personal mastery (either formally through a personal learning plan or informally) in my mid-management role	1 2 3 4 5 6 7 N
4.	Recognize that qualities of character are often tested in a mid-management role, and I am deliberate in exercising them	1 2 3 4 5 6 7 N

Senior leader responsibilities

In order to use my attributes of self to be a better leader, I

1.	Make a conscious effort to continuously surface my assumptions, values, principles, strengths and limitations; and understand them in the context of my strategic role to connect mid-managers with organizational priorities	1 2 3 4 5 6 7 N

2.	Take responsibility for managing my emotions, mindset and role expectations as they relate to interacting with executives and mid-management	1 2 3 4 5 6 7 N
3.	Systematically employ personal mastery—either formally (through a personal learning plan) or informally, to enhance my interpersonal and strategic capabilities	1 2 3 4 5 6 7 N
4.	Recognize that qualities of character are regularly tested in bridging strategic and operational responsibilities; and I am deliberate in exercising them	1 2 3 4 5 6 7 N

Executive leader responsibilities

In order to use my attributes of self to be a better leader, I

1.	Make a conscious effort to surface my assumptions, values, principles, strengths and limitations; and exercise them appropriately in my interactions with the board, media, other executives, professional groups, staff, stakeholders and the community	1 2 3 4 5 6 7 N
2.	Take responsibility for managing my emotions, mindset and role expectations as they relate to interacting with the board, media, other executives, staff, professional groups, stakeholders and the community	1 2 3 4 5 6 7 N
3.	Model personal mastery either formally (through a personal learning plan) or informally, in a process aimed at enhancing my executive capability	1 2 3 4 5 6 7 N
4.	Recognize that qualities of character are regularly tested in bridging strategic and operational responsibilities; and I am deliberate in exercising them	1 2 3 4 5 6 7 N

References

1. Bartleby.com. The sayings of Confucius, The Harvard Classics. 1909–14 XII, 7; 2019. https://www.bartleby.com/44/1/12.html. Accessed 23 Sep 2019.
2. Inceoglu I, Thomas G, Chu C, Plans D, Gerbasi A. Leadership behavior and employee well-being: an integrated review and a future research agenda. Leadersh Q. 2018;29(1):179–202. https://doi.org/10.1016/j.leaqua.2017.12.006. and Banks B, Gooty J, Ross RL, Williams CE, Harrington NT. Construct redundancy in leader behaviors: a review and agenda for the future. Leadersh Q, 2018;29(1), 236-251. doi:10.1016/j.leaqua.2017.12.005.
3. Sharma P. Moving beyond the employee: the role of the organizational context in leader workplace aggression. Leadersh Q. 2018;29(1):203–17. https://doi.org/10.1016/j.leaqua.2017.12.002. and Pundt A, Sxhwarzbeck K. Abusive supervision from an integrated self-control perspective. Appl. Psychol. 2017;00(00):1-25.
4. Optimize; 2019. https://www.optimize.me/quotes/mihaly-csikszentmihalyi/20250-to-know-oneself-is-the-first-step-toward/. Accessed 23 Sep 2019.
5. Baron L, Rouleau V, Simon G, Baron C. Mindfulness and leadership flexibility. J Manag Dev. 2018;37(2):165–77.
6. Baron L. Authentic leadership and mindfulness development through action learning. J Manag Psychol. 2016;31(1):296–311. https://doi.org/10.1108/JMP-04-2014-0135.
7. Spotlight: Interview with Ellen Langer. Mindfulness in the age of complexity. Harv Bus Rev. 2014;1:21–5.

8. Ridderinkhof A, de Bruin EI, Brummelman E, Bögels SM. Does mindfulness meditation increase empathy? an experiment. Self Identity. 2017 May;16(3):251–69. https://doi.org/10.1 080/15298868.2016.1269667.

9. Jung C, Sharma R. The monk who sold his ferrari. New York: HarperCollins; 1998.

10. Caramela S. 4 ways to unmask vulnerability and become a stronger leader. Business News Daily. 2018 Apr 9 5:08 pm EST. https://www.businessnewsdaily.com/10680-unmasking-vul-nerabilities-leadership.html. Accessed 5 Sep 2019.

11. Arbinger Institute. Leadership and self-deception: getting out of the box. San Francisco: Barrett-Koehler; 2010.

12. Zaphron S, Logan D. The three laws of performance: rewriting the future of your organization and your life. San Francisco: Jossey-Bass; 2009.

13. LohI MJ, Thomas L, Bismarck M, Phelps G, Dickinson H. Shining the light on the dark side of medical leadership—a qualitative study in Australia. Leadersh Health Serv (Bradf Engl). 2016;29(3):313–30.

14. Dickson G. Physician identity: benefit or curse. CJPL. 2015;2(2):55–7.

15. Dickson G. Anchoring physician engagement in vision and values: principles and framework. Saskatchewan: Regina Qu'Appelle Health Region 0; 2012. http://www.rqhealth.ca/service-lines/master/files/anchoring.pdf. Accessed 5 Sep 2019.

16. Carissa L, Philippi J, Feinstein S, Khalsa A, Tranel D, Landini G, et al. Preserved self-awareness following extensive bilateral brain damage to the insula, anterior cingulate, and medial pre-frontal cortices. PLoS One. 2012;7(8) https://doi.org/10.1371/journal.pone.0038413.

17. Mohapel P. Lead self. Book one of five LEADS booklets. Ottawa: Canadian College of Health Leaders 2010. https://leadscanada.net/site/books. Accessed 4 Sep 2019.

18. Marques J, Dhiman S, editors. Engaged leadership. Cham (SUI): Springer; 2018.

19. Swart T, Chisholm K, Brown P. Neuroscience for leadership. Swam{SUI: Palgrave Macmillan; 2015.

20. Pinker S. The blank slate: the modern denial of human nature. New York: Penguin; 2002.

21. Stein S, Book H. The E.Q. edge: emotional intelligence and your success. Mississauga (ON): Wiley Publishing; 2000.

22. Bar-On R. The Bar-On model of emotional-social intelligence (ESI). Psicothema. 2006;18:13–25.

23. Merriam Webster Staff. Merriam-Webster's Collegiate Dictionary. 11th ed. Springfield (MA): Merriam Webster Staff; 2004. p. 1139.

24. Kaye B. Help them grow or watch them go: a development edge gives retention results. San Fransisco: Berrett-Koehler; 2012.

25. Goldsmith M, Govindarajan V, Kaye B, Vicere A. The many facets of leadership. New York: Pearson; 2003.

26. Covey S. Seven habits of highly effective people. New York: Free Press; 1990.

27. Dweck C. Mindset: the new psychology of success. New York: Ballantine Books; 2016.

28. De Vries K, Ramo LG, Korotov K. Organizational culture, Leadership, change, and stress. Instead; 2018. https://sites.insead.edu/facultyresearch/research/doc.cfm?did=41924. Accessed 5 Sep 2019.

29. Senge P, Scharmer C, Jaworkski J, Flowers B. Presence: human purpose and the field of the future. Cambridge, (MA): Society for Organizational Learning; 2004.

30. Cromack M. A journey of leadership from bedside nurse to Chief Executive Officer. Nurs Adm Q. 2012;36(1):29–34.

31. Dickson G, Norman P, Shoop M. Self-directed learning as a strategy for improved health literacy and health human resource continuing professional education. Victoria, BC: Royal Roads University; 2007.

32. Senge P. The fifth discipline. New York: Doubleday; 2006.

33. Pearce C, Manz C. The new silver bullets of leadership: the importance of self- and shared leadership in knowledge work. Organ Dyn. 2005;34(2):130–40. https://doi.org/10.1016/j.orgdyn.2005.03.003.

34. Welch D, Grossaint K, Reid K, Walker C. Strengths-based leadership development: insights from expert coaches. Consult Psychol J: Pract Res. 2014;66(1):20–37. https://doi.org/10.1037/cpb0000002.
35. Rath T, de Vries D. StrengthsFinder 2.0. New York: Gallup Press; 2007.
36. Lombardo M, Eichinger R. For your improvement: a development and coaching guide. Lohminger: South Minneapolis; 1998.
37. Zenger J, Folkman J. Ten fatal flaws that derail leaders. Harv Bus Rev; 2009.
38. Dickson G, Tholl B, Baker GR, Blais R, Clavel N, Gorley C, et al. Partnerships for health system improvement, leadership and health system redesign: cross-case analysis. Ottawa: Royal Roads University, Canadian Health Leadership Network, Canadian Institutes of Health Research, Michael Smith Foundation for Health Research; 2014. http://tinyurl.com/qh6ogzu.
39. Anonymous. Measuring the return on character. Har Bus Rev. 2015;93(4):20–12.
40. Bass B, Steidlmeier P. Ethics, character, and authentic transformational leadership behaviour. Leadersh Q. 1999;10(2):181–217.
41. Arnold K. Transformational leadership and employee psychological well-being: a review and directions for future research. J Occup Health Psychol. 2017;22(3):381–93.
42. Ledesma J. Conceptual frameworks and research models on resilience in leadership. SAGE Open. 2014:1–8.
43. McQueen G, Bart C. Enhancing physician leadership resilience. Canad J Phys Lead. 2015:12–5.
44. Klann G, Mohapel P. Lead self. Book one of five LEADS booklets. Ottawa: Canadian College of Health Leaders; 2010. https://leadscanada.net/site/books. Accessed 4 Sep 2019.
45. Mayo Clinic. Smart management and resiliency (SMART) program attention & interpretation therapy session handout. Mayo Clinic; 2019. https://mcpa.memberclicks.net/assets/ETI2014/PresentationHandouts2014/finding%20serenity%20amidst%20the%20storm-stress%20management%20and%20resiliency%20training.pdf. Accessed 5 Sep 2019.
46. Johnston D. Trust: twenty ways to build a better country. Toronto: Random House; 2018.

The LEADS in a Caring Environment Framework: Engage Others

Graham Dickson and Bill Tholl

...no individual in our movement can change Mississippi. No one organization in our movement can do the job...alone. I have always contended that if all of us get together, we can change the face of Mississippi. This isn't any time for organizational conflicts, this isn't any time for ego battles over who's going to be the leader. We are all the leaders here in this struggle....

Martin Luther King [1]

This quote by Martin Luther King on the civil rights struggle in Mississippi could just as easily be written about health care. To paraphrase: "If we—administrators, professional clinicians, employees, community groups, family members—can just get together, we can change the face of health care." Getting together is the key. In our definition of leadership, leaders engage others—teams, organizations, patients, families, communities, systems—who get together to develop and deliver service and, in the spirit of distributed leadership, become leaders themselves.

We define engagement as: "constructive joint action between leaders and followers to achieve a shared vision of high-quality patient care." The main factor that shapes workplace engagement is the quality of its leadership [2–6]. In recognition of the importance of engagement, many organizations have added to the well-known US Institute for Health Improvement's triple aim—improving the health of populations, enhancing the experience of care for individuals, and reducing the per capita cost of health care—a fourth aim: attaining joy in work [7].

While optimal engagement is the ideal, the real degree to which an organization or group achieves engagement is on a sliding scale from "hostile engagement," typical of toxic organizations, to the highest level, found in

G. Dickson (✉)
Royal Roads University, Victoria, BC, Canada
e-mail: graham.dickson@royalroads.ca

B. Tholl
Canadian Health Leadership Network, Ottawa, ON, Canada
e-mail: btholl@chlnet.ca

© Springer Nature Switzerland AG 2020
G. Dickson, B. Tholl (eds.), *Bringing Leadership to Life in Health: LEADS in a Caring Environment*, https://doi.org/10.1007/978-3-030-38536-1_6

generative organizations. There are unfortunately numerous examples in health care of the negative face of engagement. In a report, the auditor general for the state of Victoria in Australia, put it this way:

> …health sector agencies are failing to respond effectively to bullying and harassment as a serious [occupational health and safety] risk. They are not demonstrating adequate leadership on these issues, which is illustrated by the fact that the audited agencies do not understand the extent, causes or impact of bullying and harassment in their respective organizations, even when such issues have resulted in significant media attention and reputational damage [8].

Engagement in Context

Health services to patients and citizens are delivered by providers who consume a large proportion of health care expenditures, "and earnings of health professionals have increased at a higher rate than in the general economy." [9] That money goes to pay doctors and nurses, other professionals and all the workers, from clerks to cleaners, who support them. Their services, of course, are being delivered to patients, clients, families and citizens—for whom the health system exists; and who are the focus of your efforts to engage followers.

Engaging highly educated professionals has special challenges: they are knowledge workers, often self-directed, expert in their profession, and predisposed to managing themselves rather than being managed. Their knowledge, judgment, beliefs, values and ethics will determine how well—and sometimes whether—a service is delivered, or a change will happen. Leaders who do not recognize the dynamics of knowledge workers are destined to fail at engagement with them. But engagement isn't solely an issue for knowledge workers; although its absence is egregious for the performance of their work. It is also an important issue to create healthy workplaces for all employees, regardless of their responsibilities.

Tse and colleagues [10] recommend health care leaders constantly assess their emotions and the impact they may have on followers, teams and the overall organizational climate. Successful engagement is determined by how employees' personalities, characters, knowledge and resources interact within the workplace, and with the leader. That interaction can be either enhanced or impeded by actions of the leader, the organization and the individual.

In 2013 the Mental Health Commission of Canada asked the Canadian Standards Association to outline the workplace conditions necessary for the creation of psychologically healthy and well workplaces [11]. In 2018 the *"By Health, For Health" Collaborative* (the Collaborative) led by the Mental Health Commission of Canada [12] and Healthcare*CAN*[1] asked your authors to show the relationship between the *LEADS in a Caring Environment* capabilities framework and the 13 workplace

---

[1] Healthcare*CAN* is the national voice of health care organizations and hospitals across Canada. It is a member organization, comprised of hospitals and regions across the country that deliver service to patients.

conditions[2] the Canadian Standards Association had developed. The results showed *LEADS in a Caring Environment*, if put into practice, would contribute significantly to enhancing those conditions and therefore the engagement of knowledge workers [13].

Learning Moment

Take a moment to reflect on what you learned about Lead self in Chap. 5. Can you:

1. Create a logical argument to explain why the capabilities of Lead self are germane to achieving workplace health and wellness?
2. Explain how the leader's own psychological health might impact on the psychological health of others in the workplace?

Engagement and Diversity

Any discussion of engagement—and the leadership capabilities required to achieve it—must address the growing challenges of workplace diversity. For the purposes of this chapter, we will discuss diversity in the following categories:

- Gender diversity
- Ethnic diversity
- Professional diversity

More than 80% of providers in health care organizations are women [14]. Because gender can affect both the practise and acceptance of leadership, understanding gender differences is important. The goal of ensuring women have equitable access to leadership roles remains elusive; understanding barriers to gender equity is fundamental to achieving it.

Ethnic diversity poses a similar, if more complex and multi-faceted set of issues. For example, in Canadian nursing, visible and linguistic minorities are under-represented in managerial positions and over-represented in clinical nursing roles [15]. The fact most are women simply exacerbates the gender biases mentioned above. In both Canada [16] and Australia [17] health providers of Indigenous heritage face a similar challenge. For this reason, we are exploring—specifically in Chap. 14—how the LEADS approach can be put to work in Indigenous communities and how it fits within the cultural and leadership context of First Nations, Metis and Inuit peoples in Canada.

---

[2]The 13 factors affecting psychological health and safety are: organizational culture, psychological and social support, clear leadership and expectations, civility and respect, psychological demands, growth and development, recognition and reward, involvement and influence, workload management, engagement, balance, psychological protection and protection of physical safety.

Professional diversity refers to the engagement challenges faced by people from across health disciplines. The health care provider workforce comprises more than 150 different professions: probably more than any other enterprise in society. Dr. John Van Aerde says much more about the challenge of professional engagement in Chap. 15: LEADS and the Health Professions.

The engagement of a group of employees and leaders can be measured collectively.[3] [18, 19], Research shows the level of engagement of a group affects its ability to achieve a people-centred work environment [20]. In our framework, leaders need four capabilities to engage others effectively. They are to:

- Foster development of others;
- Contribute to the creation of healthy organizations;
- Communicate effectively; and
- Build teams.

We'll look at each of them more closely now.

Foster the Development of Others

The first of the four Engage others capabilities is to foster the development of others. Leaders do that by supporting and challenging people to achieve their professional and personal goals (access to training and development is one of the eight major factors used to identify top employers in Canada and the United States). Also, fostering the development of others is directly related to four of the Canadian Standards Association's 13 workplace conditions—access to a supportive culture, growth and development, engagement, and psychological protection. Look at this positive example from Hamilton Health Sciences, in Ontario Canada:

> Learning has always been central to work and life at Hamilton Health Sciences (HHS); a commitment to it is embedded in its strategic plan. After staff and physicians indicated in the organization's engagement survey that learning and development was an important contributor to their engagement, HHS launched the Centre for People Development, with the dedicated hard work of key individuals such as Sandra Ramelli, Director, Office of the CEO, Strategy and Organizational Development and Kathryn Adams, an Organizational Development Specialist. The Centre offers a range of programs, courses and development opportunities that are relevant to the needs of the organization, to individual departments and to the development aspirations of individuals and to the community.
>
> The Centre's programs have been designed to build individual capability in the five domains of LEADS. With LEADS as the underpinning to the design, programs are offered under the broad headings of Growing Leadership, Team Success, Enhanced Performance, and Compassion and Resilience. The growing leadership stream offers many programs

---

[3] A number of instruments have been validated as methods to measure engagement. The Gallup Corporation has developed an engagement instrument, but it is not used widely in Canada given data storage issues. The Health Standards Organization (HSO) in Canada also utilizes many tools to measure organizational engagement and physician engagement. A Medical Engagement Scale has been developed and used in the UK.

including a Charge Person Development Program which offers sections on human rights, conflict resolution, health, safety and wellness and dealing with difficult people.

Other topics covered in the other streams include problem solving for continuous quality improvement, crucial conversations, building high performing teams, healthcare financial management, introduction to mindfulness, finding clarity and balance in work and life and experience-based co-design. Any staff member or physician can sign up; some are specifically tailored for certain groups.

Physician and staff participation are key measures of success. There are more doctors in programs than ever before, and HHS boasts a critical mass of physicians as change agents. Sandra Ramelli says "Enabling and empowering our people is one of our strategic pillars. At HHS, we are committed to supporting and investing in our people; we know that when our people are at their best care is at is best. Fostering the development of our staff through the Centre for People Development is something we are committed to for the long term."

Support for the Centre is also strong from the board and president and CEO Rob MacIsaac, who says on the Centre's website "Learning is more than an academic exercise at Hamilton Health Sciences. Indeed, it is foundational to delivering on the Best Care for All regardless of each of our roles" (Sandra Ramelli, Kathryn Adams, Interview, 2019 Sep 9) [21].

Leaders who don't focus on the development needs of others or aren't committed to increasing employee's abilities may discourage people from taking advantage of learning opportunities. A supervisor who discourages time off for learning, or doesn't support employees who want to pursue personal development can deflate energy and commitment, undermining engagement and accelerating employee turnover. Not recognizing achievement or failing to provide constructive feedback to help correct poor performance will also hinder employee development and engagement [22]. For example, Jennifer, a nurse, found that when the "leader exemplified passive leadership behaviours such as delayed feedback and limited communication, a negative impact on work engagement was identified." [23]

Developing others is even more vital during times of change, when failing to recognize the need for retraining can dramatically diminish peoples' enthusiasm for anything new. While you're assessing readiness for a change, you can identify factors that may help people deal with it more confidently. Preparing for change will make an organization more likely to accept it; but lack of readiness or unstable leadership can mean change is more likely to be rejected [24].

A fundamental leadership skill needed to produce change is leadership connectivity. Hurst and Hurst say leadership connectivity "is relationship-focused rather than task-focused and is a *follower-centred* approach that challenges those involved to develop observational and critical thinking skills while exploring attitudes and beliefs about leadership and site practices and habits of their organizational culture." [25] In addition to mastering tools and knowledge, people also need to be supported through the psychological demands of change. That's best fostered through a strong relationship with an empathetic and knowledgeable leader.

Leaders who think and act as coaches build engagement. Leaders who coach are confident, care about their employees and want them to succeed. Coaches are attuned to feelings of inadequacy and helplessness, and can distinguish between resistance and fear of trying [26, 27]. Delegating is another way to engage people, but leaders need to be aware of how ready individuals are for delegation [28].

Learning Moment: How Well do You Coach Others?
Research has shown that leaders who are successful coaches:

- Ask if the other person is open to receiving feedback
- Explore the other person's goals and intentions, to contextualize feedback
- Understand the impact of context on the situation as opposed to making it solely personal
- Give positive feedback immediately and publicly
- Provide critical feedback privately and in a constructive manner
- Engage the other person in a two-way dialogue (more about dialogue later in this chapter)
- Listen deeply and avoid being judgmental

Reflective Questions
1. How often do you employ these coaching skills as you work with others in your area of responsibility?
2. Which of these do you do well? Which would you like to develop?
3. Are there individuals in your workplace that would benefit from coaching? Try it!

The antithesis of coaching and the death-knell for fostering development is micro-management—trying to control every aspect of another's work. Micro-management is a pathology of poor leadership, diminishing trust, making people feel undervalued and stifling the desire to learn.

If leaders do not offer employees resources, time and personal support to learn and grow—development will be minimal or non-existent.

Contribute to the Creation of Healthy Organizations

A healthy organization is characterized by strong mental health and wellness, a sense of physical safety and achievement. Healthy organizations tend to have lower absenteeism, above-average retention and lower turnover. One study found that leaders who demonstrate high levels of authentic leadership create increased trust, greater congruence in the areas of work-life balance and fewer adverse patient outcomes [29].

Unhealthy workplaces, on the other hand, detract from optimum patient care [30]. Doctors with burnout give lower quality care, more unnecessary tests and drugs, are less empathic and have a negative impact on team satisfaction [31, 32]. Nurses with significant psychological stress can have an even more immediate negative effect on patients. High levels of anxiety, mood disorders and depression increase absenteeism, turnover, and ultimately detract from patient care [33].

Tracking measures of staff satisfaction and self-reported health can help leaders make a healthy workplace a top priority. The following example profiles the importance of that measurement, while at the same time highlighting many of the factors contributing to a healthy work environment.

Learning Moment: Eastern Health Region of Newfoundland
Eastern Health has developed a set of measures to assess the state of psychological health and wellness in the organization. The measures are a major component of Eastern Health's Healthy Workplace Priority Plan 2017—2020.

Employee Family Assistance use:	2014/15	6.2%
	2015/16	9.3%
	2016/17	10.5%

Top three referral reasons (2016/17)	Top three long-term disability claims (2015/16)
1. Mental health (39%)	1. Musculoskeletal (31%)
2. Family Issues (15%)	2. Mental health (25%)
3. Stress (14%)	3. Cancer (19%)

Rates of use of the program, referral rates for mental health and stress, and rates of long-term disability for mental health reasons can be monitored to determine the overall long-term effectiveness of the Healthy Workplace Priority Plan.

Eastern Health's Engagement Survey, done every three years, is included in the measurements. It measures engagement but also gives Eastern Health valuable program-specific insight into various dimensions of the Canadian Psychological Standards' workplace conditions for psychologically healthy workplaces [11].

Eastern Health has committed to be a pilot site for a health care survey sponsored by the Mental Health Commission of Canada. This survey adds two additional psychosocial factors specific to health care.

Information courtesy of Josee Dumas and Leslie Brown, HR Strategists, Eastern Health.

Reflective Questions
1. Can you access similar data, or equivalent data for the employees and/or clinicians in your area of responsibility? If so, how healthy are they? If not, why not?
2. If you do not belong to an organization, but are leading a community change or volunteer group, how often do they attend meetings? Participate in events?
3. What could you do to ensure that such data is available to you on a systematic basis?

Work-life data reflects health and wellness in an organization, including levels of injury and stress. Sadly, many health organizations in Canada and elsewhere are not doing well in those areas. The Canadian Health Workforce Network says "Rates of burnout and poor mental health issues among health professionals are high and rising, and rates of absenteeism, illness and disability are higher in the health workforce than any other worker group in Canada." [34] The largest and fastest growing claim area in hospital benefit plans are prescriptions for stress and anxiety. The situation is similar in Australia and the UK [8].

Leadership behaviour has a significant impact on employee behaviour, performance and well-being [35]. Narcissistic or abusive behaviour can significantly damage the mental health of employees and clinicians [36]. However, leaders can help build healthy workplaces by modelling healthy lifestyles [37] and by behaving respectfully, considerately and in a caring manner.

The mental and spiritual side of employee wellness (morale) is greatly helped when leaders are simply present in the workplace, whereas absentee leaders are seen as uncaring and distant. Remember in Chap. 3, Suann Laurent's instinct to *be there* to support her health care providers as they coped with the Humboldt crisis? Present leadership is not just physical presence—it's also emotional and psychological presence. If doors—real or mental—are closed to others, a leader may be physically present but perceived as absent [38].

If you are a formal leader, your span of control—the range of people who officially report to you—is a critical factor in your ability to build and sustain a healthy workplace. In health care, leaders have anywhere from a handful of people to more than 200 reporting to them. It's a huge challenge for a leader to connect with 200 people, especially when many health care organizations operate 24/7, but most managers work the day shift Monday through Friday [39, 40]. In a study comparing large and small spans of control of nurse managers [40] researchers found staff who reported to a manager with a large number of direct reports had higher levels of stress and more turnover. The leadership of managers with more direct reports was less positive for staff satisfaction and engagement and for patient satisfaction.

> **Learning Moment**
> When you think of the leadership imperatives of being present and modelling—how difficult is it for a nurse manager to act accordingly when she has a large span of control?
>
> 1. Please reflect and consider the impact on employee health and wellness.
> 2. What steps might you take to be more present in your workplace or community?

How decisions are made also contributes to both morale and productivity. Daniel Goleman and colleagues identified six leadership styles that reflect how a leader's emotional intelligence plays out in decision making [41]. They outline four styles of decision making that employees think enhance engagement—the authoritative or visionary style, the democratic style, the coaching style (discussed earlier) and the affiliative style. Two styles—pace-setting and coercive—are not engaging, unless used sparingly in special circumstances. A study done in 2016 showed leaders in medical education use different styles at each leadership level from junior to senior and each was adapted to address different accountabilities, so senior leaders used a broader range of styles than juniors [42].

Table 6.1 shows which leadership style works best in different situations.

Workplaces with great morale are usually highly productive. In healthy organizations, people have meaningful opportunities to contribute. They do their best in jobs they enjoy, when they feel valued, and when the environment is productive. As a leader, you can create an environment where people can contribute by ensuring:

- People can see the benefit of their work to patients or citizens or their workmates.
- People know what is expected of them.
- Barriers (red tape, unnecessary regulations) to effective work are removed.
- People receive constructive feedback through formal performance reviews.
- People's work takes advantage of their talents and skills.
- Work processes are efficient and effective.

For many health workplaces, approaches such as Six Sigma, Business Process Engineering, and Lean are being used to redesign work process to make them more efficient and effective. However, such processes often require leaders to be much more present with their staff and put a premium on the leader's ability to be proficient in the skills of dialogue and coaching.

But does gender influence how we do it? Read the next learning moment: [43] can you be the leader you need to be for followers?

Learning Moment

A recent study compared gender and personality differences in transformational leadership behaviour.

The study found personality types were equally distributed between the genders but women regarded themselves as more enabling and rewarding, and men saw themselves as more challenging. Subordinates' appraisals were consistent with the leaders' self-ratings. Essentially, women leaders are expected to be helpful, nurturing, and gentle while men are expected to be more assertive, controlling and confident.

1. Does this phenomenon play out in your workplace? With you?
2. Please reflect on the following questions: do follower perceptions of how male or female leaders should lead condition men and women to lead differently, even though their natural personality is the same? Or is it how we condition ourselves to lead? Or both?
3. Does this create a challenge for you in terms of (1) men being less able to be helpful, nurturing and gentle when they need to be; and (2) women being less able to be more assertive, controlling and confident when they need to be? If it is an issue, how might you begin to address it?

Table 6.1 Six styles of leadership

	Commanding	Visionary	Affiliative	Democratic	Pacesetting	Coaching
The leader's *modus operandi*	Demands immediate compliance	Mobilizes people toward a vision	Creates harmony and builds emotional bonds	Forges consensus through participation	Sets high standards for performance	Develops people for the future
The style in a phrase	"Do what I tell you."	"Come with me"	"People come first."	"What do you think?"	"Do as I do, now"	"Try this."
Underlying emotional intelligence competencies	Drive to achieve, initiative, self-control	Self-confidence, empathy, change catalyst	Empathy, building relationships, communication	Collaboration, team leadership, communication	Conscientiousness, drive to achieve, initiative	Developing others, empathy, self-awareness
When the style works best	In a crisis, to kick start a turnaround, or with problem employees	When changes require a new vision, or when a clear direction is needed	To heal rifts in a team or to motivate people during stressful circumstances	To build buy-in or consensus, or to get valuable input from employees	To get quick results form a highly motivated and competent team	To help an employee improve performance or develop long-term strengths
Overall impact on climate	Negative	Most strongly positive	Positive	Positive	Negative	Positive

Goleman, Daniel, "Leadership that Gets Results" Harvard Business Review March–April 2000 p. 82–83

Another way to encourage employees to contribute is to create an environment where conflict is productive, not destructive. Conflict is unproductive when it leads to entrenched views, fragmented effort and refusal to collaborate. But conflict can be productive when people disagree but learn from it to better define problems, explore root causes and come up with workable solutions. As Martin Luther King said, "We as a society have not learned to disagree without being violently disagreeable." [1] Leaders need to know how to ameliorate conflict when necessary.

Health Workplaces Demand Equity, Diversity and Inclusion (Dr. Ivy Bourgeault)

Engage others, the E in the LEADS framework, is a key area for equity, diversity and inclusion-informed leadership. Indeed, leaders committed to engaging others need to build these activities into their workdays, not try to handle them off the side of the desk. How can you do that? When you're working to engage others, whether it's to build teams or foster individual development, strive to recognize who you are and are not engaging, and develop strategies to reach out to under-represented voices.

Developing mentoring and sponsorship relationships with emerging leaders from diverse backgrounds, and focusing on equity, diversity and inclusion while thinking about succession planning are critical issues. Effective communication skills must include attention to "micro-incivilities" and "micro-aggressions" and how they are disproportionately experienced by members of equity groups. That adds to the emotional labour and burden certain team members bear and creates an unhealthy work environment for all.

Making workplaces more amenable to diverse personal and family circumstances increases inclusion. Leaders must explicitly ensure psychologically healthy and safe environments, free of violence, harassment and bullying: building on the Mental Health Commission of Canada's psychological health and safety standard. Effective, transparent communication via social media can increase access to information and a sense of community to people who might otherwise feel excluded because of distance, cost or timing.

Communicate Effectively

Communication is critical for engaging people and leading change. Communicating effectively has two dimensions: interpersonal communication and strategic communication. The former is day-to-day interactions between leaders and followers. The latter involves formal efforts to share, receive and examine information vital to organizational function.

Communication is a complicated blend of message, medium and audience. It's not one-way broadcasting, but an interchange of ideas among people that requires concentration and a true desire to understand other perspectives to be successful. What you don't say can be as important as what you do. Communicating effectively is central to your ability to influence others—and to their ability to influence you when you need to follow.

Deep Listening

"You listen deeply for only one purpose—to allow the other person to empty his or her heart." [44] Deep listening is a more receptive kind of listening, where we overcome our inherent assumptions and interests to become more open to the other person's meaning and intentions. It's a skill that enables you to understand people better and—in an ideal world—helps to create shared meaning with them. (Shared meaning is more than understanding a message, it means grasping the values underpinning the message).

When combined with probing questions, deep listening enhances the potential for shared action [45]. For example, the Webasto Group (a company that manufactures products for cars) found interpersonal and interdepartmental communication was fractured and siloed. They ran a program called "Listen like a Leader" to improve the way they behaved and interacted with one another. The result was deeper engagement and greater willingness by those who participated to engage in organizational change [46].

Leaders, like most humans, may find it harder to listen to someone they don't agree with, don't find interesting or who is challenging them in some way. In a confrontation, it's important to control your emotions and consider where the attack is coming from. What lies behind the emotion? If your behaviour caused it, accept responsibility for the behaviour, but don't accept the anger: that's the other person's responsibility. It's when you have to work with people you don't like or disagree with that emotional intelligence and sophisticated communication skills become essential for success.

Dialogue

"Dialogue" to us means the open exchange of information and ideas. It requires a desire to understand where other people are coming from; it's about building shared meaning based on the contributions of each person involved. It's essential for coaching and group work. Any kind of prejudgment will get in the way of creating something special together. As Stephen Covey says, "seek first to understand, and then be understood." [47]

American management consultant Robert Fritz says an organization is the "sum of its conversations," [48] but many groups never have good dialogues. Time and work pressure get in the way, as do the desire to control and workplace power dynamics [49] that prevent open conversations between leaders and followers [50]. Instead of dialogue, advocacy and debate take over.

Learning Moment
Megan Reitz [55] says leaders need to deepen shared understanding in order to improve our ability to create solutions to some of the major issues that we face in health care in the 21st century. She argues if we persist in

understanding leadership as positional and hierarchical, and act accordingly, our ability to have meaningful dialogue on issues of great import is severely limited. Think back on the last three weeks at work.

1. Have there been times, in meetings or interpersonal interaction or in group discussions where dialogue was needed? Reflect on why.
2. How comfortable are you in your ability to initiate and conduct a dialogue with your direct reports? How might you develop that capacity?

Don Dunoon, a leadership consultant in New South Wales in Australia, says there was a time when communicating effectively suggested a leader confidently trying to persuade others of something. In today's more fluid, complex and high-pressure health care environments, however, effective communication needs to take on a different hue. It's critical that leaders work with multiple meanings, competing priorities and different interests.

This requires recognizing and reflecting on your own mindset, exploring other peoples' ideas and finding common ground across diverging points of view. It's easy, however, to be tempted to respond to turbulence and uncertainty by holding tight to your own ideas, seeing different views as wrong, misguided or poorly motivated, and avoiding difficult topics.

Dunoon created the OBREAU Tripod to assist in situations where poor communication is causing problems [51]. OBREAU is an acronym for OBservation, REasonableness and AUthenticity (see Fig. 6.1).

- Observation means working from data and evidence as much as possible, rather than reacting or moving quickly to interpretation.

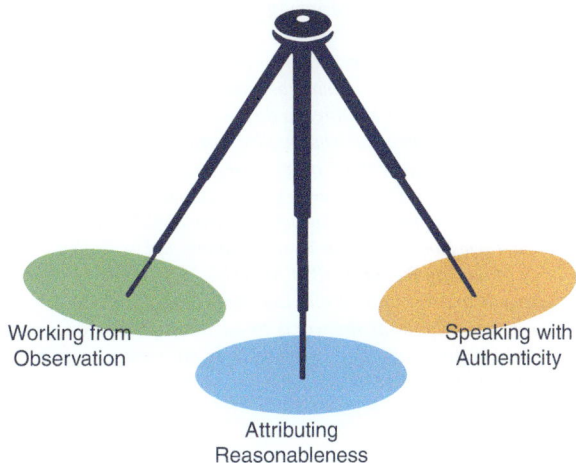

Fig. 6.1 The three legs of the OBREAU Tripod as a structure for supporting safer, authentic conversations

Working from Observation

Speaking with Authenticity

Attributing Reasonableness

- Reasonableness means assuming others are reasonable, or at least their ideas seem reasonable to them, rather than defaulting to judging them.
- Authenticity means speaking from the heart, to what is true for us, rather than dancing around.

The following story, courtesy of Don Dunoon, shows how the process can work.

Anita is a mid-career clinician leader. Over the past six months she has headed a state-wide taskforce to develop a model for service provision in her specialty. Comprising senior clinicians from around the state, her group meets monthly. Each of the past three meetings have followed the same pattern. Although the meetings have agendas, members spend the first half hour talking a lot about their own facilities, services and local needs. By the end of the meeting, Anita succeeds in getting them to adopt a state-wide perspective. But when the group reconvenes a month later, the pattern repeats.

Asked how she responds, Anita said "Early on, I find myself thinking 'here we go again.' I'll say, 'can we please focus on the agenda,' but it's like herding cats. The committee members are more interested in local issues than state-wide challenges. They're just so caught up in their own parochial needs, and incapable of looking more broadly. There's one clinician, Gerald, who tends to drive this local focus. I'd like to raise this issue with him, but don't think I could. He was a guru even when I was a student."

How can the OBREAU Tripod help Anita talk to Gerald and possibly the wider group? She can prepare for the conversation by considering each of the OBREAU Tripod legs in turn, beginning by making some observations (which are distinct from interpretations).

It's observable the group has a brief to develop a state-wide model, that the meetings have an agenda, and that the group has talked about local needs and issues in the first half hour of the last three meetings. While it may be true, it's an interpretation the group members are more interested in local issues than state-level challenges.

The benefits of starting with observation include that it may help us to see more clearly and to be more mindful. It grounds us in a specific instance, informed by evidence and makes us less prone to seizing on a single interpretation to the exclusion of others.

Moving to the second leg, attributing reasonableness, Anita's task is to imagine the story the group members are telling themselves, in a way that's consistent with them being reasonable—in the sense their actions seem reasonable to them.

Perhaps the clinicians regard the monthly meetings as an important opportunity to share experience and ideas as well as to network with colleagues from across the state. Conceivably, they're becoming increasingly attuned (as the meeting progresses) to the importance of developing a state-wide service model, but when they get back to their sites, colleagues might influence them to advocate for local issues and focus less on state-wide challenges. Possibly, committee members feel conflicted—between their state-wide responsibilities and their loyalties to their own facilities and clinician colleagues.

Seeking to imagine what reality looks like to stakeholders has the potential to help Anita stretch out interpretation of an issue and pay more attention to some of the subtleties and nuances at play. The challenge is to develop ideas about what is taking place that are consistent with assuming the others are acting reasonably. Presuming reasonableness enables us to frame better questions to test our interpretations, and to explore the relevant views of others.

Moving to the third OBREAU Tripod leg, speaking with authenticity, Anita's task at this stage is to delve into the mindset she brings to the issue. Partly, this means reflecting on her own interests, what she wants to advance, protect or avoid. In Anita's case, one interest could be to ensure that momentum is gathering for framing a state-wide service model, without excessive concern for local, site-specific matters. Anita might also usefully reflect on assumptions she holds. It seems, for instance, she assumes she can't raise with the committee the pattern she sees them slipping into.

Like all tripods, the OBREAU's strength comes from all three legs being in place at the same time. When we work from observation, maintain a view that others can be reasonable, and tap into what matters deeply to us, we can have conversations that otherwise might seem impossible.

What does this example teach us about the relationship between effective communication and engagement? First, how important high-quality, face-to-face communication is, especially in difficult situations. By high quality, we mean event-based reflective thinking combined with deep listening and authentic speaking—which is to say, observation, reasonableness and authenticity. Secondly, it shows the damage of neglecting any one of those features. Thirdly, it shows an unavoidable consequence—how relationships, both short- and long-term, hinge on the consequences of an interpersonal exchange. If individuals don't trust and respect each other, engagement can suffer dramatically.

Social Media

Social media is shaping patient and family experience through consumer apps and consumer friendly websites. It and the web have given people who were otherwise disenfranchised a voice that reaches not only the health care system, but potentially thousands of other patients and citizens. Inevitably, it is also affecting health care leaders and leadership.

E-mail, blogging, Twitter, Instagram, Facebook and all the other sites have created limitless new opportunities for conversation, gathering information and building relationships. Leaders have no option to using them and must become conversant with their strengths and weaknesses because these new media have tremendous power to enhance and enable communication to increase engagement. Think of the power to galvanize action inherent in a well-constructed documentary, a *Go Fund Me* initiative, or a well-chosen picture or tweet. Social media must be part of your personal toolbox for improving your leadership. It can assist health care leaders to learn, network, educate stakeholders in the organization and in the community [52].

Mastery of social media cannot replace other forms of communication—it doesn't help you recognize people, listen deeply to them or hold more productive dialogues. There's a risk that using social media will convert interactions into transactions and diminish the interactive skills this chapter is about. "Transactions are the way of the industrial era. They are scalable, repeatable. You can Six Sigma transactions. You can Kaizen them. None of that works with interactions." [53] Don't let yourself rely solely on social media to connect. it's still necessary to work directly with people.

Build Teams

Leaders get results through their ability to convert independent, capable, and self-motivated individuals into interdependent, well-functioning, high-performing teams. The ability to bring individuals together—whether they're professionals, executives, community members or a board of trustees—is an essential aspect of leadership. Consider the following example of putting the capability of Build teams to work:

> Lorrie Hamilton is the director of Bioethics, Patient Experience and Spiritual Care at Michael Garron Hospital in Toronto, Canada. The hospital is going through an extensive redevelopment project and all the change and stress has worn down teams and individuals. "People can articulate, with great accuracy, what they do and how they do it but in times of challenge, it's easy to disconnect from the "why" of the work they do," Lorrie says.
>
> To help them reconnect, and improve relationships among patients, families and care givers, team agreement workshops were created to help frontline teams reconnect with their purpose and each other. At the sessions, team members work collectively to write their agreements. Together, they discuss the nature and purpose of their work and create an agreement on team behaviour that embodies the culture of the organization. Then they all sign.
>
> Lorrie facilitated the Medical Device Reprocessing Department as it went through the process of writing its agreement. They began by reviewing the characteristics of high-performing teams, then talked about their team purpose—who their work reached or influenced and how it affected patient journeys through care. After that, they discussed how the values of the organization are demonstrated in the way people act toward each other and in providing care to patients.
>
> Finally, the team agreed on the terms of an agreement—including their purpose as a team and the fundamental expectations of members, and describing the team's commitment to patients, families and each other. Everyone signed it.
>
> "Seeing their relationships and passion for wanting to be respectful of each other and the patients and families they support is very meaningful to me," Lorrie said. (Christine Devine, email, 2019 Mar 11).

Lorrie's example offers a model for the teams that are found in all aspects of health care today. High-performing teams are specialized groups of individuals with complementary skills, shared values and interdependent accountabilities. They may be permanently grouped, or work together on a short-term project. Team members share responsibility for a well-defined unit of work and creating a whole, greater than the sum of the parts, to achieve it. Team work differs significantly in hospitals, primary care centres, extended care homes or the executive suite; depending on the players, the work (such as operational vs. strategic), and the clients served. As happened at Michael Garron Hospital and regardless of the context, studies have shown that without an intentional effort to create high-performing teams, most attempts to adopt a team approach fall short [54–57].

A study done by Harris and colleagues to guide deliberate teamwork in medical and related practices outlines the following principles:

- Rehearse team work as much as possible in a controlled setting; include different members and vary tasks to prepare for issues you'll encounter in the real world.
- Research and adapt evidence-based practices for effective teamwork.
- Use clear, objective, and quantifiable measures of performance and efforts to improve it; assess both human dynamics and objective performance measures [56].

Practical experience and research have spawned a significant number of books and team-building tools [58–60]. One team assessment tool we particularly like was created by Dr. Sandy MacIver, a career coach and advisor on building high performance teamwork [61]. He identifies twelve qualities that help teams become high performing, such as a clear purpose, focus on results, the ability to be creative, etc.

Team charters are also good tools to lay a foundation for excellent teamwork.

Creating a Team Charter

What Is It?
A 1- or 2-day meeting to set your team's course for the year. It's not a work plan, it's how you'll work together.

Why Should I Use It?
It's a team agreement, intended to:

- Involve all team members in setting achievable values, standards and protocols
- Clearly identify results the team is expected to achieve
- Build team spirit and enthusiasm for the group's goals
- Give a set of improvement goals against which progress can be measured

How Does It Work?

Planning
Share information with your staff about your work plans and existing charter elements if you have them. Use a facilitator.

Doing
Have the facilitator focus your team on its:

- Vision and mission statement
- Workplace values
- Collective measurable results
- Service standards
- Code of conduct

- Roles and responsibilities
- Protocols for meetings, making decisions and resolving disputes
- Access to resources: where to get them
- Skills inventory
- Team improvement goals

To develop a team charter book a meeting to discuss how you will work together. Brainstorm each subject and build a team consensus on each. Together, the consensus statements on each subject form your team charter. A half day check-up after six months will let you see how on track you are. After 12 months, have another meeting to discuss things to stop doing, things to continue doing and things to start doing.

Learning Moment

Think of teams you have been on in the past. Categorize them anywhere along a continuum from high performing to dysfunctional.

1. If high performing, what aspects of the team-charter approach did you employ?
2. If less than high performing, which of the elements of the team charter might have improved your ability to work together?
3. Where would a team charter be of value in your workplace?

Summary

There are four leadership capabilities involved in promoting engagement:

- Foster development of others
- Contribute to the creation of healthy organizations
- Communicate effectively
- Build teams

Ensuring your staff, or groups of professionals, or patients and families, can work together to meet the needs of citizens and patients is the "working together" responsibility of leadership. It's most likely to happen with leaders who promote engagement, which also contributes to psychologically healthy and productive workplaces. As you work to engage individuals and groups, remember to pay attention to the challenges of diversity, equity and inclusion.

We hope this chapter has helped to clarify the importance of building personal relationships in your sphere of influence, and using them to engage followers, clients and patients. The exercises and stories highlight how you can improve engagement and also guide you toward bringing about change with deep consideration for the welfare of others. In the next chapter we will move on to Achieve results.

Now, evaluate yourself with the Engage others self-assessment tool. Then, based on your results, identify one capability you should put energy into developing.

Learning Moment
Using the following LEADS self-assessment, assess how well you demonstrate the four Engage others capabilities. Choose the appropriate level (relative to your responsibility) to make that assessment.
    If there is one capability you would like to improve upon, what is it? Why?

Engage Others Self-Assessment (For on-line access to self assessment tool please visit www.LEADSglobal.ca)

Informal leader (patient, family member, citizen) responsibilities:
In order to engage others in working to make the health system better, I:

1.	Make a disciplined effort to assist health care providers and formal leaders to learn about the challenges and issues facing patients, families and citizens in engaging with the health system	1	2	3	4	5	6	7	N
2.	Take responsibility for acting in a manner consistent with a healthy workplace, and if asked, provide suggestions to improve workplace conditions	1	2	3	4	5	6	7	N
3.	Make a disciplined effort to listen deeply, express myself respectfully, use social media appropriately, and participate in dialogue with my fellow citizens and representatives of the health system	1	2	3	4	5	6	7	N
4.	Am a willing participant in building effective teams when the opportunity arises; I take care to know when to lead and when to follow	1	2	3	4	5	6	7	N

Front-line leader responsibilities:
In order to engage others in working to make the health system better, I:

1.	Encourage, challenge and support those I supervise by encouraging them to develop personal and professional goals, pursue those goals, and seek feedback on their achievement	1	2	3	4	5	6	7	N
2.	Monitor/measure the psychological health and productivity of people in my area of responsibility; and do my best to provide clinicians and employees with the tools required to do their work	1	2	3	4	5	6	7	N
3.	Encourage an open exchange of ideas and information through a formal communications plan; and interpersonally through active listening, respectful expression, dialogue, and appropriate use of social media	1	2	3	4	5	6	7	N
4.	Create and participate in collaborative inter-professional or inter-unit teams to achieve specified goals	1	2	3	4	5	6	7	N

Mid-manager leader responsibilities
In order to engage others in working to make the health system better, I:

1.	Encourage, champion and support the use of professional development opportunities, personal learning plans, or performance management processes to achieve personal and professional goals	1 2 3 4 5 6 7 N
2.	Monitor/measure psychological health and productivity in my area of responsibility; and collaboratively create processes that staff and clinicians feel might improve psychological health and productivity	1 2 3 4 5 6 7 N
3.	Listen well; and establish both formal and informal processes for exchanging ideas and information through conversation, dialogue, effective meetings, and appropriate media	1 2 3 4 5 6 7 N
4.	Establish and provide support for the creation of collaborative inter-professional or inter-unit teams to achieve specific goals important to the organization	1 2 3 4 5 6 7 N

Senior leader responsibilities
In order to engage others in working to make the health system better, I:

1.	Ensure there is funding, processes and procedures, and appropriate accountability for professional development, personal learning plans, or performance management processes to help staff achieve their personal and professional goals	1 2 3 4 5 6 7 N
2.	Measure the quality of psychological health, workplace wellness, and productivity in my department; and ensure action is taken—with clinician and staff input—to improve psychological health, workplace wellness, and productivity	1 2 3 4 5 6 7 N
3.	Listen well, speak respectfully; and establish strategic communication processes (using appropriate interpersonal communication, media and dialogue in meetings) to elicit open exchange of ideas, evidence and information	1 2 3 4 5 6 7 N
4.	Provide materials and support for the creation and sustainability of high-performance teams in my department, and at the senior management table	1 2 3 4 5 6 7 N

Executive leader responsibilities
In order to engage others in working to make the health system better, I:

1.	Ensure we have policies supporting personal and professional development and performance management; and monitor the implementation of those policies	1 2 3 4 5 6 7 N
2.	Systematically measure the quality of engagement in my organization, and ensure the strategic plan has explicit guidance as to how to improve psychological health, workplace wellness, and productivity	1 2 3 4 5 6 7 N

| 3. | Establish communication strategies to encourage the open exchange of ideas, evidence and information and to deal with the media; and practise effective interpersonal communication with others (deep listening; speaking respectfully; and dialogue where appropriate) | 1 2 3 4 5 6 7 N |
| 4. | Develop policy to support the creation of high-performance teams in my organization, monitor its implementation and adhere to it at the senior executive table | 1 2 3 4 5 6 7 N |

References

1. King ML Jr, Carson C, editors. The autobiography of Martin Luther King, Jr. New York: Grand Central Publishing; 1998.
2. Young S, Kulesa P. Employee experience in high-performance organizations. Toronto: Towers Watson; 2019. https://www.willistowerswatson.com/en-US/Search#q=Employee%20experience%20in%20high-performance%20organizations&sort=relevancy. Accessed 3 Sep 2019.
3. Payne D, Briscoe D. Engage others. Book two of five LEADS booklets. Ottawa: Canadian College of Health Leaders; 2010. https://leadscanada.net/site/books. Accessed 4 Sep 2019.
4. West M, Dawson J. Employee engagement and NHS performance. London: The King's Fund; 2013. http://www.kingsfund.org.uk/sites/files/kf/employee-engagement-nhs-performance-west-dawson-leadership-review2012-paper.pdf. Accessed 13 Jul 2013.
5. Malila N, Lunkka N, Suhonen M. Authentic leadership in health care: a scoping review. Leadersh Health Serv (Bradf Engl). 2018;31(1):129–46. https://doi.org/10.1108/LHS-02-2017-0007.
6. Arnold K. Transformational leadership and employee psychological well-being: a review and directions for future research. J Occup Health Psychol. 2017;22(3):381–93.
7. Feeley D. The triple aim or the quadruple aim? Four points to help set your strategy. Boston: Institute for Health Improvement (IHI); 2017. http://www.ihi.org/communities/blogs/the-triple-aim-or-the-quadruple-aim-four-points-to-help-set-your-strategy. Accessed 2 Aug 2019.
8. Victorian Auditor-General. Bullying and harassment in the health sector. Melbourne (AUS: Victorian Government Printer; 2016.
9. Canadian Institute for Health Information. Health care cost drivers: the facts. Ottawa: CIHI; 2011. https://secure.cihi.ca/free_products/health_care_cost_drivers_the_facts_en.pdf. Accessed 4 Sep 2019.
10. Tse H, Troth A, Ashkanasy N, Collins A. Affect and leader-member exchange in the new millennium: a state-of-art review and guiding framework. Leadersh Q. 2018;29(1):135–49. https://doi.org/10.1016/j.leaqua.2017.10.002.
11. Psychological health and safety in the workplace—prevention, promotion, and guidance to staged implementation. Ottawa: Canadian Standards Association (CSA) in Association with the Mental Health Commission of Canada; 2013. https://www.csagroup.org/documents/codes-and-standards/publications/CAN_CSA-Z1003-13_BNQ_9700-803_2013_EN.pdf. Accessed 20 Jan 2019.
12. MHCC is a national body, established by Health Canada, to lead the development and dissemination of innovative programs and tools to support the mental health and wellness of Canadians.
13. Dickson G. Transforming health care organizations. Ottawa: Mental Health Commission of Canada; 2019. https://www.mentalhealthcommission.ca/sites/default/files/2018-11/health care_crosswalk_eng.pdf. Accessed 16 Jun 2019.

14. Bourgeault IL, James Y, Lawford K, Lundine J. Empowering women leaders in health: a gap analysis of the state of knowledge. Can J Phys Lead. 2018;5(2):92–100.
15. Premji S, Etowa J. Workforce utilization of visible and linguistic minorities in Canadian nursing. J Nurs Manag. 2014;22(1):80–8.
16. Lambert M, Luke J, Downey B, Crengle S, Kelaher M, Reid S, Smylie J. Health literacy: health professionals' understandings and their perceptions of barriers that Indigenous patients encounter. BMC Health Serv Res. 2014;14:614–24.
17. Davy C, Cass A, Brady J, DeVries J, Fewquandie B, Ingram S, et al. Facilitating engagement through strong relationships between primary health care and Aboriginal and Torres Strait Islander peoples. Aust N Z J Public Health. 2016 Dec;40(6):535–41.
18. Corbin J. Surprising results from the 2017 Gallup employee engagement report. New York: Gallup Consulting; 2017. https://www.theemployeeapp.com/gallup-2017-employee-engagement-report-results-nothing-changed/. Accessed 4 Sep 2019.
19. Spurgeon P, Barwell F, Mazelan P. Developing a medical engagement scale (MES). Int J Clin Med. 2008;16:213–23.
20. Lowe G. How employee engagement matters for hospital performance. Healthc Q. 2012;15(2):29–39.
21. Centre for people development. About the centre. Hamilton (CA): Hamilton Health Sciences; 2019. https://centreforpeopledevelopment.ca/about-the-centre. Accessed 24 Jul 2019.
22. For further insight, see Fenwick S. and Hagge E. Effective Performance Systems. Ottawa (ON): Canadian College of Health Leaders; 2015. http://leadscollaborative.ca/document/1302/Effective_Performance_Systems_Fenwick&Hagge.pdf. Accessed 24 Jul 2019.
23. Manning J. The influence of nurse manager leadership style on staff nurse work engagement. J Nurs Adm. 2016;46(9):438–43.
24. Timmings C, Khan S, Moore J, Marquez C, Pyka K, Straus S. Ready, set, change! Development and usability testing of an online readiness for change decision support tool for health care organizations. BMC Med Inform Decis Mak; 2016;16: 24. https://bmcmedinformdecismak.biomedcentral.com/articles/10.1186/s12911-016-0262-y. Accessed 4 Sep 2019.
25. Hurst P, Hurst S. Leadership connectivity: a leading indicator for organizational culture change. ODJ. 2016;31(1):81–95.
26. Berg ME, Karlsen JT. A study of coaching leadership style practice in projects. Manag Res Rev. 2016;39(9):1122–42. https://doi.org/10.1108/MRR-07-2015-0157.
27. Backman A, Sjogren K, Lindkvist M, Lovheim H, Edvardsson D. Characteristics of highly rated leadership in nursing homes using item response theory. J Adv Nurs. 2017;73:2903–13.
28. Hersey P, Blanchard K. Management of organizational behavior: utilizing human resources. New Jersey: Prentice Hall; 1977.
29. Wong CA, Giallonardo LM. Authentic leadership and nurse-assessed adverse patient outcomes. J Nurs Manag. 2013;21:740–52.
30. Pinder RJ, Greaves FE, Aylin PP, Jarman B, Bottle A. Staff perceptions of quality of care: an observational study of the NHS staff survey in hospitals in England. BMJ Qual Saf. 2013;22:563–70.
31. Post SG, Roess M. Expanding the rubric of "Patient-Centered Care" (PCC) to "Patient and Professional Centered Care" (PPCC) to enhance provider well-being. HEC Forum. 2017;29:293–302.
32. Healthy brains at work. Creating the conditions for healthy brains in the workplace. Ottawa: The Conference Board of Canada Briefing; 2017. https://www.sunlife.ca/static/canada/Sponsor/About%20Group%20Benefits/Group%20benefits%20products%20and%20services/The%20Conversation/Mental%20Health/9187_Healthy%20Brains%20at%20Work_BR.pdf. Accessed 4 Sep 2019.
33. Wall S. Employee (dis)engagement: learning from nurses who left organizational jobs for independent practice. Nurs Leadersh. 2015;28(3):41–51.
34. Quality of worklife. Ottawa: The Canadian Health Workforce Network; 2019. http://www.hhr-rhs.ca/index.php?option=com_content&view=article&id=431&Itemid=151&lang=en. Accessed 4 Mar 2019.

35. Inceoglu I, Thomas G, Chu C, Plans D, Gerbasi A. Leadership behavior and employee well-being: an integrated review and a future research agenda. Lead Q. 2018;29(1):179–202. https://doi.org/10.1016/j.leaqua.2017.12.006.

36. Mackey JD, Frieder RE, Brees JR, Martin MJ. Abusive supervision: a meta-analysis and empirical review. J Manag. 2017;43(6):1940–50. https://doi.org/10.1177/0149206315573997.

37. Haller DK, Fischer P, Frey D. The power of good: a leader's personal power as a mediator of the ethical leadership-follower outcomes link. Front Psychol. 2018;9:1094. https://doi.org/10.3389/fpsyg.2018.01094.

38. From innovation to action: the first report of the Health Care Innovation Working Group; 2014. https://www.hhr-rhs.ca/images/stories/CoF_Health_Innovation_Report-E-WEB.pdf. Accessed 18 Jul 2019.

39. Span of control. The Economist; 2009. http://www.economist.com/node/14301444. Accessed 15 Mar 2013.

40. Doran D, McCutcheon AS, Evans MH, MacMillan K, Hall LM, Pringle D, et al. Impact of the manager's span of control on leadership and performance. Ottawa: Canadian Health Services Research Foundation; 2004. https://www.cfhi-fcass.ca/Migrated/PDF/ResearchReports/OGC/doran2_final.pdf. Accessed 15 Mar 2019.

41. Goleman D, Boyatzis R, McKee A. Primal leadership: realizing the power of emotional intelligence. Boston, MA: Harvard Business School Press; 2002.

42. Saxena A, Desanghere L, Stobart K, Walker K. Goleman's leadership styles at different hierarchical levels in medical education. BMC Med Educ. 2017;17(1):169. https://doi.org/10.1186/s12909-017-0995-z.

43. Brandt T, Laiho M. Gender and personality in transformational leadership context: an examination of leader and subordinate perspectives. Leadership Org Dev J. 2013;34(1):44–66.

44. Swendiman R. Deep listening. Acad Med. 2014;89(6):950.

45. Brown J. From new learning environments for the 21st century. Aspen; 2005. http://www.johnseelybrown.com/newlearning.pdf. Accessed 13 Jul 2019.

46. Schramm P. Listening to drive culture change. Strategic HR Rev. 2017;16(4):161–5.

47. Covey S. Seven habits of highly effective people. New York: Free Press; 1990.

48. Fritz R. The path of least resistance for managers. New York: Berrett-Koehler; 1999.

49. Rigg C. Dialogue in organizations, developing relational leadership. Action Learning: Research and Practice. 2016;13(2):192–3. https://doi.org/10.1080/14767333.2016.1170982.

50. Reitz M. Leading questions: dialogue in organizations: developing relational leadership. Leadership. 2017;13(4):516–22.

51. See Dunoon D. The Obreau Tripod: Enabling challenging conversations; 2019. http://www.dondunoon.com/the-obreau-tripod. Accessed 18 Jul 2019 and Dunoon D. Mindful OD Practice and the Obreau Tripod: Beyond Positive/Problem Polarities; 2019. http://www.dondunoon.com/articles-and-resources. Accessed 18 Jul 2019.

52. Toney B, Goff DA, Weber RJ. Social media as a leadership tool for pharmacists. Hosp Pharm. 2015;50(7):644–8.

53. Collaboration, culture, management. Transactions vs. interactions. mmitll; 2019. https://mmitii.mattballantine.com/2019/02/25/transactions-v-interactions/. Accessed 18 Jul 2019.

54. Pogosyan L, Liucero RJ, Knutson AR, Friedberg MW, Poghosyan H. Social networks in health care teams: evidence from the United States. J Health Organ Manag. 2016;30(7):1119–39. https://doi.org/10.1108/JHOM-12-2015-0201.

55. Rönnerhag M, Severinsson E, Haruna M, Berggren I. A qualitative evaluation of health care professionals' perceptions of adverse events focusing on communication and teamwork in maternity care. J Adv Nurs. 2019;75:585–93. https://doi.org/10.1111/jan.13864.

56. Harris KR, Eccles DW, Shatzer JH. Team deliberate practice in medicine and related domains: a consideration of the issues. Adv in Health Sci Educ. 2017;22:209–20.

57. Kilpatrick K, Lavoie-Tremblay M, Ritchie J, Lamothe L. Advanced practice nursing, health care teams, and perceptions of team effectiveness. Health Care Manag. 2011;30(3):215–26.

58. Katzenbach JR, Smith DK. The wisdom of teams. Boston: Havard Business Review Press; 2015.

59. Landman N, Aannestad LK, Smoldt RK, Cortese DA. Teamwork in health care. Nurs Admin Quar. 2014;38(3):198–205.
60. Onwochei DN, Halpern S, Balki M. Teamwork assessment tools in obstetric emergencies: a systematic review. Simul Healthc. 2017;12(3):165–76.
61. MacIver K. A systems-based model for team development. K. A. McIver and Associates: Victoria, BC; 2000.

The *LEADS in a Caring Environment* Framework: Achieve Results

7

Graham Dickson and Bill Tholl

> *Leadership is about not only developing and communicating a vision and setting objectives but also following through to achieve results.*
>
> McKinsey and Company, 2015 [1]

All of us want to make a positive difference when we get up in the morning. Who doesn't like checking off their to-do list at the end of the day? And, as the quote above suggests, success for health care leaders is judged not by just having a clear and compelling vision but also checking off the achieving results box in our annual or quarterly performance reviews.

Let's look at what Simon Kennedy says about making a difference. Simon was one of Canada's longest-serving federal deputy ministers of health in a generation, at just over four years from 2015-2019. He has worked in a variety of portfolios across the federal government. Here's Simon's story:

> *My minister's 2017 mandate letter [2] from the Prime Minister set a clear goal: "To engage provinces and territories in the development of a new multi-year Health Accord." In realizing a new health accord, the federal government hoped to advance the twin objectives for Canadians of achieving improved access to necessary mental health and home care services.*
>
> *While it has sometimes proven difficult for governments to find common ground on health care, I and my provincial colleagues were certainly able to start with the premise that everyone agrees on the need for a better and more accountable system. It also seemed important at the outset to acknowledge that the provinces have constitutional responsibility for health care delivery and position Health Canada as seeking to be a helpful part-*

G. Dickson (✉)
Royal Roads University, Victoria, BC, Canada
e-mail: graham.dickson@royalroads.ca

B. Tholl
Canadian Health Leadership Network, Ottawa, ON, Canada
e-mail: btholl@chlnet.ca

© Springer Nature Switzerland AG 2020
G. Dickson, B. Tholl (eds.), *Bringing Leadership to Life in Health: LEADS in a Caring Environment*, https://doi.org/10.1007/978-3-030-38536-1_7

ner—one with a clear point of view and interests, but a partner—in helping to meet the emerging health care needs of Canadians across the country. In my own view, a little humility goes a long way in finding shared solutions. Relationships are fundamental. Honesty and transparency are key to building the personal relationships needed to overcome obstacles.

A lot of hard work went into setting the table for how we would successfully work together. It seemed apparent that notwithstanding long-held institutional positions, there were many things all parties actually agreed upon, and the key was finding out how to structure an outcome that everyone felt good about. My experience from the old days working in trade negotiations was that the good negotiators gathered enough intel about the various competing interests to know where the final 'landing zone' might be.

To accomplish the two goals of improved access to mental health care and enhanced home care services, special purpose funding of an additional $11 billion spread over 10 years has been committed over and above core federal funding for health care services in that same time period. In order to help monitor and evaluate progress over this period, all jurisdictions agreed on a common set of health indicators for each of the two priority areas. I think this was a win-win for everyone: Additional funding was provided for important services outside of the core physician-and-hospitals infrastructure, and all governments agreed to an accountability mechanism that is simple and clear and could well be replicated elsewhere over time.

It always seemed to me that the most effective leaders, whether DMs or ministers or others, were those who could work in the 'here and now' and at the same time steer a course where managing these issues fits into a longer-term game plan. The urgent and the important co-exist. Short-term imperatives map against the longer-term agenda. In health care, in particular, I am under no delusions of cracking the secret over my term as deputy, however long that might be. It's clear there needs to be a longer-term game plan, vision and strategic patience. I have learned much about leadership from Indigenous leaders, who have a philosophy of taking decisions today that will have impact seven generations out! I see my role as the current DM as making it easier for those that come behind me to find the promised land.

Simon's story underscores how the four capabilities under the Achieve results domain come together. Having received very clear direction in the form of a mandate letter from the Prime Minister, Simon set about using his full bag of leadership tools, acquired over a series of different senior leadership positions outside the health sector, to deliver results. First, he was able to work with deputies from the provinces to address the needs of Canada's most vulnerable, those needing mental health and long-term care (Set direction). Then, based on this vision and on "evidence and shared values"—the need for an accountable system, respect for the constitution, and the importance of relationships based on humility, honesty and transparency—he and the provincial deputies made decisions to realize the goals of mental health and community care. Together, he and the provincial leaders then allocated resources over a 10-year time frame to take action, by employing both short- and long-term plans to achieve those goals. Finally, processes were put in place to assess and evaluate progress according to a standard set of indicators, with accountability to the Canadian electorate as a common denominator for ensuring longer-term sustainability.

Simon's story is one of many we feature in this chapter on how the four capabilities work together and how important it is to get off to the right start as a results-oriented health care leader. Before doing a deeper dive on each of the four capabilities that make up the Achieve results domain, let's take a moment to reflect on what we have learned from Simon.

Learning Moment
Take a moment to reflect on Simon's story outlined above.

- Like Simon, leaders always need to balance short-term imperatives or deliverables with longer-term results. Can you articulate the long-term results you are pursuing? What might they look like in the short term, if you were acting in a manner in keeping with those long-term results?
- Share Simon's story with a colleague. Discuss. Are there lessons in Simon's story that apply to leading your project, or organization?

As the McKinsey and Company study quoted at the beginning of this chapter suggests, "operating with a strong results orientation" is a major contributor to leadership effectiveness in both for-profit and not-for-profit sectors. From a results perspective Canada continues to lag most comparator countries, coming in ninth out of 11 countries (with the United States and France coming in behind) according to the most recent Commonwealth Fund rankings [3]. Across jurisdictions in Canada, we also see wide variations in the same performance metrics used by the Commonwealth Fund [4]. Such evidence should impel leaders—at all levels—to look for and leading practices to achieve better results. At the organization, department, or community level each of us should be translating those desired results into short- and long-term actions that align in order to contribute to their achievement.

Many health leaders' results are measured in terms of the financial sustainability of their health care systems or organizations. Bending the cost curve [5] (Jack White's phrase for reducing the rate of growth in health spending [6]) has gone to the top of the agenda. Close to 50% of total program spending by provincial governments in Canada, for example, is allocated to health, driven upward by both demographics and technology. "The sustainability of public sector health care spending has been at the forefront of a roiling policy debate for years in Canada (and abroad)" [5]. Many of the case studies featured in this book have bending the cost curve as either a constraint or an explicit public policy objective.

There are four primary factors that influence the results effective leadership can achieve. The first is that leaders need management skills to achieve results. Management practices—planning, organizing, budgeting and measuring—are rational, research-based practices that enable leaders to realize their vision. Daniel Pink describes management as technology [7] to be employed to achieve results; but it's technology that must be integrated with the people engagement approaches described in other LEADS domains [8].

A second key factor is the sea change that's happened in terms of our ability to measure results. The last 10 years have seen an "unprecedented increase in the volume and variety of electronic data related to research and development, health records, and patient self-tracking, collectively referred to as Big Data. Properly harnessed, Big Data can provide insights and drive discovery that will accelerate biomedical advances, improve patient outcomes, and reduce costs" [9]. The growing technological capacity to collect big data or real-world evidence in the moment couples with growing capacity to systematically analyze data have generated the tools to make timely and accurate evidence informed decisions. Results-oriented leaders need to design and use delivery systems that make real-time results available to decision makers.

The third factor affecting effective leadership is the ability to align effort vertically and horizontally in an organization to achieve results. Implementation science is the study of methods to encourage and promote the systematic uptake of research findings and other evidence-based recommendations into routine practice. Its goal is to improve the quality and effectiveness of health services [10, 11]. Unless decisions and activities are aligned with the desired results, the meta-values of efficiency and effectiveness cannot be achieved. Results oriented leadership is tight on results, but loose on process: leaders see the results as the goal, and adjust processes in order to get there. By employing disciplined practices to convert research knowledge to action [10, 12] and engaging in strategic planning, action planning, project management and ultimately behaviour change, the leader can logically align decisions and action with the desired vision and results.

The fourth factor is that growing data analytics capacity and clear identification of best practices for implementation have increased expectations that leaders be held accountable for delivering better results [13–15] and increasingly, in Canada, creating value-based, learning health care systems [16, 17]. Without clear evidence of how you're doing and holding yourself accountable for course corrections, progress is impossible. Consequently, accountable health care is more of a priority for leaders than ever before in Canada and many other countries. We will say more about this priority in the "Assess and Evaluate" section of this chapter.

These four factors make Achieve results the most task-oriented of the five domains of the LEADS framework. Regardless of your role—CEO, mid-manager, front-line supervisor, clinician-leader, community or informal leader—using the Achieve results capabilities will help you clarify goals, set priorities, measure your effectiveness, stay on track, deal with inevitable surprises, take appropriate action to deal with shocks and be resilient enough to get right back on track.

The Achieve results domain differs from the others in another important respect: its order matters. Much like the "Plan, Do, Study, Act" cycle [18, 19], the four capabilities of Achieve results work better together and work best when in this order:

1. Set direction
2. Strategically align decisions with vision, values, and evidence
3. Take action to implement decisions
4. Assess and evaluate

So now, and building on Simon's story, let's turn our focus to looking at the four capabilities in the Achieve results domain of the *LEADS in a Caring Environment* framework, and how together they can help focus your leadership on the task of improving health for our citizens.

Set Direction

"Would you tell me, please, which way I ought to go from here?" asks Alice.
"That depends a good deal on where you want to get to," said the Cat.
"I don't much care where–" said Alice. "Then it doesn't matter which way you go," said
the Cat. "–so long as I get SOMEWHERE," added Alice.

Lewis Carroll

To set direction is the first capability in the Achieve results domain. Leaders inspire vision by identifying, establishing, and communicating clear and meaningful expectations and outcomes. If you don't know where you are headed then any road will get you there; but you may be destined to travel it alone. Porter and Lee point out: "The first step of solving any problem is to define a proper goal. Efforts to reform health care have been hobbled by lack of clarity about the goal, or even by pursuit of the wrong goal" [15]. A vision—and related results—is the North Star for organizational or collective activity [20]. A good leader transmits a clear vision and direction, which motivates and energizes the team, especially during unsettling and difficult times [21].

Visions are leader and management-team driven and ideally, created collaboratively by engaging members of the organization and the public, which is the most effective way to win broader acceptance of a vision [22]. As we will continue to repeat throughout this book, distributed leadership is about owning what we all help create. What is also clear from our research [23] and the work of other writers [24, 25] is that visions need to be clear, compelling and inspirational. If a vision is not shared it has little power to direct collective action.

Simon's story also underlines the importance of thinking decades ahead. John F. Kennedy famously said in 1962: "I believe that this nation should commit itself to achieving the goal, before this decade is out, of landing a man on the moon and returning him safely to earth." He went on to say: "…we choose to go to the moon and do other things not because they are easy, but because they are hard" [26]. Jim Collins said inspirational leaders pursue "big, hairy audacious goals" [27] and Richard Farson said "the only vision worth pursuing is one that is impossible to achieve" [28]. In this chapter and throughout the book we encourage all health leaders to stretch themselves and, with President Kennedy in mind, to shoot for the moon.

How important is it for a health leader to have a clear and compelling vision in these extraordinarily unpredictable times? At least one study found significant relationships between visionary leadership and perceived organizational effectiveness [29]. But a vision can be hard to relate to if it's perceived as simply the purview of politicians or senior management. It must be owned by everyone who has a role in creating its results. Visions can also seem remote if it does not include a timeline and clearly defined, desired, results [30]. This is hard to overstate—it's easy these days to lose sight of where we are on a leadership journey or of the core purpose of an organization. Let us share a real story from the Canadian prairies that brings this home.

A CEO of several national health organizations, who grew up in the Canadian prairies, and happens to be one of the two co-authors of this book, is fond of telling a story about growing up in Saskatchewan. Canada, like Australia, Russia and the U.S. is a large country with vast prairies. "It is a rite of adulthood that every teenager growing up on the prairies is asked one day to take the wheel of the tractor and cultivate the field."

Dad had been making great progress. The field was half done with nice straight furrows when he said to me: "It's your turn now, Bill. Let's see what you can do!" So I took the wheel of the tractor and carefully set off down the field looking backwards to follow his furrow. I got to the end of the field and turned to see how I had done. I was crushed to see that my furrow was as crooked as a dog's hind leg. I turned to my Dad and asked "So what did I do wrong? How is it that your furrow is so straight?" He smiled and said wryly: "Well, the first problem is that you were looking backwards the entire length of the field and every time you hit a rock in the field, it set you off course and you over corrected to get back on track. The trick is to look forward, not backward."

"That's fine then, Dad, but how is it that you get back on track so quickly that your furrows look so straight?" "Well," he said. "I pick a fencepost on the horizon and I line up the tractor's smokestack with the fencepost and that helps me to get back on track quickly when I hit the rocks in the field."

The field of health care leadership, like the wheat fields of Saskatchewan, has many unexpected rocks and other obstacles. In facing them, leaders need to have a clear and compelling vision (I want nice straight furrows!) and must keep their eye on the fenceposts (results in line with the vision) and they must always be looking ahead rather than backwards as they lead the way.

Just as smaller family farms have gradually given way to large corporate ones, the health care system continues its transition from corner stores to corporations. More and more hospitals, here in Canada and elsewhere, are merging and (as detailed in Chap. 12) local regional health organizations are giving way to larger, province-wide health authorities. And, just as Saskatchewan farms are incorporating, looking to computerized equipment, even tractor drones, to improve overall efficiency and be more competitive, the health care system of 2020 is being buffeted by the technological imperatives of artificial intelligence, proteomics, precision medicine and robotics. Health leaders in 2020 and beyond will need to continue to learn, to grow and to stay ahead of what technology can do *for* them rather than *to* them. They need to be vigilant and need to beware of both negative and positive spillover effects of new technology and constantly remind themselves that technology should serve health care, not the other way around.

To take an international example of a horizon objective for health, the World Health Organization originally set the goal of "Health for All by 2000" back in 1978 [31]. Health for All 2000 garnered support from health leaders around the world. When the WHO realized it wasn't going to hit this ambitious target by year 2000, it didn't abandon the vision. Rather, it celebrated the significant progress that had been made in areas like reducing child and maternal mortality rates and, in 2000, recommitted its 191 nations to the new Millennium Development Goals, resetting the target as Health for All by 2020 [32]. This is an example of a worthy horizon objective, likely unattainable in the lifecycle of any one leader if ever (and certainly not by 2020) but worth striving for. The most recent (2015) report from WHO refines the goalposts again moving toward a broader set of sustainable development objectives [33].

Another example of pursuing a horizon objective, as mentioned previously, is provided by the U.S. Institute for Healthcare Improvement's call to action in 2006 to reduce medical errors in the system. The CEO at the time, Dr. Don Berwick, challenged health care leaders to work together to reduce deaths from preventable errors (vision) by 100,000 per year (clear, desirable result) by eliminating avoidable adverse events. The resulting *100,000 Lives Campaign* [34] took off in the United States and spread to Canada, putting health care systems around the world on a different pathway toward reducing the incidence of preventable harm in the system.

In Canada, the same movement helped spawn the creation of the Canadian Patient Safety Institute in 2003. It launched with the daunting horizon vision of creating "the safest health care in the world." However, unlike Berwick's work, specific, desirable results, in keeping with the vision, were not articulated. In their absence, can we clearly identify our progress? We are still striving to achieve an error-free health care system; patient safety has become job number one for leaders in the Canadian health care system. But how are we doing? New tools have been put in place; new pathways have been found to turn knowledge into action; and efforts to engage patients and families have grown significantly (see Chaps. 6 and 13). But without a clearly defined destination, expressed as desirable results, we may wander in the wilderness without a clear destination or GPS to guide us to it.

Strong visions have been shown to enhance organizational and system performance [35, 36] but even compelling visions expressed passionately may only inspire others for a time. When we hit those rocks in the field, when reality sets in, and people begin to be frustrated with being thrown off track, it's vitally important for a leader to identify clear and meaningful expectations and long- and short-term results, which can be measured to show that the vision is being translated into action. Measurable results, in keeping with the vision and translated into short-term measures, can give a distant goal relevance and infuse day-to-day efforts with meaning and purpose.

Learning Moment

Visions are important; but articulating desired results may be even more important. Review your organization's strategic directions document.

1. Does it clearly outline the results it wants to create with its vision and mission? If so, what are they?
2. If it does not, what metrics do you think would be appropriate measures for having achieved the vision and mission? Outline three.
3. Depending on your answer to either 1 or 2, how does your work contribute to achieving those results?

Strategically Align Decisions with Vision, Values and Evidence

The second capability of the Achieve results domain is to strategically align decisions with vision, values and evidence. "The strategic vision and values that drive the organisational culture need to be values that are meaningful and that are clearly visible to patients and staff. They have to be more than 'just words'" [20].

What do we mean by alignment? As a noun, it refers to "the degree of integration of an organization's (or local service delivery system's) core systems, structures, processes, and skills; as well as the degree of connectedness of people to the organization's (or system's) strategy. As a verb, aligning is a force like magnetism. It is what happens to scattered iron filings when you pass a magnet over them.

Visions and results; mission (purpose statements) values (organizational principles) and evidence are the forces that create aligned decisions. The key word is "decisions" because they are the domain of decision-makers and leaders, from executives to the receptionist (a.k.a. "Director of First Impressions") to the family caregiver. Decisions are how you as a leader focus, direct and maximize the use of an organization's resources to achieve its core purpose.

Figure 7.1 below shows how, in a perfect world, vision, mission, values and evidence come together to create a substantial sweet spot that defines the area of an ideal decision. The chart shows that a clear and compelling vision is necessary, but not sufficient to achieve results. The vision must align with the core mission of the organization, with the well-understood and shared values of the organization or endeavour, and the evidence that needs to be acted on for change to happen.

Fig. 7.1 Aligning mission, vision, values and evidence to make a decision

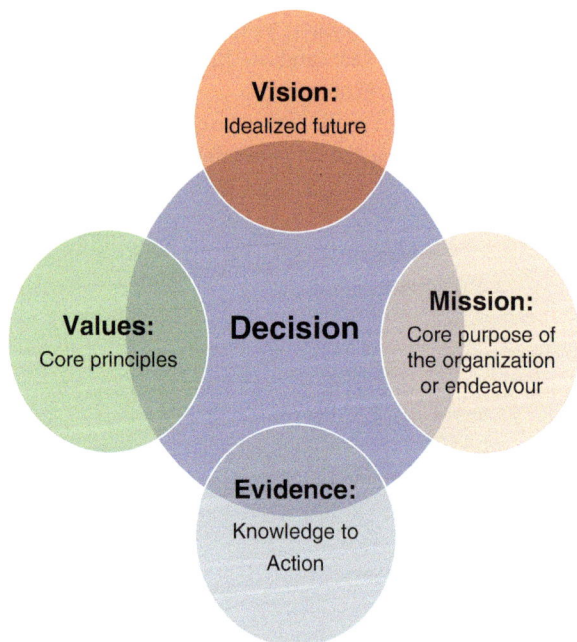

Of course, as in most leadership challenges, it's never a perfect world and there are no guarantees that it is easy to balance vision, values, mission, evidence, to create a decision. Indeed, given the dynamics of health care systems, some leaders on some days might say it is more akin to a perfect storm than a perfect fit, where unrealistic demands meet increasingly scarce resources. If decisions were purely rational, that might be the case; but given the politics of organizational life, strategic choices are not always logical, at least in the short run. In this context, leaders can only use their best judgment to make a sensible and timely decision.

In studying six Canadian health care organizations, Smith et al. [37] point out that successful leaders find effective ways to ensure executive teams actually act as teams (described in Chap. 6) to make decisions on setting priorities and allocating resources. Often, they don't: Peter Senge [38], in his discussion of organizational learning disabilities, describes executive teams as warlords who come to the table to carve up the spoils, rather than act as a fully functioning team. Smith and Mitton also stated that decision maker attitudes and behaviour were identified as a key determining factor in terms of getting commitment to a shared vision. They found that aligning structures, processes, behaviour and outcomes is critical to achieving meaningful results for high performance health care organizations.

Harking back to Simon's story, after several failed attempts under previous health accords to ensure accountability longer term, it was critical to have provinces and territories agree upon a standard set of indicators to assess both new investments in mental health and home and community care. This was necessary to ensure governments are accountable to the tax-paying public. Requiring that progress be reported regularly does set an important precedent for any future federal investments, such as discussions around introducing a universal pharmacare program for Canadians [39].

Simon's story also demonstrates the challenge of leading in the less than perfect world of health care, where real time data is often unavailable; or where data systems are not interoperable; or where data analytics are underdeveloped. Leaders are required to align multiple factors, including what other leaders are trying to do. Their collective efforts may support overall alignment but, again, they may not. For example, as an executive leader, you should try to make sure your board is "on board." Consider adding a generative role (where board members consciously think about issues in new ways to decide what they should focus on) to the board's more traditional fiduciary and strategic roles. "Given the complexities of 21st century health care, it has never been more important for boards, whether elected or appointed, to work as one" [40]. Having a board that is LEADS literate can be invaluable.

Let's now look at a case study on aligning vision, values and evidence to make a decision. One of Canada's Maritime provinces, Nova Scotia, decided to centralize its nine health regions into one province-wide authority, the Nova Scotia Health Authority (NHSA). Dr. Peter Vaughn took on the role of deputy minister of health with a mandate to create this single health authority. Here's Peter's story about some efforts to align elements of the system with the new vision and desired results (Interview with Peter Vaughn, former deputy health minister, Nova Scotia, August 15, 2019).

The overarching goal was to create an accountable health organization for all of Nova Scotia. What was a bit different for Nova Scotia compared to other provinces was that the changes had to be embedded into legislation. The intention behind legislating the account-ability framework for NSHA was to prevent possible back sliding, as it makes it more diffi-cult for subsequent governments to roll the changes back if it is the law.

In terms of lessons learned from our experience in Nova Scotia as shared right across Canada, governments tend to conflate strategy and structure. They think that changing structures is in itself a strategy and it is not. Every business school student knows that strat-egy precedes structure. Appropriate governance structures are necessary but not sufficient.

In implementing the decision to centralize the system, we pursued what I might call a "Porter-esque" value strategy. We needed to change the ministry, which most other mergers hadn't done. We also needed to build an analytical capacity that didn't really exist before that. We needed to modernize our data acquisitions, foundations, data bases and informa-tion sharing arrangements.

What many people do not appreciate, and is worth highlighting, is that we not only set up a new health authority, but we entirely redesigned the ministry to focus on data analytics and advanced analytics. This has not been done anywhere else in the country.

Peter uses the term "Porter-esque value strategy," meaning one based on the work of Michael Porter [41] who created a framework for restructuring health care systems with the overarching goal of increasing value for patients, while controlling health care costs.

We will continue Peter's story in the next section. Suffice it to say, aligning of vision, values, mission and evidence created the decision to change the ministry.

Aligning Efficiency and Effectiveness

The reference in Peter's story to the Porter value strategy highlights the importance of making decisions to strike the right balance between efficiency and effectiveness. If we become so efficient or lean that we no longer have the residual capacity to be resilient, or can no longer meet patient needs, then the organization or endeavour we are leading can crash and burn. The changes in Nova Scotia were about seeking a new approach to delivering health service that is both efficient and effective.

Demands for efficiency therefore must be aligned with demands for effective-ness, keeping them in dynamic balance. To do that we must first recognize their essential differences: being effective is all about doing the right things (such as establishing the right direction, identifying results and measuring the right things) while efficiency is all about doing things right (like use the most efficient manage-ment processes and building systems to accomplish your goals). An ideal decision aligns the two.

A good example of an over-emphasis on efficiency is how Lean, the business re-engineering process, is often used. Over the past five years we have seen an unprece-dented shift to using Lean to improve efficiency in health care. Lean uses management processes to eliminate waste and redundancy to improve overall efficiency. It seeks effectiveness by linking those processes with the value proposition you are striving for—that is, the results you desire. But what often happens is that the technical, process re-engineering dynamics of Lean are emphasized without also ensuring the leadership behaviour required of supervisors, clinicians and employees is integrated into the learning process. Lean cannot work unless people are willing to implement its discipline; they have to be able and willing to change their behaviour to set up and sustain its processes (that is, they must be motivated to do the right things). This is where the Achieve results capabilities meet the people focus of the other LEADS domains and capabilities. Dickson et al. [42] describe the symbiotic relationship that exists between Lean and LEADS, where process improvement and people engagement by necessity come together; and optimal decisions, based on vision, values and evidence can be made.

Take Action to Implement Decisions

The third capability under Achieve results is about converting decisions into action. To demonstrate this capability, health care leaders must act in a manner consistent with their organization's values to yield effective, efficient public-centred service and implement decisions that ensure changes happen to achieve results. Decisions that aren't acted on are meaningless, busy work at best; and demoralizing to your team at worst. Leadership is not simply making decisions about what should be done; in a paraphrase of Nike, it's just doing it.

Based on our research and casual empiricism, there are leaders who act or demonstrate leadership *in action* and there are those who don't, demonstrating leadership *inaction*. A decision requires new behaviour. Behaviour change is action. We have talked at length about the psychology of behaviour change in the other chapters. In this chapter we're looking at how external management practices—such as organizational or project design, action planning, measurement, and techniques such as project management—can also facilitate action. They align effort by organizing people to act together and reducing choices to a practicable level. For example, action plans create the task focus needed to achieve a common set of targeted goals and objectives and break down tasks into discrete and doable steps, which suggest clear, actionable behaviour.

Leadership in action often means overcoming system inertia and the culture of acceptance of the status quo. The decision Simon and the other provincial deputies made to invest money in mental health and improved community access, for example, will require leaders, clinicians, employees and citizens to act differently, constructing new relationships, developing new plans, engaging in new projects, allocating money appropriately, etc.

Another example comes from the context of implementing quality and patient safety decisions. Braithwaite et al. [43] identify common, reoccurring features that should be followed to generate action. They are: conducting effective and detailed

planning and project management; good communication and collaboration processes for key actors; and tools, checklists, algorithms, standards and clearly defined
roles or articulated expectations, which need to align with the goal of the decision.
The authors also emphasize the fundamental importance of engaging clinician and
stakeholders to integrate them into these actions. Without both, the quality of care
can be put at risk, and patient safety can be compromised. Leadership inaction is
often a mirror image of these action steps.

Let's now continue Peter's story about some of the actions employed—and some
that were not—to implement the decision to create a new provincial health system.

> One of the first actions we took was to downsize the ministry by 300 because under the
> legislation, our new job was to act as governors of the health care system. With the
> Accountability Framework in place it became the job of the authority, not the ministry, to
> run the health care system. Our job was to fund and oversee it centrally. We also needed to
> put in the kinds of metrics that both of us could agree would be evolved over time, which
> they would be accountable for.
>
> Physician engagement is another key to any successful accountable health organiza-
> tion. Here's where things went off the rails. We saw very clearly the need and desire for a
> co-leadership model with physicians. We did a lot of work and made a lot of good progress.
> One wild card in the change process was that the renewal of the contract with Doctors Nova
> Scotia was long overdue. This renewal coincided with the setting up of NSHA and Doctors
> Nova Scotia went outside to hire a prominent labour lawyer who worked for all the major
> unions. The government saw this as a major ramping up of union demands across the
> board, and reacted perhaps predictably. Five years later there is still a lack of physician
> engagement.
>
> It was terrible timing in terms of coming at a time when we really needed physicians on
> board to achieve the results. This was out of my hands as deputy minister and became a
> much bigger deal than we had anticipated as the dispute dragged on.
>
> A second step was to build the strategy, after the structure was in place. But as it turned
> out the provincial government, for fear of being held accountable politically decided not to
> put strategies out into public domains. This was the second wild card. We could not get the
> government to allow us to engage the public with the strategy. This was a key piece. For,
> while we were holding the NSHA to account, government was not being held to account.

As Peter's story tells us, leadership *in action* led to the restructuring of the
Ministry of Health in Nova Scotia and the creation of a meaningful accountability
framework for the new NSHA. But leadership *inaction* led to physician estrange-
ment and public disengagement. The lesson is—you as a leader must understand the
dynamics of change a decision requires and turn that understanding into action others will support. That's where the Engage others and Develop coalitions domains of
LEADS complement the capabilities of Achieve results. Results-oriented leaders
try to anticipate where the agenda is headed, recognize threats and opportunities
sooner and are prepared to seek forgiveness rather than wait for permission when
conditions warrant. People judge us not by our words but by our actions. When
there's a disconnect, our credibility suffers. With the unprecedented pace of change
in health care, dithering is increasingly dangerous. Finding the right balance of
action and inaction is an art; one based on experience, judgement and intuition of
the leader.

Learning Moment

Consider all the actions Peter had to take to implement the decision to undertake transformational change for an entire system.

1. Which ones speak to the elements we have identified as important for implementing success?
2. What kinds of wild cards or surprises have you encountered in implementing decisions?
3. Contemplate when you have seen leadership inaction in your workplace. What factors contributed to inaction? Upon reflection, are there steps that could have been taken to mitigate those factors?
4. Have you, yourself, ever over-reacted? What were the consequences? What would you do differently?

In a project or organizational context, desired action—according to our definition of leadership—is when people "work together to achieve a constructive purpose: the health and wellness of the population we serve". Health and wellness results require the implementation of policies, strategic directions, goals, action plans, and clinical services. They are the actions of "working together."

Leaders know that individuals take action not just for organizational success, but also to pursue personal values and interests. Emotions such as fear of consequences and/or the potential for conflict may restrict their willingness to act. Similarly, their own understanding of their context and role may make them disagree with a proposed action. That's why actions need to reflect an understanding of context; and to recognize people need to be given the freedom to choose the best actions to achieve the desired effect in their area of expertise, for the clients they serve. That means policies and plans must allow enough flexibility for the person acting on them to interpret them for their context; and the power to act as required. Accountability systems, compliance processes and organizational plans that don't do that will drive out initiative and promote leadership inaction.

Leaders are always asking both themselves and others to change and act differently from how they are acting now. It is one thing to take on that challenge for oneself (the Lead self domain of LEADS). It's something else to demand it of others—leaders doing that need the tools and techniques to align effort in collective endeavour. People need the conditions that enables and encourages them to act; good leaders create those conditions for them—and for themselves.

Learning Moment

Observe your colleagues and others in a particular context of the workplace (overall organization, department, unit or subsidiary site). Reflecting on your observations, answer the following questions:

1. Do people in your workplace act in a timely, energetic or committed fashion, as needed?
2. If so, what features of organizational practise facilitate that?
3. If not, what features of organization design or practise are an impediment to action?
4. If you were leading the part of the organization you observed, what would you do to facilitate greater action?

Assess and Evaluate

The fourth capability in the Achieve results domain is to assess and evaluate. We define this capability as leaders measuring and evaluating outcomes. They hold themselves and others accountable for results achieved against benchmarks and correct the course as appropriate.

The assess and evaluate capability describes the pointy edge of leadership accountability—the process of knowing whether our responsibilities have been achieved, accepting the consequences or sharing the credit. Peter and his team understood that to assess something is to measure it:

> We had clear ideas of the plans, processes and metrics to build data and analytic account-ability and capacity. Ultimately it was the metrics in the accountability agreement that formed the first element of the implementation strategy. We needed to have very clear metrics to drive resource allocations and to address the historical frustrations of political ad hoc-ery that I experienced as a CEO of a region. This was fundamental to our success.

To assess something is to measure it. To evaluate something is to determine its merit or worth. A leader may need to know, for example, how many operations are being conducted in any particular hospital: that's assessment. Knowing how efficient or effective those operations are is an evaluative process—and one that is done by designing and employing benchmarks or targets to ascribe merit or worth to that result. All leaders in health care face measurement challenges. Some things—like spending—are relatively easy to measure. Other things—like caring for a patient, for an employee, or for self—are much harder. Many of the benefits and costs of health care appear to be intangible, but they're not: it's just more difficult to find the appropriate measure. Assessment and evaluation create the need for measurement and accountability, because measurement helps us be accountable. Accountability is different from responsibility, because you can be responsible for something but not held to account for it. It's important in leadership to be accountable for what you are responsible for.

Remember Peter's story? Here is how he framed the design or creation of the new NSHA and revised Ministry of Health:

> In terms of adopting a Porter-like paradigm, we were looking to transform to a value-based, accountable organization or accountable health care organizations north. Triple aim was certainly part of the conceptual framework.

Accountable health care organizations are designed to use population outcome data to assess and evaluate performance and then generate accountability by tying provider reimbursements to those quality metrics [44, 45]. Their purpose is to use data to reduce, wherever possible, the total cost of care for an assigned population of patients (hence the reference to Porter), while targeting services to be more effective. This trend surged after the Accountable Care Act ("Obamacare") became law in the United States in 2010, and accelerated the move to accountable healthcare organizations. With more than 800 in place in the US, and the number growing, many Canadian jurisdictions are looking southward to emulate the patient-centred, co-creation philosophy behind them [46].

Two elements fundamental to effective functioning of accountable health care organizations are measurement and metrics, and accountability.

Measurement and Metrics

The NHSA put into law a set of metrics to be used to guide actions in health service delivery in Nova Scotia. Likewise, Simon's story underscores the need for common indicators or metrics to measure progress. For metrics to be useful, however, they must be:

- Valid and reliable—the technique used actually measures the phenomena it is intended to and will produce similar results each time it is used.
- Realistic—data can be accessed in a reasonably cost-effective and efficient manner.
- Expressed in a measurable range—measures express themselves in an organized sequence of variable results
- Modifiable—changeable through deliberate and constructive action.
- Independent—the collection of indicators (maximally realized) describe the desired end-state; but each measure contributes a different factor than the others.

From a leadership perspective, metrics need to measure the desired results of the vision and the decisions and actions taken to realize it. Too often people measure the wrong things because they are easy to measure and easily accessed. It's often much worse to have good measurement of the wrong thing—especially when, as often happens, it's used as an indicator of the right thing—than to have poor measurement of the right thing [47]. One of the biggest challenges leaders face is to avoid defaulting to the simplest of measures—cost—as the sole determinant of effectiveness. Cost needs to be balanced with other measures of effectiveness, such as staff turnover or the quality of patient experience, even though they may be difficult to operationalize. Similarly, process measures (i.e., flow through in an emergency ward) are too often emphasized over measures of outputs and outcomes (i.e., when they left the emergency ward, did they recover as expected?) A colleague of ours who was an assistant deputy minister of health once told us that he asked his staff to determine how many metrics the ministry measured. The answer was 1734 and of those, almost none were outcome measures.

Results oriented leaders are tight on outcomes and loose on process—that is, the end result they want to achieve is the fence post at the end of the field: it doesn't move. But the processes needed to get there can be adjusted and altered as rocks in the field are encoutered. Leaders must have the right balance between outcome metrics and process measures, or those course adjustments cannot be made.

From an organizational leadership perspective one of the fundamental principles of effective measurement systems is that they need to be integrated into all facets of the organization's operations. If the priority is safety, for example, all departments and units must understand it is a major strategic imperative and everyone has a role in making it happen, or the effort may be resisted and languish. Just as responsibilities and accountabilities cascade at all levels of the organization, so is there a logical progression of processes and procedures needed to bring a meaningful quality measurement system to life (see Fig. 7.2).

There are two measurement models you might wish to look at, the balanced scorecard created by Kaplan and Norton [48], which still has significant traction in health care [49] and, as pointed out above, the Triple Aim construct promoted by the Institute for Healthcare Improvement in the United States and by the Canadian Foundation for Healthcare Improvement [50] (The IHI has introduced a fourth aim recently; staff engagement). Both models expect the leader to go beyond measuring financial results and assess results including customer or patient satisfaction, productivity (such as clinical accomplishments), employee engagement and how well important clinical practices are being implemented. The principles and procedures in both can be applied by leaders at any level.

Once you have chosen a measure, evaluate whether performance on it is satisfactory (or not), judge whether action needs to be taken and accept responsibility for undertaking that action. And finally, the more transparent you are—particularly in the final stages of a change process—the more potential there is others will understand and support the action that needs to be taken.

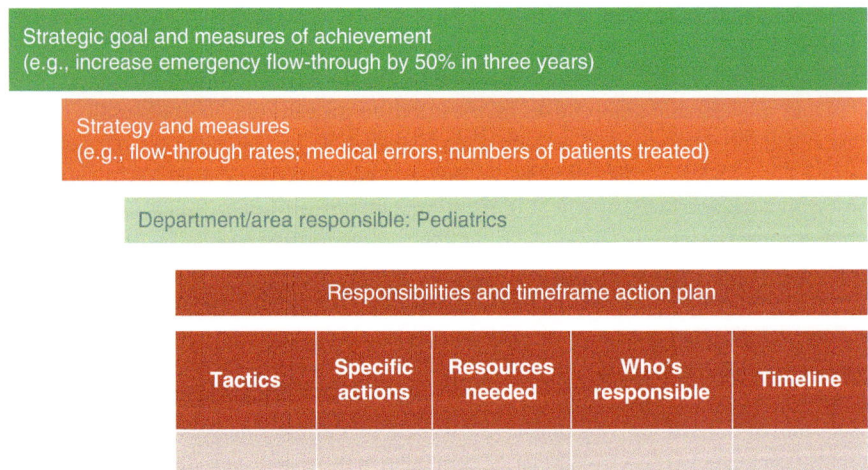

Strategic goal and measures of achievement (e.g., increase emergency flow-through by 50% in three years)

Strategy and measures (e.g., flow-through rates; medical errors; numbers of patients treated)

Department/area responsible: Pediatrics

Responsibilities and timeframe action plan

Tactics	Specific actions	Resources needed	Who's responsible	Timeline

Fig. 7.2 Aligning measures and metrics with decisions and actions

Accountability

Accountability has two forms. First, there is consequential accountability, which is accepting consequences, or being held to account for achieving your assigned responsibilities. The second is procedural accountability, which is being held to account for processes and protocols that are expected to be adhered to, such as clinical protocols or financial protocols.

Many organizations establish benchmarks, a result that sets a level of acceptable performance. These can be determined by comparing one's results to certain standards, often data from other jurisdictions. Reports then show performance relative to the benchmark on charts that make the implications of the data transparent. Many organizations have policies dictating consequences if performance is significantly below par (we elaborate on one such model below). This kind of measurement formalizes accountability: "People live up to what they write down" [51]. Holding yourself consequentially accountable for reaching benchmarks [52] means accepting responsibility to make changes to processes if the results don't stand up.

When measures suggest significant changes are required, consequential accountability may conflict with procedural accountability. It may be the process is not being followed effectively, leading to poor results; or, the process itself may be unable to achieve those results. It is your job to ensure transparent processes are put in place and followed, or to change processes that don't work to improve results. Now let's look at a health care organization that has put measurement and accountability to work. Here's Bruyère's story ((Personal interview with Amy Porteous and Isabelle Bossé 2019 Apr 15).

> Bruyère is a Catholic hospital located in Ottawa, Canada. It specializes in providing complex continuing care for the community at large.
> Bruyère's Legacy Plan was introduced in 2014, along with the adoption of the LEADS framework as a common leadership platform at the hospital. The plan includes a number of components that all work together to enhance leadership growth and long-term organizational effectiveness. Early on in its journey, Bruyère selected a few indicators to track the progress of this long-term strategy. Four main categories emerged and key metrics were identified for each (see Fig. 7.3).
> Figure 7.3 describes in some detail the four results that Bruyère was looking for from its Legacy Plan. The scorecard allows for a review of progress and shows progress relative to the four objectives set out above for staff engagement and succession planning.
> More than 100 people are engaged in the Legacy Plan at Bruyère. This represents approximately 5% of the total number of staff. Twenty per cent of them are in non-management positions and have been identified as "high potentials" by their immediate supervisors. Bruyère also keeps track of "mission critical positions" by assigning a criticality index and retirement coefficient to each leadership position. This data helps the organization prepare for future leadership vacancies.
> In terms of producing tangible results, one of the early objectives of the program was promoting from within, and 20% of individuals engaged in the Legacy Plan have been promoted into higher level positions since the beginning of the program. Also, participation in leadership development opportunities (internal and external) has more than doubled since the implementation of the plan. This is encouraging. Since embarking on this journey, Bruyère has learned three key lessons:

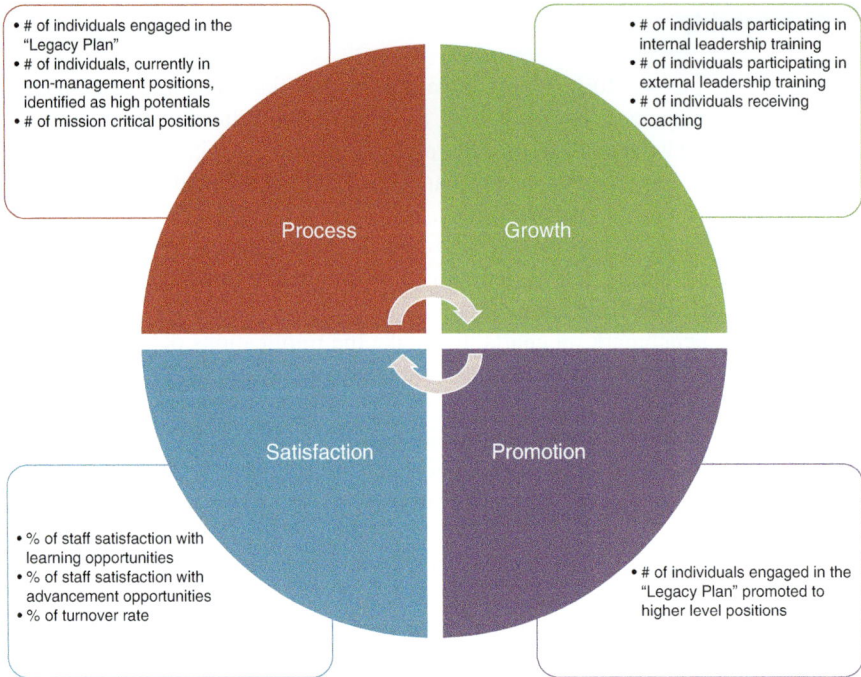

Fig. 7.3 Bruyère Legacy Plan scorecard

- *Lesson 1: Keep it simple. Aim for a simple process for identifying future leaders and, whenever possible, align it with other internal business processes (such as recruitment and performance appraisal) while building on existing metrics to avoid duplicating efforts.*
- *Lesson 2: Amp up the accountability factor. Ensure you have the right oversight and reporting mechanism for all things related to succession planning and leadership development. Not only will this help with positioning and implementing this important initiative, it will also help sustain the gains.*
- *Lesson 3: Make the technology work for you. Get a tool that will make it possible to easily track all data related to the succession plan. This will be instrumental in identifying high potential talent and developmental needs as well as determining where to focus your limited resources for maximum impact.*

Assessing and evaluating service is not straightforward. The imperatives of quality and quantity do not always align, but organizational values and culture always must. In every instance the leader must look inside (Lead self) for the guidance and fortitude to address the problem; and use the Engage others capabilities to stimulate staff and patient involvement.

Finally, in terms of accountability, leaders who thrive as opposed to just survive are acutely aware of the need to align authorities and accountabilities carefully. Having accountability for delivering on results with little or no authority over the policies or programs to get the job done is a recipe for stress and one reason for the historically high churn rate among senior health leaders. It also helps explain why younger leaders are reluctant to take on more senior roles. This has been identified recently as a fatal flaw in many efforts to regionalize responsibilities for health care decision making [53]. It's also where good leaders may turn to the serenity prayer: "God grant me the serenity to accept the things I cannot change; courage to change the things I can; and wisdom to know the difference."

Summary

This chapter provides an overview of the Achieve results domain of the *LEADS in a Caring Environment* framework and its four inter-related leadership capabilities:

- Set direction
- Strategically align decisions with vision, values and evidence.
- Take action to implement decisions
- Assess and evaluate

We have shown how, unlike the other domains, order matters—the capabilities can't be used in just any combination. Like a plan-do-study-act cycle, the four capabilities build one upon the other to help leaders Achieve results as part of a continuous improvement process.

The reader might also ask about how the four capabilities of Achieve results apply to the equity, diversity and inclusion challenges facing health organizations today:

> **Achieving Equity, Diversity and Inclusion-Informed Results**
> *The four capabilities of Achieve results are all relevant to equity, diversity and inclusion. Goal-oriented leaders who are committed to equity, diversity and inclusion will dedicate resources to address issues around them and embed the following processes in their department, division, or organization.*
>
> *First, leaders must establish a baseline of knowledge through environmental scanning and audits of data on equity, diversity and inclusion, such as staff, clients, and services if they do not already exist. Next, they must consult a diverse range of interested stakeholders in high-level meetings to reach a (near to) consensus direction for equity, diversity and inclusion initiatives that align with organizational vision and values. These plans must be resourced, implemented, and acted upon and supported with evidence-informed tools.*
>
> *One made-in-Canada toolkit, developed from the Empowering Women Leaders in Health initiative, is available on the LEADS platform. Tools include equity, diversity and inclusion-aware hiring and promotion practices and supportive organizational policies, processes, and culture. Continuous monitoring, reassessment, and evaluation to track progress towards equity, diversity and inclusion goals and resetting direction for continuous improvement must be embedded in organizational processes for optimal results.*

Each of the four capabilities of the Achieve results domain is aimed at clarifying and focusing you on the results of change, and on how to use those results to gauge progress and for course correction. This is the most task-oriented of the five domains. In our experience, the discipline required to succeed in the Achieve results domain, particularly for the capabilities of Take action to implement decisions and Assess and evaluate, is very challenging for health leaders. You need to stay focused on your fencepost and be ready for rocks in the health care field.

We certainly adhere to the adage "if you can't measure it you can't manage it." While measurement is often used effectively at the clinical level, it is used less effectively at the unit and organization levels. That may be because of rapid amalgamation of small health units into big ones, requiring the coordination of disparate and fragmented data and information systems. However, modern technology gives us the tools to collect, interpret, and use big data; and leaders need to build the information systems that are required and become capable of using them for better course correction and direction setting (in keeping with the cyclic nature or our four Achieve results capabilities).

We've also noted, with the rapid adoption of variations on the accountable health-care organizations method, traditional approaches to aligning authorities and accountabilities need to be revisited. Legislative approaches to locking in the new structures and processes can help prevent backsliding, as is the case in the United States with Obamacare and in Canadian jurisdictions including Nova Scotia and Manitoba.

Your challenge is whether you will take charge of the opportunities that assessment and evaluation provide, or wait for the government, media and the public to do it for you.

Learning Moment

To use this questionnaire, find the right category for your level of leadership, then assess how well you demonstrate the four Achieve results capabilities. Choose the appropriate level to make that assessment.

Which capability do you want to bet better at? Why?

Achieves Results Self-Assessment (for on-line access to self assessment tool please visit www.LEADSglobal.ca.)

Informal leader (patient, family member, citizen) responsibilities

In order to be a goal-oriented leader, I

1.	Contribute to direction setting (vision and results) when asked; and/or suggest new directions when results for citizens are not optimal	1 2 3 4 5 6 7 N
2.	Ensure my input into decisions, pertaining to the organization or project's direction, is in keeping with the vision, values, mission and available evidence	1 2 3 4 5 6 7 N

| 3. | Behave in a manner consistent with expectations as laid out in action plans for my area of interest and/or responsibility | 1 2 3 4 5 6 7 N |
| 4. | Participate in, or advocate for processes to measure, assess, and evaluate organizational/project performance; and monitor those results to determine course corrections | 1 2 3 4 5 6 7 N |

Front-line leaders

In order to be a goal-oriented leader, I

1.	Ensure there is a clear direction to be achieved by my unit; and that it is aligned with the organization's vision and desired results	1 2 3 4 5 6 7 N
2.	Make decisions in my area of responsibility that align with the vision, values, or mission statement of the organization; and that are consistent with the direction and available evidence	1 2 3 4 5 6 7 N
3.	Take the actions necessary to keep me and my staff focused on the desired results for my unit	1 2 3 4 5 6 7 N
4.	Assess and evaluate the desired results of my unit's work; and monitor those results to determine course corrections	1 2 3 4 5 6 7 N

Mid-level leaders

In order to be a goal-oriented leader, I

1.	Set direction for the department, in line with the organization's direction, through operational plans that outline key milestones, timelines and expected results to be achieved by all units	1 2 3 4 5 6 7 N
2.	Make decisions, relative to my department's responsibilities, that align with the vision, values, or mission statement of the organization; and that are consistent with available evidence	1 2 3 4 5 6 7 N
3.	Take the actions necessary to ensure ongoing availability of critical services in my department	1 2 3 4 5 6 7 N
4.	Ensure valid measurement tools are in place for assessing and evaluating my department's responsibilities; and that are used to improve services when necessary	1 2 3 4 5 6 7 N

Senior leaders

In order to be a goal-oriented leader, I

1.	Set direction for my portfolio, in keeping with the organization's vision and results, through strategies and metrics that will fulfill the key responsibilities of my portfolio	1 2 3 4 5 6 7 N
2.	Can clearly describe how current decisions in my strategic area align with overall organizational vision, values, mission, and relevant evidence	1 2 3 4 5 6 7 N
3.	Gain support of other senior leaders and staff for successful implementation of strategies, and for changes to those strategies when those changes are validated by new evidence	1 2 3 4 5 6 7 N
4.	Hold myself and others accountable for assessing and evaluating metrics consistent with our strategies, and monitor those results to determine course corrections and/or new directions	1 2 3 4 5 6 7 N

Executive leaders

In order to be a goal-oriented leader, I

1.	Collaborate with province, board, colleagues, and staff to create a compelling statement of values, vision, and desired results for the organization	1 2 3 4 5 6 7 N
2.	Develop strategic processes and plans that align strategies with the organization's values, vision, available evidence and desired results; and that outline decisions for organizational improvement	1 2 3 4 5 6 7 N
3.	Provide necessary support (e.g. systems, processes, resources) for implementation of the organization's strategic decisions	1 2 3 4 5 6 7 N
4.	Ensure that measures, benchmarks and targets are established to assess and evaluate desired results for the organization; and use them to course correct where necessary; or set a new direction for the organization	1 2 3 4 5 6 7 N

References

1. Feser C, Mayol M, Srinivasan R. Decoding leadership: what really matters. McKinsey quarterly. New York, NY: McKinsey; 2015. https://leadershipcoaching.com.au/wp-content/uploads/2016/03/Decoding-Leadership-What-really-works.pdf. Accessed 22 Aug 2019.
2. Minister of Health. Ministerial mandate letter. Minister of Health mandate letter. Ottawa, ON: Prime Minister of Canada; 2017. https://www.assembly.gov.nt.ca/sites/default/files/td_282-182.pdf. Accessed 22 Aug 2019.
3. Schneider EC, Sarnak DO, Squires D, Sha A, Doty MM. Mirror, mirror. Washington, DC: Commonwealth Fund; 2017. https://interactives.commonwealthfund.org/2017/july/mirror-mirror/. Accessed 22 Aug 2019.
4. Busby C, Muthukumaran R, Jacobs A. Reality bites: how Canada's healthcare system compares to its international peers. Toronto, ON: C.D. Howe Institute; 2018. ebrief 271. https://papers.ssrn.com/sol3/papers.cfm?abstract_id=3112894. Accessed 22 Aug 2019.
5. Marchildon GP, Di Mateao L. Bending the cost curve in health care: Canada's provinces in international perspective. Toronto, ON: University of Toronto Press; 2015.
6. White J. The mixed (de)merits of 'bending the cost curve'. Health Affairs. 2011. https://www.healthaffairs.org/do/10.1377/hblog20110617.011786/full/. Accessed 18 Sep 2019.
7. Pink D. Management is an outdated technology. Chicago, IL: Gaegen MacDonald; 2012. Video: 3 min. 36 sec. https://www.youtube.com/watch?.v=bgCdSnLrHJo. Accessed 22 Aug 2019.
8. Dan Pink shares 2 simple strategies for motivating employees. Business Insider, 13 Jan 2016. https://www.businessinsider.com/dan-pink-on-how-to-boost-team-performance-2016-1. Accessed 22 Aug 2019.
9. Adam NR, Wieder R, Ghosh D. Data science, learning, and applications to biomedical and health sciences. Ann NY Acad Sci. 2017;1387:5–11.
10. Weiser TG, Forrester JA, Negussie T. Implementation science and innovation in global surgery. BJS. 2019;106:e20–3.
11. Editorial. Implementation science and AOTJ's role in bridging the occupational therapy best practice – actual practice. Aust Occup Ther J. 2019;66:127–9.
12. Holtrop JS, Rabin BA, Glasgow RE. Dissemination and implementation science in primary care research and practice: contributions and opportunities. J Am Board Fam Med. 2018;31(3):466–78.

13. Sharfstein JM. Accountability for health. Milbank Q. 2015;93(4):675–8.
14. Van Kerkvoorden D, Ettema R, Minkman M. Accountability in integrated health service delivery in the Netherlands, an evidence based integrated care approach. Int J Integr Care. 2019;19(4):285.
15. Adeniran A, Likaka A, Knutsson A, Costella A, Daelmans B, Maliqi B, et al. Leadership, action, learning and accountability to deliver quality care for women, newborns and children. Geneva: World Health Organization. Bull WHO. 2018;96(**3**):222–4.
16. Porter ME, Lee TH. The strategy that will fix health care. Harv Bus Rev. 2013;2013:1–19.
17. Phipps-Taylor M, Shortell M. More than money: motivating physician behavior change in Accountable Care Organizations. Milbank Q. 2016;94(4):832–61.
18. Taylor MJ, McNicholas C, Nicolay C, Darzi A, Bell D, Reed JE. Systematic review of the application of the plan–do–study–act method to improve quality in healthcare. BMJ Qual Saf. 2014;23:290–8.
19. Canada Foundation for Healthcare Improvement. CFHI quality improvement primer. Ottawa, ON: Canadian Foundation for Healthcare Improvement. https://www.cfhi-fcass.ca/sf-docs/default-source/on-call/primer-videos/qi-primer-pdsa-e.pdf?sfvrsn=368ad744_2. Accessed 22 Aug 2019.
20. Kollenscher E, Eden F, Ronen B, Farjoun M. Architectural leadership: The neglected core of organizational leadership. Eur Manag Rev. 2017;14:247–64. https://doi.org/10.1111/emre.12108.
21. Nightingale A. Developing the organisational culture in a healthcare setting. Nurs Stand. 2018;32(21):53–63.
22. O'Connell D, Hickerson OK, Pillutla A. Organizational visioning: an integrative review. Group Organ Manag. 2011;36(1):103–25. https://doi.org/10.1177/1059601110390999.
23. Dickson G, Tholl B, Baker GR, Blais R, Clavel N, Gorley C, et al. Partnerships for health system improvement, leadership and health system redesign: cross-case analysis. Ottawa, ON: Royal Roads University, Canadian Health Leadership Network, Canadian Institutes of Health Research, Michael Smith Foundation for Health Research; 2014. http://tinyurl.com/qh6ogzu. Accessed 22 Aug 2019.
24. Kaplan R, Norton D. The execution premium. Boston, MA: Harvard Business School Publishing; 2008.
25. Lipton M. Demystifying the development of an organizational vision. Sloan Manag Rev. 1996. http://sloanreview.mit.edu/article/demystifying-the-development-of-an-organizational-vision/. Accessed Aug 2013.
26. Kennedy JF, John F. Kennedy moon speech. Houston, TX: Rice University; 1962. https://er.jsc.nasa.gov/seh/ricetalk.htm. Accessed 26 Aug 2019.
27. Collins J, Porras JI. HAG—big hairy audacious goal. Jim Collins Articles. 2019. https://www.jimcollins.com/article_topics/articles/BHAG.html. Accessed 20 Aug 2019.
28. Farson R. Management of the absurd: paradoxes in leadership. New York, NY: Touchstone; 1996.
29. Taylor C, Cornelius CJ, Colvin K. Visionary leadership and its relationship to organizational effectiveness. Leadership Org Dev J. 2014;35(6):566–83.
30. Hoog E, Lyshom J, Garvare R, Weinehall L, Nystrong ME. Quality improvement in large healthcare organizations. J Health Organ Manag. 2016;30(1):133–53. https://doi.org/10.1108/JHOM-10-2013-0209.
31. World Health Organization. WHO called to return to the Declaration of Alma-Ata. Geneva: World Health Organization; 2019. https://www.who.int/social_determinants/tools/multimedia/alma_ata/en/. Accessed 20 Aug 2019
32. World Health Organization. WHO 2000 millennium development goals. Geneva: World Health Organization; 2019. https://www.who.int/topics/millennium_development_goals/about/en/. Accessed 20 Aug 2019.
33. World Health Organization. WHO from MDGs to SDGs, WHO launches new report. 2015. https://www.who.int/en/news-room/detail/08-12-2015-from-mdgs-to-sdgs-who-launches-new-report. Accessed 20 Aug 2019
34. Wachter RM, Pronovost PJ. The 100,000 lives campaign: a scientific and policy review. Jt Comm J Qual Patient Saf. 2006;32(11):621–7.

35. Kantabutra S, Avery G. The power of vision: statements that resonate. J Bus Strategy. 2010;31(1):37–45. https://doi.org/10.1108/02756661011012769.
36. Mayfield J, Mayfield M, Sharbrough WCIII. Strategic vision and values in top leaders' communications: motivating language at a higher level. Int J Bus Commun. 2015;52(1):97–121.
37. Smith N, Mitton C, et al. High performance in healthcare priority setting and resource allocation: a literature- and case study-based framework in the Canadian context. Soc Sci Med. 2016;162:185–92.
38. Senge P. The fifth discipline: the art and practice of the learning organization. New York, NY: Random House; 2006.
39. Government of Canada. A prescription for Canada: achieving Pharmacare for all; 2019. https://www.canada.ca/en/health-canada/corporate/about-health-canada/public-engagement/external-advisory-bodies/implementation-national-pharmacare/final-report.html. Accessed 2 Aug 2019.
40. Dickson G, Waite G. Leading from the boardroom: bringing LEADS in a caring environment to Canadian healthcare boards. Ottawa, ON: HealthcareCAN; 2016. http://www.healthcarecan.ca/wp-content/themes/camyno/assets/document/Reports/2016/HCC/EN/Leading%20from%20the%20Boardroom%20mongraph_FINALv5.pdf. Accessed 22 Aug 2019.
41. Harvard Business School. Value-based health care. Boston, MA: Harvard Business School, Institute for Strategy and Competitiveness; 2019. https://www.isc.hbs.edu/health-care/value-based-health-care/Pages/default.aspx. Accessed 2019.
42. Dickson G, Mutwiri B, Blakley B. The symbiotic relationship between Lean and LEADS. Ottawa, ON: Canadian Health Leadership Network; 2015. https://chlnet.ca/wp-content/uploads/LEAN-and-LEADS-Comparison-for-CHLNet-May-2015.pdf. Accessed 23 Aug 2019.
43. Braithwaite J, Marks D, Taylor N. Harnessing implementation science to improve care quality and patient safety: a systematic review of targeted literature. Int J Qual Health Care. 2014;26(3):321–9.
44. Shortell SM, al e. Accountable health organizations: the national landscape. J Health Polit Policy Law. 2015;40(4):647–68.
45. Saliba GN. Accountable care organizations. NJ Bus. 2014;60(9):41.
46. Canadian Patient Safety Institute and Health Standards Organization. The Canadian quality and patient safety framework for health and social services. Ottawa, ON: CPSI and HSO; 2019. https://static1.squarespace.com/static/5c42463a372b96e73b4ff935/t/5c6ffea0104c7b6ae28b05c4/1550843555878/CPSI01_DraftFramework_EN_F4.pdf. Accessed 20 Aug 2019.
47. Schryvers P. Bad data. New York, NY: Prometheus Books; 2019.
48. Kaplan R, Norton D. The execution premium: linking strategy to operations for competitive advantage. Boston, MA: Harvard Business School Publishing; 2008.
49. McDonald B. Bob McDonald profiles the extensive use of the Balanced Scorecard in numerous health jurisdictions in Australia and other developed nations. A review of the use of the balanced scorecard in healthcare. Inver Grove Heights, MN: BMcD Consulting; 2012. http://www.bmcdconsulting.com/index_htm_files/Review%20of%20the%20Use%20of%20the%20Balanced%20Scorecard%20in%20Healthcare%20BMcD.pdf. Accessed Aug 2013.
50. Bisognano M, Kenney C. Leadership for the triple aim. Healthc Exec. 2012;27(2):80.
51. Cialdini R. The uses (and abuses) of influence, putting the pieces together. Harv Bus Rev. 2013;91:76–81.
52. Relias Media. Toyota situation is no reason to abandon Lean, say experts. Atlanta, GA: Relias Media; 2010. https://www.reliasmedia.com/articles/19507-toyota-situation-is-no-reason-to-abandon-lean-say-experts. Accessed 22 Jul 2012.
53. Waddell K, Moat KA, Lavis JN. Evidence brief: preparing emerging leaders for alternative futures in health systems across Canada. Hamilton, ON: McMaster Health Forum; 2019.

The *LEADS in a Caring Environment* Framework: Develop Coalitions

8

Graham Dickson, Bill Tholl, and E. Hartney

Alone we can do so little; together we can do so much.

Helen Keller

Introduction

The quote from Helen Keller applies to individuals working in teams. It also applies to teams of organizations who wish to work together. In recent years, working in collaborative partnerships across multiple sectors (such as primary and specialist care, hospitals and community care or public health, education, and urban planning) has become critical for accomplishing larger system- or policy-change goals [1].

Relationship dynamics *between* (as opposed to *in*) organizations add a layer of complexity to the practice of leadership [2]. The Develop coalitions capabilities offer a level of sophistication that recognizes that complexity, describing what strategic leaders do to build productive relationships between organizations that serve the needs of patients, families and citizens.

This chapter begins by describing what coalitions are, their potential benefits and the challenges associated with building them. It's our position that strategic leaders can't develop coalitions without drawing on all the other domains of LEADS, which have to be integrated with the four Develop coalitions capabilities. We'll look at

G. Dickson (✉)
Royal Roads University, Victoria, BC, Canada
e-mail: graham.dickson@royalroads.ca

B. Tholl
Canadian Health Leadership Network, Ottawa, ON, Canada
e-mail: btholl@chlnet.ca

E. Hartney
Royal Roads University, Victoria, BC, Canada
e-mail: Elizabeth.Hartney@royalroads.ca

© Springer Nature Switzerland AG 2020   147
G. Dickson, B. Tholl (eds.), *Bringing Leadership to Life in Health: LEADS in a Caring Environment*, https://doi.org/10.1007/978-3-030-38536-1_8

examples of coalition-building from a variety of national contexts to show how
LEADS can be put to work to build productive inter-organizational action.

What Are Coalitions?

A coalition is: *any formal inter-organizational collaboration dedicated to achieving
a common purpose.* Carpooling is a good metaphor for a coalition, because when
you're carpooling you need to be sure you:

1. *Share the same destination.* When you're carpooling, the first question you need
   to ask is, where are we going? If you don't share a destination, you'll get to the
   first intersection and one of you will be severely disappointed.
2. *Share the same values.* You might also want to ask whether the carpool is smoke
   free and whether speeding is acceptable. When you're building a coalition, be
   sure you share the same core values, such as honesty, integrity, openess and consensus decision making. Formally agree to expectations and speak to your partners if you think core values are being breached.
3. *Share the load.* As a carpooler, you may want to share the cost of gas, share the
   driving and even share payment for speeding tickets. You certainly want to be
   clear on who's doing the driving. Coalitions need to agree on how to share in the
   financial, legal and the (often underestimated) risk to personal and organizational reputation.
4. *Share knowledge.* If you need a map to chart a route, share it. If there's something the driver should know to stay safe, or evidence to show one route is
   quicker than another, share that as well.
5. *Share the credit.* When you reach the destination, don't claim to have driven all
   the way alone. Credit should be shared, too. It's infinitely divisible. And, as your
   mother always said, it's always better given than taken.

Let's now look at how this carpooling approach was used to create a coalition
around advancing the health of children: the formation of the Kids Health Alliance
in Ontario. In 2017, the CEOs of the three freestanding children's hospitals in
Ontario were discussing opportunities around how to improve access to safe, coordinated, high-quality care for children. The three hospitals were Sick Kids in
Toronto; Holland Bloorview Kids Rehabilitation Hospital (also in Toronto) and the
Children's Hospital of Eastern Ontario (CHEO) in Ottawa. Using the carpooling
metaphor, the conversation went something like this (Lauren Ettin, Executive
Director, Personal Communication, 2019 Jul 26):

> Mike says to Alex and Julia, *"We've been working together informally for some time now
> and we all want what's best for our kids: access to high quality, consistent safe care as close
> to home as possible. The system needs to achieve better, tangible results. What do you think
> about forming an alliance to reach out to specialty and non-specialty pediatric providers to
> advance the care being delivered to children and youth?"* (Share the destination).
>   Julia: *"I love the idea. We do need to step up our game, including working more closely
> with community hospitals, since 85 per cent of children's emergency department visits are
> to local community hospitals."*

Alex: "This is a great idea. As the specialty children's hospitals, we can certainly band together to get the network going. To be successful, we need to be inclusive, partnering with like-minded organizations who share the same vision and goals."

Julia: "I agree. The network needs to be member driven. Hospitals can opt-in or not, with all members co-designing joint approaches and with shared accountability, transparency of data, and responsibility for the alliance." (Share values).

Mike: "I like where this is headed. In terms of moving the idea forward, we'll have to work together to find the resources to support the alliance. We will also want to look at finding better ways to share best practices, evidence, and lessons learned in real time. There will be a lot that we can all learn from each other. And, of course, we will have to establish a small core team that will work with our partners." (Share risks and information).

Julia, Mike and Alex in unison: "Kids Health Alliance it is. Let's make this happen".

Fast forward. Two years after this seminal conversation among three CEOs, the Kids Health Alliance had six community hospital partners embrace an All Teach, All Learn model to implement, monitor and sustain shared goals and outcomes. The opt-in, member driven model underscores the Kids Health Alliance's goal of building excellence and expertise together in pediatric care, with a vision to expand across the continuum of care. The model is not about assessment or evaluation of partners or taking credit.

The Kids Health Alliance, with its shared ownership and shared responsibilities recorded in a participation agreement, is a useful example of how to carpool and of the power of "leadership without ownership." In less than two years the alliance and its partners are showing results. We will certainly continue to follow its progress [3]. (Sharing credit).

Benefits of Coalitions

Why are coalitions important for modern health care delivery? Because they can be a means to apply concerted, creative, coordinated, resource-rich thinking and action to address complex systemic challenges. Coalitions can catalyze innovation and change, which might otherwise bog down in traditional bureaucratic organizations. Coalitions allow people to explore different configurations of organizing people and resources to service patients better [1, 4, 5]. Coalition-building is the manifestation of distributed and collaborative leadership in the arena of strategic leadership. "Because alliances often consist of a diverse set of individuals from the community, many of whom are leaders in organizations that operate in the community, the leadership activities are often distributed across a broader range of individuals" [6].

Modern health leaders recognize health care is *not* a system but *should* be [7] if our goal is health and wellness, with patients, families and populations at the centre of our work. It's time to integrate the disparate efforts of multiple organizations for optimal results—especially as diminishing resources provide a strong incentive to seek out collaborations that will make improving services and creating efficiencies possible.

Challenges of Coalition Building

Coalitions offer many benefits; but their appeal is not without risk. Coalition building has unique issues that must be anticipated and dealt with—a particular challenge because building coalitions often needs a mindset, world view, and strategic thinking very different from those needed for effective organizational management.

The first challenge of coalition building is to overcome some traditional mental models. We've been conditioned to see other organizations as competitors, fighting for money, talent and reputation. It's natural in that context to fetishize one's organization, seeing it as special and better than others. That's not an attitude to bring to coalition building, where you need to be open to recognizing what other organizations do better and see them as special in their own way—potential partners that will enhance efforts to solve common problems.

There are also structural and cultural challenges to coalition building. Launching a coalition is a notoriously slow process, because it takes time to gain and build trust, understand where partners are coming from and develop clear direction and purpose. Initial enthusiasm can flag as individual egos and the security of staff in each organization feel threatened. Sometimes the leaders who championed the coalition depart, leaving a vacuum at the top. Without careful effort and attention, chasms develop between the strategic champions of the coalition and the operations leaders.

Leaders as Coalition Builders

As a leader, you need to be aware of the benefits and challenges of coalitions if you want to make one work. A quick first step is to ask the carpool questions, and keep them in mind as you begin the process of coalition building.

Coalition leaders need to be a catalyst, fostering relationships to get the work done, rather than directing it or even trying to do all the work themselves—although they may have to take on a variety of roles to build collective capacity for change [1]. They see boundaries as permeable rather than rigid and closed, giving rise to the term *boundary spanners,* used to describe effective coalition builders. Boundary spanners take time to understand partners and their priorities and are attuned to the internal dissension that might arise in their own organization [8].

Paradoxically, the first step a leader should take in boundary spanning is to strengthen his/her organization's own boundaries [9] to give staff a stronger sense of identity and purpose, which will help them develop a clearer sense of the value their organization would bring to a coalition, and enhance understanding of their distinct specialties, roles and responsibilities. Staff will feel greater elasticity and strength. They will become aware that openness can be a strength, not necessarily a weakness.

A leader who wants to build coalitions and overcome the challenges of building and maintaining them requires "…a sophisticated set of skills, knowledge, and abilities to envision, form and implement change" [10]. In the Develop coalitions domain, leaders have four capabilities. They are:

- Purposefully build partnerships and networks to achieve results.
- Demonstrate a commitment to customers and service.
- Mobilize knowledge.
- Navigate socio-political environments.

> **Learning Moment**
> Reflect on the metaphor of carpooling:
>
> 1. Contemplate the key strategic goals of your unit, department, or area of leadership responsibility.
> 2. Are there potential partners—other organizations, other individuals, outside your area of formal responsibility, with whom you could carpool to improve results for patients? Families? Communities?
> 3. Identify one potential partner. Review the carpool checklist: how might you develop a working relationship with this partner?

Purposefully Build Partnerships and Networks to Create Results

As Cikaliuk and Tholl point out: "Successful coalitions do not just *happen* and they do not just *remain* successful. They are made up of individually successful people who do the right things, at the right time, with the right structures and processes, in the right context, for the right purpose" [11]. The word *purposefully* is chosen to suggest that whatever form of coalition is chosen, it's done in an intentional, deliberate manner, with a clear purpose in mind.

For example, when partners join the Kids Health Alliance, they agree to a common partnership agreement, which describes the alliance's principles and values and areas of focus. The agreement is the foundation for collaboration, building trust and a shared understanding of what they hope to achieve together. All partners commit to sharing data, resources and lessons learned across the network through forums including communities of practice and working groups, to accelerate success through support and reciprocity.

Success depends on a shared understanding of what the alliance will achieve, clear roles and responsibilities and support for the value proposition (see Fig. 8.1 below).

The Canadian Alliance on Mental Illness and Mental Health, an alliance of 16 mental health groups, was established in 1998. Here's the story of how members refocused their vision to create one voice to advocate for improving the lives of those living with mental illness.

Through several strategic discussions in 2015 and 2016, members of the Canadian Alliance on Mental Illness and Mental Health (CAMIMH) committed to a shared goal: speaking with a single voice when they made recommendations to the federal government on how it could improve the lives of those living with mental illness. The timing was particularly opportune, because federal, provincial and territorial (FPT) discussions about a 2017 health accord were accelerating and it was a good time to try to have an impact.

The leaders of CAMIMH convened several somewhat contentious group discussions about what policies should drive their work, which someone would have to draft into policies and positions they could all get behind. It had to be someone who understood the

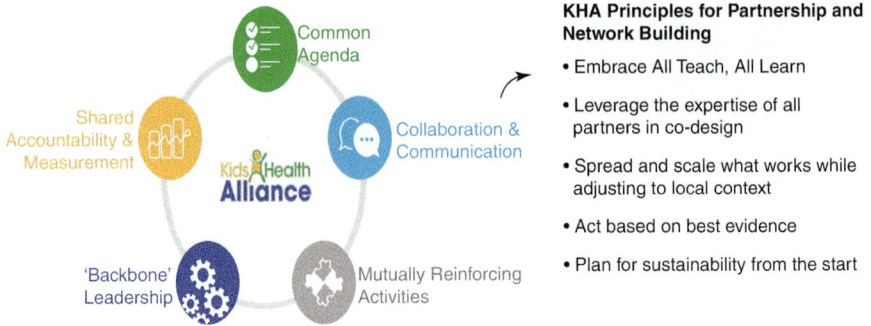

KHA Principles for Partnership and Network Building

- Embrace All Teach, All Learn

- Leverage the expertise of all partners in co-design

- Spread and scale what works while adjusting to local context

- Act based on best evidence

- Plan for sustainability from the start

Fig. 8.1 The Kids Health Alliance Model is underpinned by five first principles or concepts. (Concepts adapted from The Collective Impact Framework) [12].

members of the alliance and what they wanted to do; mental health policy needs and gaps; and the complex FPT context. They considered hiring an external consultant, but had a limited budget so agreed that two of their own, Glenn Brimacombe of the Canadian Psychiatric Association and Dr. Karen Cohen of the Canadian Psychological Association, would begin drafting a document, with each draft reviewed by all the members. The members of CAMIMH would need to take the final draft back to their respective boards for approval before the alliance as a whole could approve it.

It's important to note Glenn and Karen already had a strong working relationship as past co-chairs of HEAL (Organizations for Health Action) and in 2016 had led the development of a consensus statement on the role of the federal government in accelerating innovation and improving performance in the health system. Mutal trust was key. Their ability to work together to a tight deadline was crucial.

In getting consensus from members, the writers needed to understand the mental health landscape through the eyes of each member and how each perspective could be incorporated into a comprehensive and cohesive policy brief. Not unexpectedly for a large group of assertive advocates, discussions were lively and there was significant give and take as each draft was developed, reviewed and revised by the group, but organizational self-interest was trumped by the collective priority. Through the process, the group did not stray from its clear focus—making a policy contribution to improve mental health outcomes for Canadians. They needed to speak with one voice on key policy messages to be delivered to the federal government.

After reviewing and refining the issues to be addressed, the members chose five to focus on: ensure sustainable funding for access to mental health services; accelerate the adoption of proven and promising mental health innovations; measure, manage and monitor mental health system performance; establish an expert advisory panel on mental health; and invest in social infrastructure.

What resulted was Mental Health Now! Advancing the Mental Health of Canadians: The Federal Role [13]. Its recommendations were evidence-informed calls for action. CAMIMH recognized good intentions were not enough to have a policy impact. They needed to mobilize the evidence to compel policy change and support their work with an effective communications plan. In early 2017, following much discussion with the provinces and territories, the federal government committed to investing $5 billion over 10 years for mental health (and $6 billion for home and community care). CAMIMH's ability to seize the moment and speak with one voice through Mental Health Now! contributed to the federal government's decision to invest in mental health over a ten-year period.

The story about the genesis of the Canadian Alliance on Mental Illness and Mental Health illustrates purposeful re-positioning of an alliance to achieve an important shared vision—in this case, improvements to the health and wellness of mental health patients in Canada. In Chap. 7 we learned how important it is to have a clear and compelling vision. In a study dedicated to determining the sustainability of coalitions, Hearld et al. found "Respondents [associated with alliance organizations] who reported more positive perceptions of alliance leadership, decision-making, and conflict management were more likely to report higher levels of vision, mission, and strategy agreement, and in turn perceived the alliance as providing more value and were more likely to report changes in their home organizations" [14].

Being purposeful about developing trust is also necessary when building a coalition. In the Canadian Alliance on Mental Illness and Mental Health example, Glenn and Karen had grown to know and trust one another because of their previous experience of working together. Leveraging personal relationships is one way to build trust. Beyond Glenn and Karen, however, there was also the need to build trust among the alliance's members. Collectively, they invested time and energy to allow members to share perspectives, engage in dialogue and shape a consensus on what they should work on.

The literature on organizational and inter-organization trust says these things are needed to build trust: [15–18].

- Space: Create space for frequent and meaningful interaction among key partners.
- A compelling cause: Define a clear common cause that transcends individual interests and is supported by all.
- Interpersonal bonds: Show consideration for each other's needs, demonstrate integrity and fulfill commitments.
- A balance of autonomy and interdependence: Agree to a work structure that gives each organization discretion in how they do their share of it; don't try to manage each other.
- Time: Spend the time to get to know each other and each others' organizational culture and needs.
- Contracts: Set out the terms of the coalition in formal or informal agreements, and stick to them.
- Good will: Look for the best in all parties, assume their motivations align with yours and their commitment goes beyond contracts.
- Competence: Demonstrate the skills and knowledge that make you valuable to the coalition and allow other people the chance to demonstrate theirs.
- Commitment: Deliver on promises, do the work required, and help others as necessary to achieve the common goal.

Trust can be lost in an instant if you put your personal or organizational interests ahead of shared goals. Like a windshield, once broken trust is difficult to reconstruct. In short, "trust management is about managing risk" [19]. The deeper the level of trust in a coalition the better its performance and less the risk.

Another success factor for building purposeful coalitions is reciprocity. Working together means everyone must give slightly more than they take. Reciprocity reflects the philosopher David Hume's concept of "enlightened self-interest" or economist Adam Smith's "invisible hand" for market economics [20, 21]. Coalition members must put in more than they take out or the coalition will collapse. Similarly, if bigger players try to dominate smaller players, the coalition will fail. Coalitions are often judged by how the weaker members are treated. Mutual respect is not a function of size, but there is no room for freeloading. Everyone must contribute.

Forms of Coalitions

The structure of a coalition should be chosen to respect the needs of the partners and to facilitate achieving its goals. There are many different forms of coalitions and which form is appropriate depends on three central factors: the degree of control and centralization needed to achieve the desired results, the degree of autonomy each organization needs to make their maximum contribution for success, and the degree of coordination and administration needed to ensure the people doing the work can use their skills and abilities to best effect. These three factors can be operationalized as alliances, consortia, cross-organizational projects, public-private partnerships, networks, mergers, and partnerships. Popp et al. provide a very good overview of these and other defining features of constructive networks and dark networks [22]. Leaders need to engage in honest, serious discussion to determine the structure best suited to their coalition's needs.

Alexander et al. [23] and Tsuchiya et al. [1] studied the sustainability of coalitions over a period of change. In order to sustain coalitions, leaders must constantly communicate the vision, mission and desired results for the coalition. They must monitor both the internal dynamics of their organization to see if dedication to the coalition's challenges is being maintained and check to see if the coalition's other leaders are doing the same. They need to measure whether the desired results are being achieved and if not, correct the course or reconsider the value of the coalition. If the original purpose of the coalition has been met, partners must engage (as CAMIMH leaders did) to either design a new purpose or, if the coalition has run its course, dissolve it.

Learning Moment
Take a moment to reflect on the capability of purposefully building partnerships and networks to achieve results.

- What leadership qualities from the Lead self, Engage others and Achieve results domains would be helpful to build a clear destination for a coalition?
- Can you provide an example of a coalition that has outlived its value? Is that because it truly accomplished its goal, or because it does not have the capacity to adapt and adjust to new and emergent challenges that its member organizations should address?

Demonstrate a Commitment to Customers and Service

The second capability of the Develop coalitions domain is that collaborative leaders demonstrate a commitment to customers and service. They facilitate collaboration, cooperation and coalitions among diverse groups aimed at improving service. The words "customers" and "service" are used to suggest a people-centred purpose—which means meeting the health needs of family and care givers as well as citizens seeking care.

It may seem redundant to reiterate the importance of person-centred care at this point, since we have already emphasized you must have a purposeful vision for a coalition. But is that vision person-centred or self-serving for the organizations? Has it mutated—in the process of working together over time—into purposes that stray from the client- and customer-centred core? The health and wellness of patients and citizens' needs should be in the foreground of all coalition activity.

Let's look at another story of the power of one ultimately leading to the power of many—a coalition that launched the creation of a Youth Mental Health program dedicated to customers and service, across three health regions in Alberta, Canada. Dr. Suzanne Squires was inspired by a deep, passionate commitment to the customer, youth and the service, mental health support. This is her story:

> I'd been in family practice in Spruce Grove for 13 years and my practice was full of mostly young families. I noticed an increase in demand for children's mental health services. Families were asking for help with challenging issues they were seeing in their kids. Depression, anxiety, anger outbursts and even homicidal or suicidal thoughts or attempts were troubling kids and their parents. Wait times for existing services were increasing exponentially and now parents weren't able to get help in a timely manner, and problems worsened. The anxiety of just waiting to get help and not knowing how to get it was becoming a part of the problem.
>
> I was encountering the same scenario with my own daughter who was struggling with anxiety at school. She had always been an anxious child, but now the teachers were calling and saying she was "spacing out" in class and having freeze attacks. Suddenly I was attending parent conferences and trying to get the help we needed. I knew first-hand what it was like to sit in a doctor's office, feeling helpless to know how to help my child get through her day.
>
> I would complain about issues with wait times and challenging case presentations to my colleagues, and I heard they were facing the same problems. Eventually I tired of just complaining; I really felt like something more needed to be offered in our community. As primary care doctors in a suburban community, we practiced cradle to grave medicine. We deliver these children, watch them grow, see their parents and grandparents, and care for them until life's end. I knew this community cared about their children; yet, did we know how many families were really struggling with these difficult issues?
>
> I made a promise to myself that if I continued to complain about the problem, I would advocate to someone who could make a difference. I became a board member of the Westview Primary Care Network and started bringing up the lack of adequate service for children's mental health in our community. I found out other board members had similar struggles getting care for their own children and patients as well, and the board was very supportive in us engaging with other community members. Our first visit was to school counsellors at a local Catholic high school. I heard similar levels of frustration from the counsellors encountering teenagers presenting in crisis, suicidal, depressed, anxious. Sometimes they would send them to emergency. The teenagers would return the next day with a long wait to see a local counsellor, if any follow-up at all. Many times, they would leave without even being seen. The counsellors were as burnt out and frustrated as I was feeling.

Suzanne's experience—and her willingness to engage others in a dialogue about the needs of customers and the inadequacy of service—created a shared purpose or shared destination. She now needed to mobilize that diffused and recently articulated need in a shared vision statement to drive action. Her story continues.

> The Westview Primary Care Network board engaged our physician membership and we came up with a mental health vision statement: "Westview PCN must make every effort to work with our community partners to ensure every person who asks for help with their mental health gets the right help they need, at the right place, at the right time, from the right resources."
>
> We initially shared this vision statement with our health care partners at Alberta Health Services. We reached out people in our community from education, social services, RCMP, parents, teens, tech companies and youth groups.
>
> Fortunately, through a request from our Westview board chair, we were able to secure a project support lead—Alison Connors, from Alberta Health Services. She provided the backbone support we would need to organize and communicate with our growing coalition, the Parkland Region Partners for Youth Mental Wellness.
>
> Through discussions at coalition meetings, we learned about each other, including personal and professional struggles and triumphs with mental health. Titles and mandates began to disappear, and we built trust, relationships and a shared vision to co-create a better mental health system for youth and families who needed and deserved it. Every time we met the coalition grew. This customer service driven group, newly formed, applied for a grant to learn more about starting an integrated youth mental health hub from Policywise, [an Alberta- non-profit organization that uses evidence to promote better public policy for children, families and communities].
>
> A group of local physicians attended CanREACH Healthy Minds, Healthy Children training in pediatric mental health, and we opened a youth mental health clinic through our primary care network, operating one day per week. We worked alongside a social worker, a psychologist, and a community connector who helped reach out to youth between visits and get them involved with other community resources. We started using a referral technology that allows the schools to directly refer to our clinic.
>
> We have now formed a Tri-Region Youth Hub Steering Committee, and we are working towards securing funding to operationalize an integrated youth hub that would be open five days per week, serving the mental health and addiction needs of youth aged 11- to 24-years-old.

As the above story suggests, youth mental health and the suffering of those affected by it is felt deeply by many. Coalitions can begin with one person's passion and when the cause is shared, thrive. The services were designed by the parents and youth who came on early and worked for advancing youth mental health services. They converted need into a shared vision and continue to monitor results to measure achievement of the vision. They had early shared successes (quick wins) that fuelled their ongoing commitment [24]. They built structures and service delivery models into existing infrastructure but dedicated to the needs of their specific client group.

The commitment to customers and service are palpable in this example of a coalition at the service level. In Suzanne's words, "There have been challenges, but the belief we are in this together and we can make a positive difference in the lives of youth and families keeps us moving forward."

Giving Voice to the Voiceless

Another role leaders can play in demonstrating a commitment to customers and service is to ensure that the voices of the marginalized, disadvantaged, and powerless groups in society are heard. Formal leaders—people in positions of authority within the health system—can and should seek out informal leadership allies in the local community who can speak for the interests of people who may not know how to exercise their voice, are fearful in coming forward with their voice, or simply cannot fathom a process in which they will be heard. For example, as part of the Strategy for Patient-Oriented Research (SPOR) work being sponsored by the Canadian Institutes for Health Research across Canada, processes were employed to enable people with lived experience of substance use to collaborate with academic researchers as leaders of a collaborative research project, which was focused on improving primary care for the larger population people who use substances [25]. These patient allies helped health care professionals who otherwise would fail to understand or accept fundamental aspects of the medical condition of addiction, believing that people who use substances could simply discontinue use at any time. These misunderstandings undermine proper patient care, making the patient perspective most important in shifting practice to better meet the needs of this population. Leadership in this situation created the conditions for otherwise marginalized people to be heard in meeting their health needs.

In keeping with the commitment to customers and service physicians and researchers sometimes need to step in, where necessary, to become the voice of the unheard who need to be heard. One example of giving voice to the voiceless is a non-Indigenous physician who spoke up on behalf of Indigenous community members and leveraged her leadership within the Coroner's Service to change the process by which newborn babies lost to First Nations families through sudden infant death syndrome could be examined without the required autopsy, a process which violated the community's ability to practice burial and grieving in a culturally appropriate manner.

Dr. Elizabeth Hartney, a health leadership researcher at the Centre for Health Leadership and Research at Royal Roads University in Victoria, Canada, describes, the "allyship" role for leaders, this way:

> In matters concerning First Nations communities, there is an allyship role for everyone working in the healthcare system, because such profound system change is needed to fully meet the health care needs of Indigenous peoples. Leadership by Indigenous individuals is of paramount importance, yet the current system is not organized to enable this; therefore, non-Indigenous allies have a role in creating space and opportunities for Indigenous leaders to step in.
>
> This can be accomplished through engaging First Nations communities and recruiting Indigenous individuals into leadership positions. It is supported through creating opportunities for training the next generation of Indigenous healthcare leadership, which was a key strategy in the DESTINED project [26]. This project was conceived when a First Nations community reached out to a health authority to communicate the need to better serve their Elders in the emergency department of the hospital.

Elders were finding the emergency health care experience so traumatizing that they were avoiding essential health care services altogether. In order to engage the community, an Indigenous community member was recruited to lead the engagement within the community, enabled through a Canadian Institutes for Health Research grant. She was able to use the data she collected and analyzed as the basis for her masters' thesis [27] which supported her career development as a health leader and Indigenous ally; and that provided recommendations of how to improve the relationship between Indigenous Elders and the hospital.

The LEADS framework has tremendous potential to guide leaders in being effective allies. Being an ally means you are aware of a specific patient need, that is not being met in the current system, and use your privilege as a leader to advocate, empower, or create space for that patient need to be met. Allies can work on many different levels: from a family member at a patient's bedside to a CEO with leadership of an entire health authority, allies can take many forms.

Learning Moment

Can you think of a coalition that is truly patient-, family- or citizen-centred?

1. Is the patient or citizen purpose clearly articulated in the vision? If not, how might you alter the vision statement to make it clear?
2. Do all members of the coalition actively support, through their decisions and actions, the people-centred purpose of the coalition? If so, how? If not, what more could they do?

Are there individuals or groups, in your realm of leadership influence, that you should be enabling to be heard? If so, how might you give them voice?

Mobilize Knowledge

The third capability in the Develop coalitions domain is your ability to mobilize knowledge. Alison Powell describes the challenge of knowledge mobilization. She argues that as the complex technological, demographic and economic challenges health care leaders face "multiply and become more acute, so too does the need to bring a range of types of knowledge to bear in addressing these challenges: combining political, cultural and contextual awareness with theoretical knowledge, empirical knowledge from research and the experiential knowledge of practitioners, service users, policy-makers and citizens" [28].

One major function of coalitions is to mobilize knowledge across organizational boundaries to create new value that benefits all partners. Homel et al. describe efforts by Griffith University in Australia to work with schools and government-funded community services to mobilize knowledge. This is done in the service of a respectful partnership between frontline professionals and academics to bring evidence-based collaborative action to improve children's wellbeing in local communities. Through the Prevention, Translation and Support System, they have developed a technological portal to assist in knowledge transfer and employ community workers called collective change facilitators, "who act as a 'human bridge' between the worlds of research and practice" [29].

Communities of practice, such as employed in the Kids Health Alliance, are another means of mobilizing knowledge and improving performance in coalitions [30]. LEADS Canada (see Chap. 11) has developed a community of practice to support people and organizations learning about LEADS, and also to mobilize knowledge to improve leadership learning by LEADS facilitators and organizational partners [31].

Because coalitions are often seen as a trusted, neutral source of information and creative practice [32] they can move and combine knowledge about what works across boundaries to stimulate innovation (sometimes called knowledge mobilization).

In the prevention project described earlier, Griffith University has developed a Coalition Wellbeing Survey. All coalition members can use it to consider what is going well, where they could improve, and what is needed to make those improvements [26]. These changes are targeted both at the coalition efforts themselves, but also practices in each organization that might have an impact on the coalition's success.

Once a coalition is established, there are four actions leaders can take to mobilize knowledge effectively:

1. Make explicit the implicit assumptions coalition leaders bring to the task of knowledge mobilization.
2. Make mobilizing knowledge a formal intent of the coalition.
3. Focus on gathering and sharing knowledge that will help leaders work together.
4. Assess each organization's capacity to absorb knowledge and put it to good use.

The collective ability of a coalition to mobilize knowledge depends on the willingness of each member organization to transfer knowledge to other coalition partners [33] and its own capacity to absorb or use knowledge [34]. Sometimes organizational members withhold knowledge because they fear losing control and influence, because they might be invading another's territory, or because they fear others using it to invade their own domain [35]. This suggests strategic leaders need to assess others' willingness to share or hoard knowledge before engaging in knowledge mobilization activities.

Mobilizing knowledge effectively also requires insight into the dynamics that limit or enhance each organization's ability to embrace innovation. One factor that determines a coalition partner's propensity for innovation is its ability to translate external ideas into its practices in a way that makes sense to employees. Another is its cultural flexibility—can people adapt their mindset and practice to an innovation? A third factor is whether an organization has the technological capacity to use the same technology implicit in the external innovation's success.

Here's an example of knowledge mobilization in support of a coalition called Connect2Care, where Holland-Bloorview Kids' Rehabilitation Hospital collaborated with physicians and families and built an electronic portal to support youth to develop the capacity to manage their own care.

Holland Bloorview partnered with Canada Health Infoway and its family clients to create an electronic portal. The proposed portal would enable physicians to communicate with families and share information from electronic health records, through a secure two-way messaging function. Although there were multiple issues around privacy and risk to be dealt with, the project has created a portal and related processes for using it that meet stringent guidelines established by the College of Physicians and Surgeons in Ontario, as well as the Ontario government. Internal knowledge transfer between three departments—Information Systems, Client and Family Integrated Care and Collaborative Practice, was paramount to success.

To enhance absorptive capacity there was frequent and consistent engagement of clinicians through representation on committees and through broad engagement of technical groups at clinical practice council meetings, program meetings and staff forums. A campaign was launched to improve physician willingness and ability to use the messaging functionality of the portal. From a customer perspective, authentic and continual client and family engagement was employed throughout the implementation. The project leaders purposefully included consumers at all levels of the decision-making and employed their voice as a means of informing the product as well as a powerful force of change for clinician perceptions and behaviour.

By 2016 there were 1,060 clients and families enrolled and their repeated use of the portal (over 6,500 sessions) speaks to the enduring value the portal offers. Use of the portal has grown beyond their expectations [36].

Learning Moment
Reflect on the willingness to share knowledge between units or departments in your organization—or across coalition boundaries, if you're part of one.

1. How willing are your colleagues to share knowledge with you? You with them?
2. If the knowledge sharing is not optimal, what might the reasons be?
3. Is certain information "off limits"? Why?
4. What is your organization's absorptive capacity? What could be done to improve it?

Navigate Socio-Political Environments

The fourth capability in the Develop coalitions domain is an essential one for health leaders: navigating socio-political environments. Collaborative leaders must be politically astute, able to rally support and negotiate conflict in the politically divisive and controversial world of health and health care. In Chap. 2 we discussed some of the power challenges inhabiting politics—these are pronounced in coalition-building because of the multiple players and groups that are part of the health care world.

The broad socio-political environment is inhabited by many stakeholder and interest groups not just from health care, but from cultural, social, educational and public-service systems. This context teems with politics.

One of your authors—Bill—needed to engage Indigenous community leaders in a temporary coalition project. Bill was the CEO of HealthCareCAN, which was partnering with the Canadian College of Health Leaders to put on a new program at the National Health Leaders Conference in 2016, called the Great Canadian Healthcare Debate.

As part of this program, Bill thought it was important to partner with the leaders of a national coalition called the Indigenous Health Alliance to present—as part of the debate— a resolution calling on all health leaders to designate closing the Indigenous health gap as the number one priority for the coming year. Bill was passionate about the importance of this issue and saw it as vital for the future of health care in Canada.

Bill wanted to work with indigenous leaders to generate a compelling and strong case for improving indigenous health across Canada. Months before the conference, the report of The Truth and Reconciliation Commission of Canada [37] had been released including 23 health-related calls to action to address longstanding gaps between the health of Indigenous peoples and the settlers of Canada.

On the night before the conference, Dr. Alika LaFontaine, a member of the Indigenous Health Alliance (and co-author of Chap. 14 in this book) reminded Bill that a good carpool means being clear that everyone in the car is moving towards the same destination. Dr. LaFontaine said a number of grand chiefs and vice-chiefs who were attending the conference were looking for assurance that if they "got in the car", Bill would be moving to the same goal: serious consideration of the indigenous health issue by conference participants. He asked Bill to meet with the chiefs later that evening.

To ensure the meeting went as hoped, Bill knew he had to show his commitment and passion for Indigenous issues and model respect and consideration for these Indigenous leaders. He phoned his sister, Cheryl Mantei—who had worked with the Treaty 4 First Nations of Saskatchewan for many years—for some advice.

Cheryl noted that if the meeting is in a hotel, the tables would likely be set up in a hollow square. This, she stressed, is not in keeping with First Nations' culture. She said the best way to respect the culture is to form a learning circle with just chairs and no "head" of the table. Also, she said, it is very important to accept you're a "settler" and acknowledge you're meeting on unceded aboriginal territory. Next, you should recognize the most senior elder in the room to start the meeting and the meeting isn't over until the senior elder has had the last word. The last and most important piece of advice Bill received from his sister was that every word counts: listen very carefully.

Bill heeded his sister's advice. A circle of chairs was formed with over a dozen chiefs and senior advisors or "technicians" in the room. Bill acknowledged the meeting was being held on the ancestral lands of the Algonquin People. He then called upon Chief Ted Q, the most senior elder in the room, to begin the meeting. Chief Ted initiated a round of storytelling (as Chief Ted Q said, the stories behind the statistics) to show the true challenges of improving indigenous health.

Two hours later after a frank, honest and caring dialogue, a Vice-Chief, Bob Merasty used a Plains Cree term, 'Wicihitowin', to describe the 'spirit' in the room. When asked what Wicihitowin means, Bob said it means "Leading from the heart." Other chiefs and senior advisors nodded approvingly.

At the conference the next day—with all the grand chiefs and senior advisors in the room—the vote was no contest. The Closing the Gap resolution won approval from an overwhelming 89 per cent of the 700-plus delegates in the room. Alika thanked the delegates, thanked the chiefs and thanked the sponsoring organizations for working together in the spirit of Wicihitowin.

Bill's story shows how forming a carpool of Indigenous leaders and one non-Indigenous leader made it possible to navigate a socio-political environment. Initially, Bill and Alika created the conditions to build trust—Alika, by reaching out to Bill, and Bill by recognizing the importance of respecting a different culture. Together, they clarified their destination, shared the driving (Alika's presentation), shared knowledge and shared the map. The story also shows how important the human, cultural element of trust-building is to a successful coalition; and how that element can be enhanced through sensitivity and structure (how the meeting was organized, with attention to who took the lead, when and so on). Although this was a short-term coalition with a specific purpose, it highlights key elements all coalitions need to be successful.

Small-p Politics

Small-p politics are the micro-politics of everyday life; described as "the minute-by-minute choices and decisions that make us who we are…about the politics of identity and place…about small triumphs and defeats… (and) it is about winners and losers, haves and have-nots" [38]. Small-p politics arise from the interplay of shared values, conflicting interests, cultures, and rules, the personal relationships between visible power brokers and invisible ones. Some see politics as a necessary but unsavoury endeavor; others the stuff of life. Regardless, they cannot be expunged from human interactions. You must be politically astute to build coalitions.

Leaders need to be aware of and ready to manage small-p politics when implementing change, which involves developing and using forms of political skill and being politically savvy. Political skills are context specific. We encourage you to use the following attributes as required:

- Personal skills: exercising self-awareness and emotional intelligence.
- Interpersonal skills: influencing the thinking and behaviour of others, especially when you don't have formal authority.
- Sincerity: being authentic.
- Networking: identifying, seeking out and engaging people in personal relationships.
- Reading people and situations: understanding the dynamics among stakeholders and recognizing wider social systems and processes.
- Building alignment: promoting collaboration by aligning different interest and motives.
- Thinking long term: thinking strategically and having a sense of purpose and direction [39–41].

Learning Moment

Read, once again, Bill's *Wicihitowin* story. Reflect on the following questions:

1. Which small-p political skills did Bill use?
2. What did you learn about the importance of adapting your preferred approaches for engaging stakeholders to connect with them better?
3. Are there groups, individuals, or enterprises that you need to understand better, to help make your interactions work more effectively?
4. How might you go about learning about the ways those people and organizations work?

Conflict is inevitable in politics and coalitions create many potential sources of conflict that need to be thought through and anticipated. Figure 8.2 summarizes them succinctly.

We also recommend developing, at the outset of forming a coalition, a formal process for resolving conflicts when they arise (which they will). Realistically,

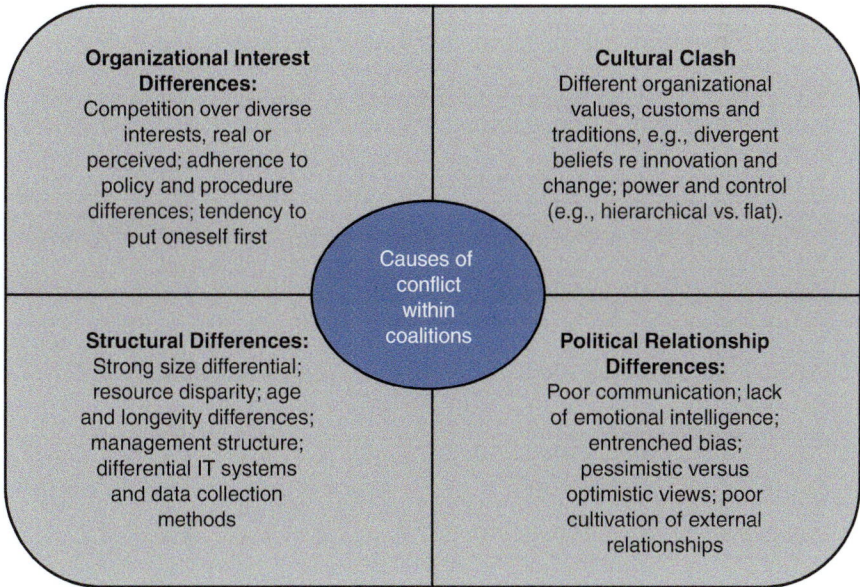

Organizational Interest Differences:
Competition over diverse interests, real or perceived; adherence to policy and procedure differences; tendency to put oneself first

Cultural Clash
Different organizational values, customs and traditions, e.g., divergent beliefs re innovation and change; power and control (e.g., hierarchical vs. flat).

Causes of conflict within coalitions

Structural Differences:
Strong size differential; resource disparity; age and longevity differences; management structure; differential IT systems and data collection methods

Political Relationship Differences:
Poor communication; lack of emotional intelligence; entrenched bias; pessimistic versus optimistic views; poor cultivation of external relationships

Fig. 8.2 Sources of potential conflict in a cross-sectoral collaboration [42]

coalition members need to identify potential conflicts in the partnership and
organize a process in order to mitigate them. Astute leaders understand coalitions
can fail over time; some of the reasons and related political actions are outlined
in Table 8.1.

Table 8.1 Potential sources of coalition conflict and amelioration tactics

Factors leading to failure	Mitigating political actions
• An inability of one partner to rise above self-interest and remain dedicated to the collective interest	• Constant reinforcement of the 'patient/citizen-centred' purpose of the collaboration • Provide support to another partner if his or her self-interest is taking them away from the coalition
• Leadership drift: turnover, and new priorities, cause one or more partners to drift away from commitment to the initial purpose of the collaboration	• Ensure the vision of the collaboration is well understood, repeated and valued by other leaders, so the loss of an individual can be mitigated • Encourage each partner organization to refer to the coalition in its strategic plan
• Lack of trust amongst the partners and a heavy reliance on legalistic mechanisms to guide action; becoming bogged down in proceduralism	• Create enabling agreements, but resist spelling out how every aspect of the work will be done • Build robust relationships based on the factors outlined earlier. Such relationships build trust and reduce the need for policies to become more detailed when trust erodes
• Lack of a clear stewardship structure to maintain oversight (note we are not talking about *governance,* which is not necessarily appropriate for networks or project teams)	• Create an appropriate structure to oversee both strategic and operational functions. Ensure meetings do not put off important decisions for internal issues
• A disconnect between operational needs (to fuel collaborative action) and strategic support for the coalition	• Hold regular meetings of both operational and strategic partners with linked agendas; attend each others' meetings
• A lack of the dedicated time, energy, and financial resources from participants	• Make people accountable for the success of coalitions they are part of and build its needs into their plans
• A lack of collaborative skill among participants	• Provide relationship and political skills training to people involved in coalitions
• Cultural differences create confusion	• Acknowledge cultural differences before starting. Don't enter into a coalition where cultural differences are so profound, they will endanger collaboration • Take action to discuss and ameliorate cultural differences that might prevent working together
• An inability to anticipate and address conflict (see Fig. 8.2 above for potential sources of conflict)	• A conflict resolution process agreed in advance by all partners

Large-P Political Astuteness

Large-P political astuteness is the skill to maneuver through governments and party systems. For example, the Canadian Alliance on Mental Illness and Mental Health coalition had to take the ideology of the federal governing party into account when it was lobbying for targeted federal funding to flow toward mental health services. Few of us deal directly with the inner workings of the political process, but it's important for all of us to understand some leaders do and it helps us to understand the challenges they face.

Ultimately, large-P decisions affect leadership at all levels. Any CEO in Australia who has recently been involved in regionalization knows the importance of dealing with state and municipal politics as hospital services are rationalized. CEOs of regional health authorities in Canada also know the challenges of dealing with provincial and municipal politics. There are a number of strategies to enhance your large-P political astuteness:

- Be aware of election cycles. If your coalition is intended to last over more than one term, time its launch and any strategic reviews of its work to coincide with elections; it's easier to get politicians' attention when they are looking for votes.
- Build relationships on a non-partisan basis with politicians. Most health organizations or regions have numerous municipalities and several provincial or federal parliamentary representatives in their geographical boundaries.
- Know your communities. Each community has a unique economic and social context and therefore unique health needs. Seek out data and information on them.
- Remind yourself of the demands of long-term change. Most significant change takes much longer than an election cycle to accomplish. Your coalition will need strategies to maintain momentum and protect your work from political shifts.
- Don't necessarily rely on government funding. If your coalition relies unduly or entirely on financial support from government, you're vulnerable to changing political priorities. Look for other sources of support.

Summary

Coalition-building is extremely important for health care because coalitions are an integral part of the connections and relationships that can transform health care organizations into a system. More and more, the challenges of meeting the needs of patients and families mean traditionally disparate organizations must begin to work together to develop integrated services that are motivated by, and can meet, the needs of our citizenry.

Leaders need to be able to create and sustain coalitions. We need to be able to:

- Purposefully build partnerships and networks to create results.
- Demonstrate a commitment to customers and service.
- Mobilize knowledge.
- Navigate socio-political environments.

Ivy Bourgeault discusses the relevance of Develops coalitions capabilities from an equity diversity and inclusion perspective:

Considering Equity, Diversity and Inclusion in Building Coalitions
Considerations of equity, diversity and inclusion should inform the leadership capabilities needed for your discipline, group or organization. They are equally important as you Develop coalitions, the D in the LEADS Framework. Collaborative leaders can develop coalitions to create awareness of equity, diversity and inclusion issues, and achieve goals for improving equity, diversity and inclusion across disciplines, groups and organizations. Partnerships can be purposively built to improve equity, diversity and inclusion, if sufficient time and attention are given to creating ongoing relationships of trust. (This may involve coming to terms with broken trust from past interactions, a key lesson from the Truth and Reconciliation Commission Calls to Action [37]). Collaborative leaders demonstrate a commitment to coalitions with diverse groups and perspectives to learn how to improve access to services and cultural safety and acceptability. Knowledge of equity, diversity and inclusion in and across organizations should mobilized towards those ends. A purposeful effort to bring people with different voices, experience and forms of power to the table and encouraging mentoring up, in and across organizations helps leaders navigate complex socio-political and cultural environments.

Many individuals—some part of the coalitions highlighted in this chapter—have told us they wish they had known about the Develop coalitions capabilities before they undertook to build a coalition themselves. Others have said knowing them in advance might not have resonated with what they knew at the time, but now provide a great checklist for evaluating the effectiveness of their leadership and determining what will move their coalition forward. Building on the metaphor of car pooling, this chapter gives ideas to maximize your odds of successfully developing coalitions: share the same destination; share values; share knowledge; share the risks and benefits; and share the credit.

Learning Moment
To use this questionnaire, find the right category for your level of leadership, then assess on how well you demonstrate the four Develop Coalitions capabilities.
Which capability do you need to improve on? Why?

Develops Coalitions: Self Assessments (for on-line access to LEADS self assessment, please visit www.LEADSglobal.ca)

Informal leader (Patient, Family Member, Citizen) Responsibilities: As a collaborative leader, I:

1.	Champion and/or support coalitions that have a clear, well-articulated purpose; and participate where and when I have something to offer	1	2	3	4	5	6	7	N
2.	Demand that coalitions I am involved with have a clear, compelling commitment to clients and service	1	2	3	4	5	6	7	N
3.	Take steps, in my role and responsibility, to facilitate the sharing and use of knowledge across coalition boundaries	1	2	3	4	5	6	7	N
4.	Demonstrate political astuteness in my efforts to influence coalition actors and activities	1	2	3	4	5	6	7	N

Front-Line Leaders: As a collaborative leader, I:

1.	Actively work on projects with experts, specialists and front-line leaders representing outside organizations that are partnered with ours	1	2	3	4	5	6	7	N
2.	Interact with patients, family members and citizens to determine their needs in relation to the partnership project	1	2	3	4	5	6	7	N
3.	Share knowledge and evidence shaping the practices of the partnership project and ensure fidelity to that evidence is maintained	1	2	3	4	5	6	7	N
4.	Resolve emergent conflict with coalition representatives through pro-active planning and personal conflict resolution skills	1	2	3	4	5	6	7	N

Mid-management leaders: As a collaborative leader, I:

1.	Work collaboratively with other managers from coalition partners, internal and external to the organization, on projects consistent with a shared patient or citizen mandate	1	2	3	4	5	6	7	N
2.	Actively integrate knowledge of the desired quality of results for the customer into the coalition's operational plans	1	2	3	4	5	6	7	N
3.	Develop processes to integrate knowledge and evidence from a variety of sources into work practices, as appropriate to the task at hand	1	2	3	4	5	6	7	N
4.	Demonstrate an awareness of the key players influencing a given situation (their vested interests and competing priorities), and can negotiate through conflict	1	2	3	4	5	6	7	N

Senior leaders: As a collaborative leader, I:

1.	Bring together multi-organizational groups to develop coalition infrastructure and build connections consistent with the service mandate of the coalition and my organization	1	2	3	4	5	6	7	N
2.	Actively support and develop processes to involve or seek input from customers when planning changes that may affect the customer (patient, family or citizen)	1	2	3	4	5	6	7	N
3.	Develop processes to encourage the gathering, interpretation, and dissemination of quality evidence and knowledge to influence coalition action	1	2	3	4	5	6	7	N
4.	Maintain strong political support for the coalition from required individuals and organizations; and engage in a process to resolve emergent conflicts	1	2	3	4	5	6	7	N

Executive leaders: As a collaborative leader, I:									
1.	Develop strategic frameworks for formal and informal coalitions that are in the best interest of patients, citizens and my organization	1	2	3	4	5	6	7	N
2.	Ensure the vision and mission for the coalition reflects a clear people or patient need; and monitor the actions of the coalition so it adheres to its purpose	1	2	3	4	5	6	7	N
3.	Ensure the work of the coalition is based on relevant evidence and knowledge; and uses it to keep the coalition on track	1	2	3	4	5	6	7	N
4.	Demonstrate advanced small-p and large-P political skills in building and leading the coalition	1	2	3	4	5	6	7	N

References

1. Tsuchiya K, Caldwell CH, Feudenberg N, Silver M, Wedepohl S, Lachance L. Catalytic leadership in food & fitness community partnerships. Health Promot Pract. 2018;19(1):458–548.
2. Roy DA, Litvak E, Paccaud F. Population-accountable health networks rethinking health governance and management. Montreal, QC: The Point Publishing; 2013. (translated by The Canadian Foundation for Health Improvement).
3. Kids Health Alliance. A network of care for children and youth. Ocala, FL: Kids Health Alliance; 2019. http://www.kidshealthalliance.ca/en/about-us/. Accessed 23 Jul 2019.
4. Alexander JA, Hearld LR, Shi Y. Assessing organizational change in multisector community health alliances. Health Serv Res. 2015;50(1):98–115.
5. Spring M, Araujo L. Indirect capabilities and complex performance implications for procurement and operations strategy. Int J Oper Prod Manag. 2014;34(2):150–73.
6. Hearld LR, Alexander JA, Shi Y. Leadership transitions in multisectoral health care alliances: implications for member perceptions of participation value. Health Care Manag Rev. 2015;40(4):274–85.
7. Lewis S. A system in name only – access, variation, and reform in Canada's provinces. N Engl J Med. 2015;372(6):497–500.
8. Williams P. The life and times of the boundary spanner. J Integr Care (Brighton). 2011;19(3):26–33. https://doi.org/10.1108/14769011111148140.
9. Lee L, Horth DM, Ernst C. Boundary spanning in action tactics for transforming today's borders into tomorrow's frontiers. Greensboro, NC: Center for Creative Leadership; 2013. p. 1–24.
10. Kanter RM. Collaborative advantage the art of alliances. Harv Bus Rev. 1994;72:96–108.
11. Cikaliuk M, Tholl W. Develop coalitions. Book four of five LEADS booklets. Ottawa, ON: Canadian College of Health Leaders; 2010. https://leadscanada.net/site/books. Accessed 4 Sep 2019.
12. Hanleybrown F, Kania J, Kramer M. Channeling change: making collective impact work. Stanf Soc Innov Rev. 2012;2012:1–8. https://ssir.org/pdf/Channeling_Change_PDF.pdf
13. eCAMIMH. Mental health now! Ottawa, ON: Canadian Alliance on Mental Illness and Mental Health; 2016. http://www.camimh.ca/wp-content/uploads/2016/09/CAMIMH_MHN_EN_Final_small.pdf. Accessed 23 Jul 2019.
14. Hearld LR, Alexander JA. Governance processes and change in organizational participants of multi-sectoral community health care alliances: the mediating role of vision, mission, strategy agreement and perceived alliance value. Am J Community Psychol. 2014;53:185–97.

15. Zak PJ. The neuroscience of high-trust organizations. Consult Psychol J. 2018;70(1):45–58.
16. Zak PJ. The Neuroscience of Trust. Harvard Bus Rev. 2017;95(1):1–8.
17. Den Hartog F, van den Esker FG, Wagemakers A, Vaandrager L, van Dijk M, Koelen MA. Alliances in the Dutch BeweegKuur lifestyle intervention. J Health Educ. 2014;73(5):576–87.
18. Trujillo D. Multiparty alliances and systemic change: the role of beneficiaries and their capacity for collective action. J Bus Ethics. 2018;150(2):425–49.
19. Huxham C, Vangen S. Researching organizational practice through action research: case studies and design choices. Organ Res Methods. 2003;6(3):383–403.
20. Smith A. Wealth of nations. London: Methuen &Co; 1776.
21. Hume D. A treatise of human nature. Oxford: Clarendon Press; 1739.
22. Popp J, MacKean G, Casebeer A, Milward HB, Lindstrom R. Inter-organizational networks: a critical review of the literature to inform practice. Washington, DC: IBM Center for The Business of Government; 2015. p. 93–6. http://www.businessofgovernment.org/sites/default/files/Management%20Popp.pdf. Accessed 23 Jul 2019.
23. Alexander JA, Hearld LR, Shi Y. Assessing organizational change in multisectoral health care alliances. Health Serv Res. 2015;50(1):98–115.
24. DAunno T, Hearld L, Alexander JA. Sustaining multistakeholder alliances. Health Care Manag Rev. 2019;44(2):183–94.
25. Urbanoski K, Pauly B, Inglis D, Cameron F, Haddad T, Phillips J, et al. Reducing stigma and building cultural safety in primary care for people who use(d) substances. CISUR bulletin #18. Victoria, BC: University of Victoria; 2018.
26. Hartney E, Antoine A, Joe E, Hastings H. Developing elders' support through trauma informed emergency departments (DESTINED). Healing our spirit worldwide. Sydney, NSW: The Eighth Gathering Conference; 2018.
27. Joe EA. focus on wellness: supporting development of trauma informed emergency care at West Coast General Hospital. Master's thesis. Victoria, BC: Royal Roads University; 2019.
28. Powell A, Davies HT, Nutley SM. Facing the challenges of research-informed knowledge mobilization: 'practising what we preach'? Public Adm. 2018;96(1):36–52.
29. Homel R, Branch S, Freiberg K. Implementation through community coalitions: the power of technology and of community-based intermediaries. J Prim Prev. 2019;40:143–8.
30. Ranmuthugala G, Plumb J, Cunningham F, Georgiou A, Westbrook J, Braithwaite J. How and why are communities of practice established in the healthcare sector? A systematic review of the literature. BMC Health Serv Res. 2011;11:273–89.
31. Canadian College of Health Leaders. LEADS community for practice. Ottawa, ON: Canadian College of Health Leaders; 2019. https://www.leadscanada.net/site/communityforpractice. Accessed 23 Jul 2019.
32. Hearld L, Alexander JA, Wolf LJ, Shi Y. Dissemination of quality improvement innovations by multisector health care alliances. J Health Organ Manag. 2019;33(4):511–28.
33. Kang S-W. Knowledge withholding: psychological hindrance to the innovation diffusion in an organisation. Know Manag Res Prod. 2016;14:144–9.
34. Zobel A-K. Benefiting from open innovation: a multidimensional model of absorptive capacity. J Prod Innov Manag. 2017;34(3):269–88.
35. Kwan LA. The collaboration blind spot. Har Bus Rev. 2019;2019:67–73.
36. CHA Learning. CHA learning change leadership certificate (CLIC) [requires course payment]. Ottawa, ON: CHA Learning; 2019. https://www.chalearning.ca/programs-and-courses/leadership/change-leadership-certificate/. Accessed 4 Sep 2019.
37. Truth and Reconciliation Commission, Government of Canada. Honouring the truth, reconciling for the future. Ottawa, ON: The Truth and Reconciliation Commission of Canada; 2015. http://www.trc.ca/assets/pdf/Honouring_the_Truth_Reconciling_for_the_Future_July_23_2015.pdf. Accessed 23 Jul 2019.
38. Janks H. The importance of critical literacy. Engl Teach Pract Cri. 2012;11(1):150–63.

39. Waring J, Bishop S, Clarke J, Exworthy M, Fulop N, Harley J, et al. Healthcare leadership with political astuteness (HeLPA): a qualitative study of how service leaders understand and mediate the informal 'power and politics' of major health system change. BMC Health Serv Res. 2018;18:1–10.
40. Comber S, Wilson L, Crawford KC. Developing Canadian physician: the quest for leadership effectiveness. Leadersh Health Serv (Bradf Engl). 2016;29(3):282–99.
41. Ferris G, Treadway DC, Kolodinsky RW, Hochwarter WA, Kacmar CJ, Douglas C, et al. Development and validation of the political skills inventory. J Manag. 2005;31(1):126–52.
42. Moore C. The mediation process: practical strategies for resolving conflict. 3rd ed. San Francisco, CA: Jossey-Bass; 2003.

The *LEADS in a Caring Environment* Framework: Systems Transformation

Graham Dickson and Bill Tholl

The complex nature of health care organizations requires distributed leadership to ensure successful system transformation. Many individuals must assume leadership roles within their individual units.

Baker and Axler [1]

Leading transformation change is not easy. And, as the quote from Baker and Axler suggests, it will take a full court press to achieve the transformational changes required to meet the health care challenges we face. Our goal is to get to a deeper understanding of critical success factors for successful system-wide change: the degree of change needed, the leadership practices to achieve it and how to implement these practices to achieve health and wellness for the populations we serve.

We use the term *system* in three ways. First, to denote the social enterprise called health care. Second, to describe the type of people dynamics that leaders must deal with as they practise leadership (i.e., patterns of thinking; culture and belief). And third, to refer to the efficient and effective operations leaders use to achieve their goals (i.e., information systems).

The word transformation is defined as "a complete change in the appearance or character of something or someone, especially so that thing or person is improved" [2]. Used with respect to health care systems, "transformation" tells us the result of change will be a different kind of system [3]. It's different from other synonyms for change—improvement, reform, innovation—which imply adjustment more than revolution.

G. Dickson (✉)
Royal Roads University, Victoria, BC, Canada
e-mail: graham.dickson@royalroads.ca

B. Tholl
Canadian Health Leadership Network, Ottawa, ON, Canada
e-mail: btholl@chlnet.ca

© Springer Nature Switzerland AG 2020
G. Dickson, B. Tholl (eds.), *Bringing Leadership to Life in Health: LEADS in a Caring Environment*, https://doi.org/10.1007/978-3-030-38536-1_9

Health care systems are complex, confusing, multi-actor entities, sometimes described as "VUCA" environments: volatile, uncertain, complex and ambiguous [4–6]. They are a leadership challenge in which the systems scientist Alexander Laszlo says the right kind of leader can foster a positive VUCA world based on vision, understanding, clarity and agility [4].

Theories of leadership—distributed, change, systems and contextual—all emphasize the interconnectedness of effective leadership interventions as leaders interact with followers and other dimensions of context [7]. These changes in practise embrace all of the concepts we have discussed in the previous LEADS chapters, including mental models (Lead self); relationships and connections (Engage others, Develop coalitions, and this chapter: Systems transformation); and policies, practices and resource flows (Achieve results) [8].

The story of Canterbury Health in New Zealand is an example of leadership in a VUCA environment—one where LEADS-style practices can create systems transformation.

> Canterbury Health, on New Zealand's South Island, has been pursuing transformational change since 2006, when it became clear its business model could not sustain modern, people-centred care. They calculated continuing without radical reform would require a new 500-bed hospital and 8,000 additional employees—completely unaffordable.
>
> They tried different ways of improving efficiency, including two groups, each of 40 staff, learning Lean, Six Sigma and other techniques for improving efficiency. Then, at an event called Showcase, those 80 people were invited to meet in a warehouse, where they were walked through scenes that set out what the system was facing and asked questions such as How would you like to be treated? How would you transform the system? In turn, members of the group of 80 invited others to go through the same process. An event originally planned to last a fortnight ended up running for six weeks, with more than 2,000 out of Canterbury's 18,000 employees joining in.
>
> Out of this work came a vision captured by the phrase "one system, one budget."
>
> It was the participants' way of saying that despite the number of parties delivering health and social care, there is only one budget and the system should be organized to reflect that. In short, the constituent parts of Canterbury health—the hospitals, the general practices, community and laboratory contractors, social care—needed to work together in new ways as a single integrated health and social care system if patient services were to improve and the budget be balanced.
>
> A key component of the transformation process has been formal learning. There has been continued, sustained investment in building the managerial and innovation skills needed to achieve the new vision. More than 1,000 staff have now taken part in these programmes. As well, contractors participate in these programs.
>
> There was natural resistance in some areas to innovation but there are clear signs of success: Waits for elective surgery went down, and general practitioners were given direct access to a range of diagnostic tests which shortened waits for them, dramatically in some cases. Treating many conditions in primary care that were previously treated purely or mainly in hospital has also increased efficiency. And fewer patients are entering nursing homes as more are supported in the community [9].

We're opening this chapter with the Canterbury example because its key leadership practices exemplify the capabilities we'll be describing in it (as well as other domains of LEADS). In this chapter we have three goals. First, to emphasize the construct of learning—personal, organizational, and system-wide—as a metaphor for natural adaptation and productive change, and the importance of systems thinking as vital to creating conditions for learning. Second, to provide an overview of contributions from recent literature to our understanding of the four Systems transformation capabilities. And third, to update some of the models and approaches leaders can use to operationalize effective systems-informed change.

Please take time to review the following learning moment [10].

Learning Moment

Remember the parable of the five blind men and the elephant? Each exploring a different part—trunk, leg, tail, etc.—and describing the elephant accordingly, but showing that all perspectives needed to be connected to understand the elephant holistically?

Hugh MacLeod, the former CEO of the Canadian Patient Safety Institute in Canada, and a former senior official with the Province of Ontario, described his knowledge of systems dynamics in the following way:

> *My time as lead of the Government of Ontario Climate Change Secretariat expanded my thinking about inter-relationships and contradictions between complex systems. Each and every week I witnessed separate conversations about climate change, economy and health. Convention dictated that there is something called health care, something called environmental protection and something else again called the economy. Yes, they look at different issues, use different language and depend on different types of expertise. Yet, I was beginning to see how they were connected and was also beginning to see that we will never fully optimize progress in any of these domains unless we begin to think of them holistically.*
>
> *How we live, where we live and how we make our living are so tightly integrated that it is impossible to think of one without the other two. If we think of health care in isolation, we can easily focus on curing people of disease. Yet a reduction in infant mortality is of limited value if it means more children survive disease to die of poverty and starvation. If we think of the environment in isolation, we can expend huge efforts to preserve the wilderness yet remain heedless of the human destitution just outside the borders of wildlife sanctuaries. If we think of the economy in isolation, we will focus on growth as the only measure of human development but ignore its effects on resource depletion, pollution, an overindulgent life-style and even mental stress.*

Reflect on your current role and responsibilities as a leader.

- How many different social systems—like health—interconnect with your system or area of responsibility?
- When there's an issue in your system, why might it be valuable to consider it in the context of the larger system?
- We talked earlier about the power of one—how an individual can make a big difference if s/he intervenes to change a system. Leaders more often feel they are being captured by the system; immobilized by its multiplicity of tentacles and red tape. Which of these descriptions describes your approach to leadership?
- What attitudes and approaches to leadership are consistent with the notion of distributed leadership: i.e., the power of one, as one of many?

Learning, Leadership and Change

> In systems such as contemporary society, evolution is always a promise and devolution always a threat. No system comes with a guarantee of ongoing evolution. The challenge is real. To ignore it is to play dice with all we have. To accept it is not to play God—it is to become an instrument of whatever divine purpose infuses the universe [4].

We saw the importance of strategic learning in the transformation example from Canterbury Health in New Zealand. The above quotation shows the strong connection between the concepts of learning—ongoing evolution, in Laszlo's words—and leadership: becoming an instrument of divine purpose. In our case, health and wellness are the purpose. John Kennedy, quoted in Chap. 1, said: "Leadership and learning are indispensable to each other." Why? Because they both speak to change—the first as the instrument of change, the second, the ideal process of change.

A learning health care system [11] is defined by the Institute of Medicine as a one where "science, informatics, incentives and culture are aligned for continuous improvement and innovation, with best practices seamlessly embedded in the delivery process and new knowledge captured as an integral by-product of the delivery experience" [12]. In learning health systems, the parts speak to each other, share resources, provide information, and connect action across boundaries. Leadership needs to create the conditions for learning health systems.

Health care leaders create the conditions for learning through the coalitions they build and the methodologies they employ to catalyze change across the broader health care system. Figure 9.1 shows how strategic learning and systems leadership create better health and wellness outcomes system wide.

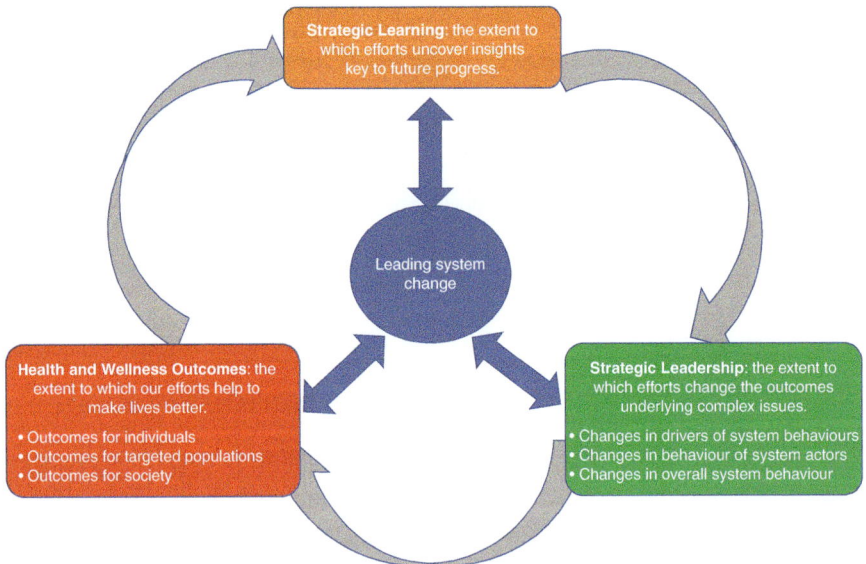

Fig. 9.1 Systems transformation through strategic learning and systems leadership [13]

Strategic learning catalyzes systems leadership, which creates changes in three forms: drivers of system behaviour (policies, procedures, resource allocation, innovative practices, etc.), mental models and the behaviour of individual leaders at all levels; and changes in overall system behaviour (by creating opportunities for people in systems to behave differently). Strategic leadership then works to improve health and wellness outcomes system-wide.

To create winning conditions for change, leaders need to use LEADS capabilities. For example, policies, practices and resource flows reflect the capabilities of the Achieve results domain of LEADS. The relationships and connections, and power dynamics of overall system behaviour are represented by the Engage others, Develop coalitions and Systems transformation domains of leadership. And the mental models and behaviour of system actors for change relate directly to the Lead self domain of LEADS.

Now let's explore each of the four capabilities of Systems transformation. These capabilities work with the other domains and capabilities to create strategic leadership for system-wide change. Systems leaders:

- Demonstrate systems and critical thinking
- Encourage and support innovation
- Orient themselves strategically to the future
- Champion and orchestrate change.

Demonstrate Systems and Critical Thinking

Health care issues increasingly preoccupying leaders include: chronic disease, obesity, drug, alcohol and other addictions and mental health. Why are these of growing interest? Partly because they suggest a shift in focus from acute illness to chronic conditions, partly because they appear to be beyond the influence of any one of us to change. But it's also because addressing them effectively requires critical and systems thinking [14].

In our definition of leadership, we said changing system outcomes requires commitment not just from the providers of health care but also from patients, families, and citizens. A doctor cannot effectively treat a patient who refuses to quit smoking, for example. The relationship is interdependent: if patients cannot lead themselves, then doctors can't engage them in their treatment. If a health authority doesn't deliver mental health services that meet the needs of patients, those patients may end up in conflict with police. Welfare Wednesday—when social-assistance cheques go out—spikes opioid overdoses, which in turn raises psychological distress in first responders and the community at large. Eventually these interconnected conditions lead to acute conditions over-taxing our hospitals.

Earlier we said leaders must use both forms of systems thinking to conceptualize and act as a strategic leader. There are two kinds: organic and mechanistic. Organic systems thinking means looking at a system through the lens of the people in it—what patterns of belief, capacity to act and motives drive their actions? Mechanistic thinking focuses on the logical, rational side of human behaviour, applying our organizational and planning skills to complement our work with people. We need to explore each a little further.

Interconnectedness is a fundamental principle of organic systems thinking [15]. For change to happen in large systems, changes in personal, organizational and broader health system behaviour need to align. A second fundamental principle of organic systems thinking is "the power of one." (See Chap. 7). Individuals make a difference *because* of interconnectedness. A third principle of organic systems thinking is behavioural variability—a well-functioning system is greater than the sum of the parts, so that non-linear dynamic interactions can emerge among individuals, organizations and across different dimensions of health care systems [16]. A fourth principle is self-organization—a process where something unpredictable arises from multiple interactions among variables in the system.

A strategic leader must also understand the contribution of mechanistic systems thinking—the application of reason, logic and linear causal chains to create efficient and effective technical solutions to problems. It's the foundation of information systems, communication systems, organizational design and project plans. Many of our management practices derive from mechanistic thinking, which works well in predictable, stable conditions. Once the context for an activity is stable, a business process can be designed to work in it.

Complexity Leadership

Because the dominant delivery of health services is a person-person interaction, health care systems at the regional, provincial/state or national level exhibit many of the qualities of an organic system, often described as a complex adaptive system [17, 18]. Complexity leadership is a term describing how to lead in a complex adaptive system. A scoping study [19] dedicated to understanding complexity leadership suggests that leaders acknowledge change is not a linear process and requires risk taking, trust and permission to make mistakes. Because the root causes of the problems are often uncertain, leaders should encourage testing solutions and continuous learning. It's the leader's job to set boundaries, ask the right questions and guide but not steer. To deal with the uncertainty inherent in this approach, leaders need to engage in self-management. We will discuss some of the disciplined practices leaders can employ to work on large complex problems in the "Champion and Orchestrate Change" section of this chapter.

Critical Thinking

Critical thinking leaders first determine the nature of the problem or issue they are dealing with. Ronald Heifitz and colleagues analyzed the challenges strategic leaders face in modern health care systems. Based on the thought processes of both organic (people) systems and mechanistic (technical) systems thinking,

Table 9.1 Two forms of leadership change challenges: technical and adaptive [20]

	Technical challenges, i.e. payroll issues	Adaptive challenges, i.e. culture change
Distinctions	• Solved by experts • Logic & intellect • Often quick & easy solutions • Easy to identity	• Cannot be solved by experts • Changes in values, beliefs, behavior, roles, relationships, & approaches to work • Difficult to identify & easy to deny
Nature of Solution	• Requires change in one or few places, often within organizational boundaries • Solutions can be implemented quickly – often by edict • People generally receptive to technical solutions • Locus of work: AUTHORITY	• Changes in many places, often across organizational boundaries • Solutions often require experiments & new discoveries • Implementation often takes time & cannot be done by edict • People often resist adaptive solutions • Locus of work: STAKEHOLDERS
Role of leader/ authority	• PROBLEM SOLVER: solve or delegate to experts to solve • Implement solutions by edict, resource assignments, etc. • Focus on SOLUTION	• CONVENER: bring the people together with the problem to do the work of solving it • Allow for long term outcomes • Communicator: transparency • Focus on PROCESS
Strategy	FIX IT!	• Convene conversations necessary for group thinking (i.e. relationship-building, mutual understanding, possibilities, action) • Allow for experiments that explore opportunities or test assumptions • Prototype & scale up what works; share learning from what doesn't
Learning required	• INFORMATIVE learning • Bringing into mind new ideas, skills & content • Basic perception of self & world remains the same	• TRANSFORMATIVE learning • Changing whole mind—perspective, perception, orientation • Feels unfamiliar, outside of comfort zone, risky • Requires courage & growth

he suggested there are essentially two kinds of strategic challenges leaders face (see Table 9.1) [20].

This table shows the important and necessary distinctions a critical-thinking leader must make between change challenges of a technical nature and those that are adaptive. Technical challenges are addressed by applying science but adaptive change challenges can only be solved by changing behaviour and culture. Large-system challenges fall into the latter category and often demand significant (some-times painful) shifts in people's habits, status, role, identity and ways of thinking.

Critical thinking leaders also recognize that human beings act in their own self-interest as they see it. In this context, human behaviour—emotions, irrational fears and drives—sometimes supplant logic and reason. That's why leadership involves adapting to the beliefs and actions of the follower. From a change perspective, leaders are encouraged to think critically, not just to understand the logic of change, but also the human dynamics of change.

Critical thinking includes the ability to analyze a situation to better understand its parts and how they contribute to a whole; to discriminate among alternative actions; and to find connections and interdependence among variables that are not obvious, or clear. Challenging the *status quo*, identifying issues, attempting to resolve them and designing and implementing new processes require a sophisticated form of critical thinking.

From a large-scale change perspective, critical thinking leaders must also look inside to determine their own need for control and recognize when indulging that need may get in the way of strategic leadership. In his book *Humanizing Leadership*, Hugh MacLeod described the challenge of letting go in the following way:

> Letting go and becoming the leader within allowed me to see that my leadership vision was often constrained by my personal shackles: my ego, the facade of being 'all knowing,' the avoidance of my vulnerabilities, ignoring my limitations, and failing to utilize the aid and greatness of those around me. An organization is much more than any one particular individual. Through experiences, I learned firsthand that the more you let go, the stronger you become. Very simply, leadership is about looking within and all around you. We must lead and inspire by example, by personifying the qualities of honesty, integrity, resilience, and confidence, demonstrating how leadership, too, is a process of self-development, not an ultimate arrival. Leadership starts with, and is elevated by, a solid relationship with self [10].

Many of the practices associated with strategic leadership require leaders to relinquish personal control vested in authority and replace it with control vested in process, where a disciplined approach is required to engage multiple actors in change. Systems change models attempt to balance giving people some freedom to create the future, but not so much as to generate a confusing space for change in which people's efforts are, and feel diffused and chaotic.

Learning Moment
Reflect on your current role and responsibilities as a leader.

- How willing and able are you to let go of control?
- Reflect on the last six weeks at work. Did control issues emerge? How did you handle them?
- Pair up with a colleague. Explore the notion of technical versus adaptive problems as you experience them in your organization. Do the methods you employ to solve them reflect the distinct differences of approach as described in Table 9.1?
- If you are facing an adaptive problem, what approaches (which may require you to give up your traditional notions of control) might be employed to lead others?

Encourage and Support Innovation

Transformations take time—moving from one state to another is a process [21]. On the other hand, innovations, small local changes that contribute to transformation, can be quick. Leaders who want to achieve systems transformation should support innovative health care practices and promote them because innovation creates cultural receptivity for, and is, a catalyst for large-scale change.

Lean is one approach to innovation in health care thought to have great potential for meaningful innovation [22–25] but empirical studies show implementing Lean is highly localized and brings small successes, rather than transforming large systems [26, 27]. The following story shows the importance of putting LEADS to work to sustain Lean practices and their contribution to transformation longer-term.

> In 2012 the Saskatchewan Ministry of Health committed to a multi-million dollar investment in using Lean methodology as an innovation tool to improve the province's health system. The deputy minister of the day called it a 50-year project and one of the largest experiments of its kind in health care [28].
>
> Was Lean successful? Debate raged in 2016, as the Lean contract with the American consultant came to an end early in the process. Some argued that Lean had a profound positive impact. An article in the Saskatoon Leader Post outlined many benefits: cardiac patients going to Regina by ambulance are now registered while in transit, so they receive diagnostic care 95 percent faster when they arrive at hospital; prescriptions for chemotherapy patients are being filled more quickly; mental health clients in Regina have faster access to services and in Prince Albert, follow-up care has improved [29]. However, one study found no evidence to prove the quality of health care was improved by it and said Lean had a statistically significant negative effect on nurse engagement [30]. It's clear efforts to use Lean as a transformative tool were genuinely well intended and brought many small examples of successful innovations but in other situations, Lean didn't achieve its promise.

We became interested in the Lean experiment because of the theme of this book: putting LEADS to work. Did the leadership practices in jurisdictions that used Lean successfully (such as Canterbury), differ from the practices in those that did not?

Saskatchewan's experience with Lean highlights many factors needed for innovation to trigger transformation of a system. First, it takes sustained effort over time. The deputy minister who initiated Lean in Saskatchewan envisaged a 50-year time frame, but would political processes around health care allow that to happen? Second, was there the critical mass of small, successful Lean innovations necessary for transformation to take place? In Saskatchewan it's hard to determine whether Lean's reach was sufficient to create that critical mass because we don't know how many innovations were successful and how many weren't. Third, did the leaders introducing and implementing Lean provide the space for staff and community members to adapt it to their unique context?

We don't know if the right leadership was provided to sustain changes, either provincially or locally. The use of the kind of leadership capabilities we have in LEADS—problem solving, empowering, communicating, supporting, being democratic, organizational learning and clearly identified wins–were needed to complement the logical discipline of Lean [31]. Did unit managers implementing Lean display those leadership qualities? [32]

Table 9.2 Innovation techniques often used in health care

Approach	Purpose	Innovation approach
Lean	Lean is a core methodology for redesigning health systems. Lean aims to improve the value proposition to the patient, and on eliminating waste. Many health systems adapt Lean to a variety of contexts.	Lean is a process redesign involving staff at the front line reviewing all processes and procedures in light of desired outcomes and streamlining them. It creates expectations for ongoing dialogue between management and front-line staff to identify new ideas for continuous improvement.
Six Sigma	Six Sigma seeks to improve process by identifying and removing causes of defects and minimizing variability in clinical care practices.	Six Sigma's methodology for innovation is to define a problem, collect data, and use statistical methods to determine sources of variation and opportunities to improve. Processes are then adjusted to remedy the problem, and data are collected and analyzed multiple times to check for improvement in error rates.
PDSA cycle	This model tests incremental improvement in rapid cycles in a discrete component of a system, usually related to quality and safety.	The PDSA cycle creates innovation through creating continuous cycles of incremental change. It is an action research methodology. The four steps are: Plan the work; Do the work; Study whether the outcome was achieved and Act on change by adjusting effort as needed; then repeat.
Positive Deviance	The concept of positive deviance is that no matter how intractable a problem, there is almost always a community that has individuals whose practices or behaviour lets them find better solutions to problems than their neighbours.	Positive deviance creates innovation through a disciplined process to discover unique and uncommon successes in one setting; examine the conditions for that success; and attempt to replicate them in other settings.

Innovative health practices are numerous (see Table 9.2). The LEADS capabilities can be employed to surround and support their strategic use and to facilitate embedding them in organizational culture.

Braithwaite and colleagues state there are four pivotal systems factors important for innovation to occur. These are: one, "the innovation itself, and its characteristics; two, the system's propensity, or its readiness, for change; three, the journey of implementation process; and four, the external or outer context" [33]. All four factors played into the Saskatchewan Lean example presented earlier—either with respect to an individual department or unit undergoing Lean transformation, the region or the province. Without the capacity to bring individual innovative practices together—to see them holistically and generate enthusiasm for scaling up innovation—the few pockets that are successful will never be strong enough to catalyze transformation.

For multiple innovations to stimulate transformation, it takes an actionable innovation agenda stewarded by an entity charged with encouraging, identifying, documenting, and connecting innovations across traditional boundaries to facilitate the use of innovation for transformation [34]. The report of the 2015 Canadian Federal

Advisory Panel on Healthcare Innovation, chaired by Dr. David Naylor, recognized this deficiency. The report said many excellent ideas and inventions are never translated into saleable or scalable innovations and recommended the federal government exercise leadership to "create the healthcare innovation agency of Canada to work with a range of stakeholders as well as governments to…set healthcare innovation goals" for the health care system [35]. These recommendations have yet to be fully acted upon, although the Canadian government has announced in 2019 the creation of a New Frontiers in Research Fund, which has been deemed "Naylor lite" by some.

There are some examples of efforts to spread innovative practices in quality and safety improvement in Canada and elsewhere. One is the Partnership for Patients in the USA—an initiative that applies a systems approach to innovation in safety for hospital patients [36]. The Canadian Patient Safety Institute (CPSI) also established a consortium consisting of over 50 health enterprises dedicated to spreading innovative practices in quality and safety improvement [37]. Yet these initiatives—while successful on a limited scale—have not yet succeeded in embedding quality and safety as Job 1. Scaling and spreading innovations in quality and safety still happens more by accident than design. "Leadership is central to this and *compassionate* leadership in particular is a fundamental enabling factor that will create a culture of improvement and radical innovation across health care" [38].

Organizational Culture and Innovation

The key to transforming into a person-centred system, customized to individual need, may lie in the ability to change social and organizational culture. In general, culture is either receptive or resistant to innovation. A recent study in Italy showed how leadership can use existing culture to create greater receptivity to innovation [39]. It describes two efforts—the first a failure and the second a success—to implement an innovative new accounting change in a large health region. The study says the first attempt (2005–2009) was top-down, driven by a desire to comply with mandated policies and procedures; and lacked clarity of purpose and transparency of desired outcomes. It was also superficial. It left the core values of the organization unchanged but didn't link the change to those values. In contrast, in the second approach (2010—2013) the leadership did more communicating to encourage staff to feel ownership of the goal. They fostered cooperation among stakeholders, including clinicians; and worked on promoting the core values through discussion. This approach did bring about a change in practice. "This was possible thanks to cooperation and dialogue that took place for the accounting change and thanks to the accounting change" [39].

Leaders can learn systems-thinking skills to enhance innovation through simulation activity. The following story highlights the power of simulation.

> *Phil Cady is a systems thinking expert who uses experiential systems approaches to engender organizational innovation. "Time and time again," Phil says, "living an experience through simulation or experiential activity deepens people's understandings and helps them learn systems concepts in ways their brain on its own just wouldn't do for them."*

Phil developed two game sessions to apply systems thinking to optimize organizational performance in an Emergency Room setting.

Phil has also seen significant behaviour change. "Participants' behaviours changed quickly. First, I noticed a desire to immediately challenge assumptions and mental models about what can and cannot be done. Second, I noticed increased whole system awareness and a jump in collaborative capacity. Conducted in a workplace setting, I have seen transfer of these behaviours beyond the simulation itself into day-to-day practise." (Personal email, 2019 Apr. 16).

Leaders who use continuous improvement methods and leadership practices consistent with LEADS can encourage and support innovation. To achieve long-term benefits, you'll have to be conscious of aspects of culture that may affect innovation and continuous improvement.

Orient Themselves Strategically to the Future

Leaders see the future faster, scanning the environment for ideas, best practices and emerging trends that will shape the system. Then they weigh them against their organization's history and values, and their personal value system. It's a bit like being the Roman god Janus [40], who could see the past and future at the same time. Janus is a great metaphor for leadership in systems transformation—except he didn't have to collaborate with a bunch of other gods to make things happen (Fig. 9.2).

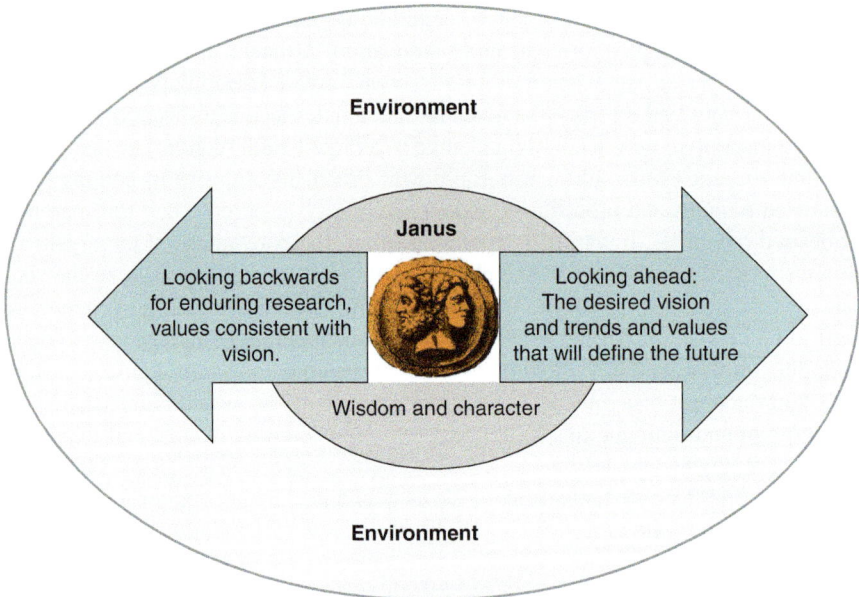

Fig. 9.2 The Janus approach

Like Janus, you too must find creative ways to reconcile competing trends and forces that will define the future with evidence and values from the past that must endure. It is your wisdom and character that will determine what transformational strategies will move you toward your future vision [41, 42]. Listen again to Hugh MacLeod:

> You can find yourself on the face of a transformation-change wave. If you are too far ahead, the wave will crash down and you will be at the mercy of its violent surge. If you are tentative and fail to harness the available energy, you run the risk of being left behind. If you place yourself in perfect trim and continue to make adjustments, you can actually ride the wave.... As the transformational waves peak and subside, the leader needs to chart the course, ride each wave with finesse and conviction, and ultimately stay focused on the end game. Flexibility and dexterity are required to conquer the waves of change and to navigate a new course if necessary.

To "ride the wave," wise strategists constantly probe the environment looking for emerging trends and values, then use systems and critical thinking skills, grounded in personal experience and their character, to determine what value patterns they should pay attention to and which are passing fads. Doing this lets leaders see the limitations of a purely scientific or research-based approach to leading change. It allows them to distinguish which waves of change to ride; and which to safely ignore.

Inherent in the challenge of strategically orienting yourself to the future is the need to deal with contradictions and dilemmas that emerge from attempting to reconcile past experience with future needs. We counsel health care leaders to be evidence-based but not evidence-bound. By definition, the research that generates evidence is knowledge of the past and seldom definitive. Will it fit the context of the future?

Leaders who strategically orient themselves to the future must constantly review the context of emerging trends and patterns that evidence will be placed in. This is much easier to do in small, discrete stable contexts; but when you are in a VUCA environment, it's the collective wisdom of you and your team that will determine whether evidence is suitable for handling the situation you're experiencing. There's always a risk with co-creative systems approaches, because there's no blueprints or guarantees when you work with others. Wisdom allows you to assess which factors (such as values, ethics and innovation) should help shape your decision.

The dilemma of evidence-based decision-making highlights the inherent uncertainty in a complex adaptive system like health care. Dilemmas are problems that cannot be solved but must be managed. These problems sometimes appear as either-or choices but the apparent contradictions simply reveal the tension between two opposites that cannot be resolved in favour of one or the other, and must be kept in dynamic equilibrium. One of those dilemmas in health care is balancing the demands of acute care with population health. The solution will lie in a continuum between two poles, not an either/or choice. A balance point needs to be maintained between the two that meets the needs of the population; and this balance point may be in constant flux. A strategic leader needs to regularly monitor the current state between the two competing perspectives as best s/he can and take action when needed to ensure that pursuit of the long-term future vision of health and wellness is maintained (remember the mindset described in Chap. 5, of pursuing the 100-year vision in the immediate moment?) As Roger Martin says, "whenever you're faced with an either/or proposition, look for an and!" [43].

How does a strategic leader balance the poles of a dilemma? Peter Schulte [44] describes how to manage polarities. First, identify the two poles or opposites you tend to move between. Second, create a list or a map of the advantages and disadvantages of each of the poles. This depiction should be filled with the symptoms and indicators of when you are experiencing these advantages or disadvantages. In the next step, you commit to continuously sensing which of the advantages and disadvantages you are experiencing in any given movement. If you are experiencing a disadvantage of one pole, you take steps to move toward the other. Once you start experiencing the disadvantages of the opposite pole, you move back toward the other.

Remember: the poles aren't the goal, rather you should constantly move between the poles in an upward spiral toward perfect balance between the two. The goal is *between* the poles. You put processes in place to avoid the disadvantages and maximize the advantages of both simultaneously; you invite discussion and analysis of where you are in this tension and where you need to be right now. You accept that that answer might be different tomorrow and different yet again the day after.

Complex adaptive systems, as mentioned earlier, are rife with human dilemmas and polarity challenges. On the other hand, complex adaptive systems can have positive effects, such as breakthroughs in innovation because of a confluence of ideas and technology. For example, one who is tuned into the 'customization' of consumer health devices might be excused for thinking that such a breakthrough might spin the traditional health care system into a completely new form. What would such a system look like, and how would we as leaders react to it?

Learning Moment
1. Search the internet for all the examples you can find of consumer devices/ tools/techniques that are being touted as potential ways of helping citizens manage their own health. Identify three that have potential to be used in the health system.
2. Do you think there would be "polar reactions" if these tools were proposed for use in the health care system?
3. Create a polarity map to describe the dynamics that might occur if such tools were introduced.
4. Do any of the tools—or the tools taken together—have the potential to completely transform health care? If so, how?

So, what else can you do to help balance polarities and enhance your leadership capability of orienting yourself strategically to the future? First, increase your environmental awareness. Focus on figuring out what trends, events or movements in the environment can't be ignored. Use informal meetings, discussions and encounters to assess what others believe is important. Then use your wisdom to discern factors that can be used to achieve your vision. Rely on your formal and informal networks. Finally, use the wide variety of tools and techniques available for scanning the environment and gathering intelligence [45, 46].

Scenario planning is a systems-thinking process that enables you to orient yourself strategically to the future. See the example below:

> *For many years the federal department of health, Health Canada, had encouraged pan-Canadian health organizations (PCHO) to find better ways to work together to service Canadians* [47]. *The CEOs of those organizations, however, found it difficult to collaborate. In 2018, Dr. P-G Forest and Dr. Danielle Martin were commissioned by Health Canada to explore and recommend measures to maximize the efficiency and effectiveness of eight national healthcare organizations that are funded by the federal government.*
>
> *Forest and Martin used scenario planning, a systems thinking process, to shape their recommendations. They stated that "a successful PCHO suite must be designed to support the emergence of health systems of the future across Canada. Therefore, before recommending a future set of PCHOs, we endeavoured to understand what these 21st century systems will look like." Martin and Forest employed four scenarios to explore the future of the pan-Canadian organizations* [48]. *All four scenarios ended up proposing fewer agencies that needed to be more focused on the infrastructure for learning health systems, consistent with the earlier section in this chapter on strategic learning.*

A second way to orient yourself strategically to the future is to develop your information and communication networks so you can engage and consult outside groups quickly and often. New technology lets us enter exchanges with stakeholders and the public in ways never dreamed of.

A third way to orient yourself to the future is to contemplate the future in terms of the systems principle of interdependence—the idea that everything is connected, with mutual, rather than linear, cause and effect. Here's an example from one of Canada's largest health authorities. A patient came to the emergency ward in a large city hospital 10 times in a year, four times winding up in the intensive care unit, with total costs of $400,000. When an administrator (seeing her for the eleventh time) looked into why she came to emergency so often, he learned she could not afford the $30–40 a month her medication cost, and social services would not cover it. The administrator persuaded the health system to pay for the medication, the woman no longer had to come to emergency and the health system saved almost $399,500. Just as in this example, future-oriented leaders ask how social, economic and political events are connected, how they interact and what happens if they do?

Champion and Orchestrate Change

"I need to be seen as a credible champion for my people and taking what they say seriously" says a senior Australian health leader [49]. To champion something is to advocate, support and fight for it. To orchestrate change involves shaping and combining its parts to achieve a desired effect. Both verbs emphasize behaving differently, in tune with all the LEADS capabilities.

Most of the time our leadership actions should be based on parking personalities and engaging people in a disciplined way to achieve change. As another Australian senior health leader recently stated, "It's very, very easy to see people in the workplace and go 'Well, they're an ally' or 'They're an enemy.' As soon as you've compartmentalized people that way, I think you're on thin ice…I'm a lot more successful at dealing with so-called 'difficult' or 'prickly' people because I have that ability now, I think, to identify the things that are irritating me and then park them to one side and go 'They really don't matter'" [49].

We are not so naïve as to think coercion and force are never necessary. But knowing the difference between being irritating and being power hungry is what matters; if it's the latter, a leader must act. Those that seek power for power's sake, rather than to serve the health interests of the population, need to be challenged. Indeed, one of the most important leadership abilities might be knowing clearly who your adversaries are and have the inner strength to deal with them.

How do you apply these notions to championing and orchestrating change? First by recognizing that most people are not power hungry and if appealed to in the right way have a social conscience and want a better world for others. Second, by seeing the power in collective action and sharing power to achieve results. Third, by employing a discipline to harness collective action. We'll now expand on each of these in turn.

Inspiring People's Social Conscience

In the process of writing this book we had discussions with leaders from across Canada, Australia and the United Kingdom about the challenge of redesigning large, complex health systems. They consistently told us the key to getting collective action for change is to appeal to people's social conscience. Co-creation—letting go of traditional authority and engaging people in change—demands trust and faith. As one senior Australian leader said of medical leadership:

> As far as I'm concerned, I don't care what the doctor has a passion for, so long as it's something that can be translated into better health care: let them be a leader in that. That's where they will achieve some of the aims that they have and the organization have, simply because they really care about it [49].

If we look back at the Canterbury story, we see people behaved in accordance with the vision of *one system, one budget*. Why? Because senior leaders had faith that given appropriate learning opportunities, middle, clinical and front-line leaders would be guided by their social conscience and character and the shared vision. Rather than prescribing actions that people had to take, they provided opportunities for learning that encouraged them to act according to first principles and enabled them to act [50]. They also set out to ensure services would "enable people… (patients and consumers)…to take more responsibility for their own health and well-being" [9].

Learning Moment

1. Think back on the policies, processes and procedures that are employed in your organization to engage people in change. Do they demand compliance? Or are they structured to enable people to judge for themselves what's appropriate and act accordingly?
2. What happens when people do act according to their judgement—and the results are not effective? Are they punished? Shamed? Or is the response "we must learn from our mistakes and move on"? Which response is consistent with enabling others to act?

Seeing the Power of One as One of Many

Leadership is the ability to overcome the natural tendency of human endeavours to fragment; dissolve into entropy. Collective action—of leaders, in and across organizations, working together to generate change—is an antidote to entropy; and helps bring about large-scale change [51]. We have made this point numerous times in previous chapters including when we talked about engaging diverse populations. No matter what role you play in the health system, it's only by working with other leaders at multiple levels that you'll effect large-scale, lasting change. As another Australian leader stated,

> I can't think of any part of the health care system at the moment, whether we're talking about the operating theatre or the admissions system or clinical care, that can be done by any single individual… I've always believed that I have to have a team, that it was pointless trying to do it by yourself [49].

Other leaders include informal care-giver leaders and others from the larger community, captured in the people-centred standard the Health Standards Organization of Canada [52] is building into its leadership and governance standards (see Chap. 13).

Shared leadership is not easy. In general, most CEOs struggle to get collective action in their own organizations, much less across a system. They also compete for resources with other organizations including, for example, face time with the minister or deputy minister when dealing with government. We need new ways of working together, of forming coalitions and strategic partnerships, to see more coordinated action on large-scale change.

Interestingly, the individuality and power implicit to some in the word 'leader'—qualities that attract some people to leadership—are the very things that limit the ability to share leadership with others for systemic change. But if you're too wrapped up in your own role, you're at risk of overlooking what others have to offer in creating system change (as we discussed in Chap. 8). Hubris is the ultimate downfall of all too many leaders [53]. Collaboration can achieve change where a lone leader falls short [54, 55]. Collective action is what makes a system a system, both vertically (from micro- to macro-levels) and horizontally—across departments, organizations, and jurisdictions (such as community agencies and institutions).

Depending on your vintage and where you've worked you may feel the demands of collective action are overwhelming. However, like other aspects of leadership, collective action can be catalyzed through coordinated development initiatives based on a common vocabulary of leadership—such as LEADS, Health LEADS in Australia, or through the NHS framework. As we discussed in Chap. 4, any leadership development or succession-planning program should emphasize systems awareness through interaction among participants from a variety of roles.

Employing a Disciplined Approach to Harness Collective Action

There are many models and approaches for carrying out large-scale change based on the principle of collective action. Many embody the 20 LEADS capabilities. They bring a disciplined approach, embracing all partners, mobilizing available knowledge and generating shared ownership of the change process. Putting LEADS to work is not the sole job of any one person or department in an organization. It takes a critical mass to bring system change to life. The following story from Alberta Health Services provides an example of how one such model was used to generate large-scale change.

> Alberta Health Services (AHS) is a fully integrated health system that serves more than 4 million people who live in the Canadian province of Alberta. It has more than 110,000 employees, more than 14,300 volunteers, an extensive network of community partners, and provides programs and services at over 650 facilities.
>
> AHS takes an intentional approach to systems change. In 2014, for example, it gathered almost 700 human resources staff in Edmonton to identify "things to pay attention to" to get the best value possible from a centrally driven human resources department.
>
> The meeting used a professional facilitator and a modified open space forum (a type of self-organizing approach where participants at a meeting help decide who speaks and what topics are discussed) so everyone gets input from everyone on what was working well and what should be done differently. Based on the systems- and critical-thinking capability of frontline leaders, AHS developed its "People Strategy."
>
> Since then, a group of AHS staff has organized meetings where social systems leadership learning could be applied directly to organizational issues around patient care. They used organic systems framework strategies (Phil Cady for Elaine Watson, Personal email, 2019 Apr. 19).

There are many other models of collective action for large scale change in the health sector [46, 56–58]. Large-scale change approaches allow issues such as culture and sub-cultures to be examined for their impact and can create shared meaning among participants on vision, purpose, and direction of change. They allow you to determine which groups and individuals are resisting change because they don't understand it, as opposed to those whose values are at odds with the change. The right model can identify resources, help you align participants' efforts and help create momentum for a long-term process of change. The more organizations and groups that get involved, the harder it is to get going—and the harder it will be to stop the change process. Accomplished change leaders provide arenas for gathering intelligence, developing a shared vision, and engaging in strategic planning.

Finally, the decision to use a large-scale change model prompts us to recall a fundamental principle of systems thinking: there is no blame. When change is not happening on the scale we think it should or resistance is holding it back, we all tend to blame someone—politicians, the public, doctors. But we need to remember systems are comprised of interconnected people, so each of us is part of blocking progress. What is happening is no one's fault, or it's the fault of all of us. It's system failure. The point of large-scale change activities is to help us design the path forward together.

Summary

The Systems transformation domain of LEADS in a Caring Environment framework has four leadership capabilities:

- Demonstrate systems and critical thinking
- Encourage and support innovation
- Orient themselves strategically toward the future
- Champion and orchestrate change

This is how our equity, diversity, and inclusion lens on leadership puts the systems transformation capabilities to work:

Equity, Diversity and Inclusion-Informed Systems Transformation
Successful leaders think systemically to help achieve Systems transformation, the S in the LEADS framework. Systems transformation is not only focused on the health system, but also on the human patterns of thinking and behaving within it that perpetuate inequity, lack of diversity and exclusion within the health system, be that sexism, racism, ableism, classism, ageism or settler colonialism.

This can be daunting for health leaders, but it builds on the previous elements of the LEADS framework. The first capability, systems thinking, can be augmented through tools such as Gender-Based Analysis Plus (GBA+), where the plus refers to other equity, diversity and inclusion dimensions of visible minority and Indigenous status, and disability, among others. A GBA+

*perspective encourages leaders to be cognizant of the forms of differentia-
tion, to challenge commonly held assumptions (that is, unconscious bias)
and to apply it consistently and transparently across all leadership activities.
The federal Department for Women and Gender Equality (formerly Status of
Women Canada), hosts a number of GBA+ tools as a starting point.*

*Equity, diversity and inclusion-informed transformation requires leaders
to move beyond their own journey and develop capabilities to strategically
assess which key societal structures pose the strongest barriers to equity,
diversity and inclusion and to strategically orient themselves to the future
to support innovation and champion change. Keeping gender, diversity and
inclusion in the forefront of their minds, and leading from where they are, successful leaders can champion and orchestrate systemic change.*

Together, the Systems transformation capabilities—and the approaches associated with them—can assist leaders to achieve large-scale, systemic change in health
care. In essence, these capabilities describe a process of strategic learning: an ability
to adjust and adapt to external forces in a productive manner.

Yet it's clear that Canadian and other international systems remain fragmented,
despite the best actions of leaders. Is that because we adhere to the old models of
leadership emphasizing control over the fiefdom? Is it because we don't believe others are as committed as we are? Or because we have difficulty embracing behaviour
and practices that facilitate innovation and change? Or is it that complex adaptive
systems are not responsive to linear, step-by-step change processes?

Learning Moment
Use this tool to assess how well you demonstrate the four Systems
transformation capabilities. Choose the level appropriate for your level of
responsibility.
If there were one capability you would like to improve on, what is it? Why?

Systems Transformation Self Assessment (For on-line access to self assessment tool, please visit www.LEADSglobal.ca)

Informal leader (patient, family member, citizen) responsibilities
In order to help transform the health system, I

1.	Employ systems and critical thinking skills to learn about the challenges and issues facing patients, families, citizens, and providers, in transforming to a people-centred health system	1	2	3	4	5	6	7	N
2.	Take responsibility for encouraging and supporting innovation in patient, family and citizen practise; and to support providers to embrace innovations consistent with improving people-centred care	1	2	3	4	5	6	7	N

3.	Make a disciplined effort to orient myself to the future of a people-centred health system: I am able to manage the contradictions and changes such a view requires of me	1	2	3	4	5	6	7	N
4.	Am willing to champion and orchestrate change, in collaboration with others, to achieve a people-centred system	1	2	3	4	5	6	7	N

Front-line leader responsibilities
In order to help transform the health system, I

1.	Use critical/systems thinking to ensure our practices are consistent with people-centred care, the vision of my organization and the broader system	1	2	3	4	5	6	7	N
2.	Support the innovation required improve quality, and use my creativity to influence practices aimed at improving service to patients and clients	1	2	3	4	5	6	7	N
3.	Model and encourage people I interact with to think about trends and enduring values of importance to the organization and system. I anticipate issues and consider how to change practices accordingly	1	2	3	4	5	6	7	N
4.	Champion change approaches being employed in my organization or the larger system, orchestrate them, and change my personal practices to be consistent with them	1	2	3	4	5	6	7	N

Mid-manager leader responsibilities
In order to help transform the health system, I

1.	Within my area of responsibility, use critical/systems thinking to improve service to patients or citizens, consistent with the people-centred focus of my organization and the broader system	1	2	3	4	5	6	7	N
2.	Within my area of responsibility, create an environment supportive of innovation so people can see and use innovation and creativity to achieve efficient and effective service for patients and clients	1	2	3	4	5	6	7	N
3.	Enable people in my area of responsibility to think about trends, issues and enduring values presented to us by the future; and consider how to change practice accordingly	1	2	3	4	5	6	7	N
4.	Communicate a compelling rationale for change and orchestrate approaches to it that are consistent with the large-change approaches being used in the organization or larger system	1	2	3	4	5	6	7	N

Senior leader responsibilities
In order to help transform the health system, I

1.	Use critical/systems thinking to identify issues and practices that could improve service to patients or clients in my program or department, and consistent with the person-centred focus of my organization and the broader system	1	2	3	4	5	6	7	N
2.	Create an environment in my program or department where innovation and creativity are valued as sources of tactical and strategic improvement	1	2	3	4	5	6	7	N
3.	Encourage people to look into the future to anticipate problems our department will face; identify opportunities; and create solutions in line with the values of our organization and system	1	2	3	4	5	6	7	N
4.	Champion and orchestrate the use of small- and large-system approaches to change consistent with the organization's strategies to achieve a people-centred purpose	1	2	3	4	5	6	7	N

Executive leader responsibilities								
In order to help transform the health system, I								
1.	Encourage and employ strategic critical/systems thinking practices to analyze system needs and identify practices that could improve service to the patients or clients organization-wide	1 2 3 4 5 6 7 N
2.	Create an environment in my organization and the broader system where strategic practices utilize innovation and creativity to improve quality and efficiency organization/ system wide	1 2 3 4 5 6 7 N
3.	Encourage people in my organization and partner agencies to identify future trends, anticipate issues, and create strategic solutions in line with our own and system values	1 2 3 4 5 6 7 N
4.	Champion person-centred system change and employ large-system approaches to implement changes required in our organization or broader health system	1 2 3 4 5 6 7 N

References

1. Baker GR, Axler R. Health system reconfiguration. Creating a high performing health care system for Ontario: evidence supporting strategic changes in Ontario. Toronto, ON: Institute of Health Policy, Management and Evaluation. University of Toronto; 2015. https://www.oha.com/Documents/OHA%20High%20Performing%20Healthcare%20System%20Paper.pdf. Accessed 22 Aug 2019.
2. Cambridge University Press. Cambridge dictionary. Cambridge: Cambridge University Press; 2019. Transformation. https://dictionary.cambridge.org/dictionary/english/transformation. Accessed 10 Apr 2019
3. Randhawa M. Is transformation in the NHS really transformational? The Kings Fund. 2018. https://www.kingsfund.org.uk/blog/2018/02/transformation-nhs. Accessed 2 Aug 2019.
4. Laszlo A. Leadership and systemic innovation: sociotechnical systems, ecological systems, and evolutionary systems design. Int. J. Sociol. 2018;3:380–91. https://doi.org/10.1080/03906701.2018.1529076I.
5. Bennett N, Lemoine GJ. What VUCA really means for you. Harv Bus Rev. 2014;2014:27–8.
6. Rodriguez A, Rodriguez Y. Metaphors for today's leadership: VUCA world, millennial and "Cloud Leaders". J Manag Dev. 2015;34(7):854–66.
7. Dinh J, Lord R, Gardner W, Meuser J, Liden R, Hu J. Leadership theory and research in the new millennium: current theoretical trends and changing perspectives. Leadersh Q. 2014;25(1):36–62.
8. Kania J, Kramer M, Senge P. The water of systems change. FSG. 2018. http://efc.issuelab.org/resources/30855/30855.pdf.
9. Timmins N, Ham C. The quest for integrated health and social care: A case study in Canterbury. The Kings Fund: New Zealand; 2013. https://www.kingsfund.org.uk/sites/default/files/field/field_publication_file/quest-integrated-care-new-zealand-timmins-ham-sept13.pdf. Accessed 2 Aug 2019.
10. MacLeod H. Humanizing leadership. Vancouver: Friesen Press; 2019.
11. Agency for Health care Research and Quality. Learning health systems. Rockville, MD: Agency for Health care Research and Quality; 2019. https://www.ahrq.gov/learning-health-systems/index.html. Accessed 20 Jul 2019.

12. LHS. Learning healthcare systems. Newcastle: LHS; 2019. The Learning Health Care Project. http://www.learninghealth careproject.org/section/background/learning-health care-system. Accessed 20 Jul 2019.

13. Tamarack Institute. This diagram is adapted from a diagram in Cabaj M. Evaluating systems change results: an inquiry framework. Waterloo, ON: Tamarack Institute; 2019. https://www.tamarackcommunity.ca/hubfs/Resources/Publications/Paper%20Evaluating%20Systems%20Change%20Results%20Mark%20Cabaj.pdf and Kania J, Kramer M, Senge P. The water of systems change. Foundations Strategy Group; 2018; http://efc.issuelab.org/resources/30855/30855.pdf. Accessed 20 Jul 2019.

14. Egger G, Dixon J. Beyond obesity and lifestyle: a review of 21st century chronic disease determinants. BioMed Res Int. 2014; https://doi.org/10.1155/2014/731685.

15. Hurst P, Hurst S. Leadership connectivity: a leading indicator for organizational culture change. Org Dev J. 2016;34(1):81–95.

16. Van Wietmarschen HA, Wortelboer HM, van der Greef J. Grip on health: a complex systems approach to transform health care. J Eval Clin Pract. 2016;24(1):269–77.

17. Tan J, Wen J, Awad N. Health care and services delivery systems as complex adaptive systems. Commun ACM. 2005;48(5):36–44.

18. Sturmberg JP, O'Halloran DM, Martin CM. Understanding health system reform – a complex adaptive systems perspective. J Eval Clin Pract. 2012;18(1):202–8. https://doi.org/10.1111/j.1365-2753.2011.01792.x.

19. Belrhiti Z, Giralt AN, Marchal B. Complex leadership in health care: a scoping review. Int J Health Policy Manag. 2018;7(12):1073–84.

20. Heifetz R, Laurie D, Heifetz R. Adaptive work. In: Goethals G, Sorenson G, Burns JM, editors. Encyclopedia of leadership. Thousand Oaks, CA: SAGE Publications; 2004. https://doi.org/10.4135/9781412952392.n4.

21. Newman D. Innovation vs. transformation: the difference in a digital world. Forbes. 2017. https://www.forbes.com/sites/danielnewman/2017/02/16/innovation-vs-transformation-the-difference-in-a-digital-world/#6be15f2565e8. Accessed 15 Jul 2019.

22. Camgöz-Akdağ H, Çalişkan E, Toma S. Lean process design for a radiology department. Bus Process Manag J. 2017;23(4):779–91. https://doi.org/10.1108/BPMJ-02-2017-0025.

23. Danese P, Manfe V, Romano P. A systematic literature review on recent Lean research: state-of-the-art and future directions. Int J Manag Rev. 2018;20:579–605.

24. Conference Board of Canada. Current state of Lean in Canadian health care. Ottawa, ON: Conference Board of Canada; 2014. https://www.conferenceboard.ca/temp/dc8e5843-765d-45ab-9e95-1cdab3d23858/6448_CurrentStateOfLean_CASHC_(PUB3437)-BR-FR.pdf. Accessed 23 Aug 2019.

25. Australia has an organization dedicated to Lean Health care, called the Australasian Lean Health care Network (ALHN), while Canada does not appear to have an analogous enterprise although Lean is used extensively. The AHLN (http://www.leanhealth.org.au/) is affiliated with Lean Enterprise Australia a not-for-profit organisation devoted to the spread of knowledge and information about Lean Thinking and its applications (http://leanaust.com/services/lean-health-care)

26. Hallam C, Contreras C. Lean health care: scale, scope and sustainability. Int J Health Care Qual Assur. 2018;31(7):684–96.

27. This may well be due to the mechanistic methodology of Lean; its application in a discrete context in which variables appear to be finite; and the cause and effect linear mapping involved in the process. In large scale change, as we noted in the previous section, the multitude and unknowable nature of many variables within a complex system may not interact well with the simple system foundation of Lean.

28. Dickson G, Mutwiri B, Blakley B. The symbiotic relationship between Lean and LEADS. Ottawa, ON: Canadian Health Leadership Network; 2015. https://chlnet.ca/wp-content/uploads/LEAN-and-LEADS-Comparison-for-CHLNet-May-2015.pdf. Accessed 23 Aug 2019

29. Shaw S, Kendel D. Lean improvement process making positive impact on Saskatchewan health care. Regina Leader Post; 2016. https://leaderpost.com/opinion/columnists/lean-improvement-process-making-positive-impact-on-saskatchewan-health-care. Accessed 23 Aug 2019.
30. CBC News. New report 'final straw' for Lean, Sask. NDP says. Toronto, ON: CBC; 2016. https://www.cbc.ca/news/canada/saskatoon/new-report-final-straw-for-lean-ndp-says-1.3429291. Accessed 20 Jul 2019.
31. Maijala R, Eoranta S, Reunanen T, Ikonen TS. Successful implementation of Lean as a managerial principle in health care: a conceptual analysis from systematic literature review. Int J Technol Assess Health Care. 2018;34(2):134–46.
32. As in described in chapter 12, and subsequent to our story, in 2017 Saskatchewan joined the growing ranks of province-wide, integrated regional health authorities.
33. Braithwaite J, Churruca K, Long JC, Ellis LA, Herkes J. When complexity science meets implementation science: a theoretical and empirical analysis of systems change. BMC Med. 2018;16(63):1–14. https://doi.org/10.1186/s12916-018-1057-z.
34. Snowdon A. A blueprint for innovation to achieve health system transformation. HealthcarePapers. 2017;16(3). https://www.longwoods.com/content/25086/healthcarepapers/a-blueprint-for-innovation-to-achieve-health-system-transformation. Accessed 10 Jul 2019.
35. Naylor D, Girard F, Mintz J, Fraser N, Jenkins T, Power C. Unleashing innovation: excellent health care for Canada. Report of the Advisory Panel on Health care Innovation. Health Canada: Ottawa, ON; 2015. http://tinyurl.com/qx2cf8z. Accessed 12 Jul 2019.
36. Conway P. Partnership for patients: innovation and leadership for safer health care. J Healthc Manag. 2017;62(3):166–70. https://doi.org/10.1097/JHM-D-17-00039.
37. Canadian Patient Safety Institute. Vision and results. Evaluation of the national patient safety consortium & integrated patient safety action plan: final report. Ottawa, ON: Canadian Patient Safety Institute; 2018. https://www.patientsafetyinstitute.ca/en/toolsResources/Evaluation-National-Patient-Safety-Consortium/Documents/National%20Consortium%20Executive%20Summary%202018.pdf. Accessed 1 Aug 2019.
38. West M, Eckert R, Collins B, Chowta R. Caring to change: how compassionate leadership can stimulate innovation in health care. London: The Kings Fund; 2017. p. 1–40. https://www.kingsfund.org.uk/sites/default/files/field/field_publication_file/Caring_to_change_Kings_Fund_May_2017.pdf. Accessed 1 Aug 2019.
39. Spano R, Caldarelli A, Ferri L, Maffei M. Context, culture and control: a case study on accounting change in an Italian regional health service. J Manag Govern. 2019:1–44.
40. Encyclopedia Mythica; Encyclopedia mythica; Janus; 1997. www.novareinna.com/festive/janus.html. Accessed 15 Jul 2019.
41. Nonaka I, Takeuchi H. The wise leader. Harv Bus Rev. 2011;1:58–67.
42. Barbuto J, Millard M. Wisdom development of leaders. IJLS. 2012;5(1):233–45.
43. Martin R. The opposable mind. Boston, MA: Harvard Business School; 2009.
44. Schulte P. Polarity management 101: the solution to unsolvable problems. Triple Pundit. 2016. https://www.triplepundit.com/story/2016/polarity-management-101-solution-unsolvable-problems/20846. Accessed 15 Apr 2019.
45. Nauheimer H. The change management toolbook: a collection of tools, methods and strategies. 2019. https://docs.wixstatic.com/ugd/83f877_c338c6f644484749a0f962d0456b0fda.pdf. Accessed 5 Jul 2019.
46. Holman P, Devane T, Cady S. The change handbook: the definitive resource on today's best methods for engaging whole systems. San Francisco, CA: Berrett-Koehler; 2007. NOTE: A revised edition of the Change Handbook (Holman, Devane and Cady) is in the process of being published in 2019.
47. The eight organizations are: The Canadian Foundation for Health Improvement (CFHI), The Canadian Agency for Drugs and Technology in Health (CADTH), The Canadian Patient Safety Institute (CPSI), The Canadian Centre on Substance Use and Addiction (CCSA), The Canadian Institute for Health Information (CIHI), The Canadian Partnership Against Cancer (CPAC), Canada Health Infoway (Infoway), and Mental Health Commission of Canada (MHCC).

48. Forest PG, Martin D. Fit for purpose: findings and recommendations of the external review of the pan-Canadian health organizations – summary report. Ottawa, ON: Health Canada; 2018. https://www.canada.ca/en/health-canada/services/health-care-system/reports-publications/health-care-system/findings-recommendations-external-review-pan-canadian-health-organization.html. Accessed 5 Jul 2019.
49. In 2016, one of your authors interviewed a series of senior Australian medical leaders as part of a commissioned project for the Royal Australasian College of Medical Administrators. This—and subsequent quotations in this chapter—are found in unpublished interview transcripts. While permission to use the interviews was gained for the project, it was impossible to do so for this book: hence, none of the interviewees are identified by name.
50. Enabling others to act is one of five dimensions of effective leadership based on the research profiled in Kouzes J, Posner B. The leadership challenge. How to make extraordinary things happen in organizations. Hoboken, NJ: Wiley and Sons; 2017.
51. It should be emphasized that relationships and connectedness is a fundamental principle underpinning the LEADS framework, the NHS framework, and the Australia HWA framework, referenced in chapter 3. It is also a major theme in almost all leadership works; after all, the leader-follower dynamic is a relationship.
52. Health Standards Organization. HSO 76000: integrated people-centred systems (IPCS) standard. Health Standards Organization Ottawa, ON 2018. https://healthstandards.org/ipcs/. Accessed 2 Aug 2019.
53. Collins J. How the mighty fall. Jim Collins Articles. 2009. https://www.jimcollins.com/books/how-the-mighty-fall.html. Accessed 20 Aug 2019.
54. Montgomery A, Dacin P, Dacin M. Collective social entrepreneurship: shaping social good. J Bus Ethics. 2012;111:375–88.
55. Currie G, Spyrdonidis D. Sharing leadership for diffusion of innovation in professionalized settings. Hum Relat. 72(7):1209–33.
56. Sustainable Improvement Team and the Horizons Team. Leading large scale change: a practical guide. London: NHS England; 2018. https://www.england.nhs.uk/wp-content/uploads/2017/09/practical-guide-large-scale-change-april-2018-smll.pdf. Accessed 20 Jul 2019.
57. McCannon CJ, Schall MW, Perta RJ. Planning for scale: a guide for designing large-scale improvement initiatives. IHI Innovation Series White Paper. Cambridge, MA: Institute for Health Care Improvement; 2008. http://www.ihi.org/resources/pages/IHIWhitePapers/PlanningforScaleWhitePaper.aspx. Accessed 20 Jul 2019.
58. Cheuy S. Small actions, big change: pathways for system impact. Tamarack Institute: Waterloo, ON; 2016. http://www.tamarackcommunity.ca/latest/small-actions-big-change-pathways-for-system-impact. Accessed 20 Jul 2019.

Putting LEADS to Work as a Change Leadership Model: Integrating Change Leadership and Change Management

10

Graham Dickson and Bill Tholl

The best way to predict the future is to create it.

Peter Drucker [1]

It is trite but true to say that the only constant in health care in 2020 is change. Leaders have no real purpose unless they are trying to create, as Drucker suggests, the changes needed to create a better future.

This chapter picks up where Chap. 9 leaves off. It describes how LEADS can be used as a change model. Of course, there is a bevy of change management models out there to choose from [2–5], each with its own strengths and weaknesses. A recent comparative assessment of three models of change—Kotter, the PROSCI model and LEADS—found, while each has its relative strengths, it is by combining approaches to fit distinct leadership challenges that we see the most success [6].

Three of the advantages we see in LEADS as a preferred change model are: (1) a major function of leadership is to create change; (2) the framework has already gained widespread purchase in Canada as a by health, for health model; and (3) it combines many concepts and ideas from a multitude of change models across its five domains.

We were only beginning to realize back in 2014 that the real leadership challenge of advancing the health agenda in Canada and comparable countries was to find a better, more reliable way of not just managing but leading small- and large-scale change. In this chapter, we profile three case studies where LEADS is being used as a change leadership tool or model. We asked our case study writers to use an after-action review process [7], and by doing so, we explore how exactly LEADS is

G. Dickson (✉)
Royal Roads University, Victoria, BC, Canada
e-mail: graham.dickson@royalroads.ca

B. Tholl
Canadian Health Leadership Network, Ottawa, ON, Canada
e-mail: btholl@chlnet.ca

© Springer Nature Switzerland AG 2020
G. Dickson, B. Tholl (eds.), *Bringing Leadership to Life in Health: LEADS in a Caring Environment*, https://doi.org/10.1007/978-3-030-38536-1_10

197

being put to work as a model of change. The process asked three key questions: What were the expectations going into the change process? What surprises or wild cards were encountered and what corrective actions were taken? What can we learn from the change process going forward?

Living LEADS: Aligning the Gears

One of the big surprises in writing this second edition is how the framework has changed the way leaders embrace LEADS personally as well as how it is being used as a model of change. For example, here's a story from Ellen Melis, an experienced LEADS facilitator and coach (personal interview 2019 Apr 8).

> When I ask community leaders: "What's your biggest challenge?" they often say "We're too small to make a difference." LEADS is a big equalizer because it gives voice to everyone on the team, from the C-suite to the front line. It is empowering in that it encourages everyone to think big and to think about the system. It's enabling because it encourages all of us to lead from where we are, from our relative strengths and in our own way. It allows everyone on the team to see the bigger picture.
>
> I first start my conversation about change guided by the need to "Listen, listen, listen— and listen most closely to those working at the front line." Change only happens when leaders can take ideas and strategies and put them to work. And this requires a change in mindset, which in turn requires a change in culture. The leader shift required is to understand the critical coming together in the middle, those that can see both the leadership opportunities and the health care delivery and management challenges.
>
> In putting LEADS to work as a change model, I start with Mintzberg's [8] principle of starting from the middle out rather than the top down or bottom up. I always see the change leadership process as involving three gears. The smallest gear is associated with the senior executives of any organization. They certainly can help create an environment that encourages system thinking around the needs of the patient and/or their families, but they cannot make change happen. It takes a lot of rotations to move the next gear.
>
> It is the middle gear, like in a three-speed bicycle, that is critical to converting ideas into action. Again, it takes many revolutions for this middle gear to turn the biggest gear. And, of course, it is the biggest gear—the front-line providers—that make the difference in the care experience. And, once this big gear begins to move, the momentum for lasting change begins. I call this a "feed forward" process and it is the only way to create lasting change in complex systems. The beauty of this metaphor is that it can also work in reverse. By giving voice to the front lines, small changes initiated by the biggest gears can really speed up the attainment of strategic objectives. But this requires a real shift in mental models; a real shift in the culture of an organization.

Ellen's three gears metaphor provides a powerful image, as it reinforces what we all know: real change only happens when the actions of multiple players line up (the goal of the Achieve results domain). Her story also reminds us that most people in management roles see themselves first as managers and second, as leaders of change. That's why change management seems so comfortable to all of us; it is simply an extension of our role as a manager, and why we all too often think leadership is something we can do from the side of our desk. One of the main objectives of this chapter is to support our contention that "leaders need to think and act like change masters." [9]

Ellen's three gears also remind us of Jim Collin's Flywheel Effect [10]. Collins describes just how challenging it is to initiate change and then sustain momentum, how it seems almost impossible in the early going to even begin to move a big, heavy flywheel like the health care system. Gradually, however, the flywheel gets moving to the point where the change agenda is unstoppable. Probably one of the best examples of this phenomenon is Obamacare in the USA: a change that so far, despite the best efforts of the Republican Party, has not been dismantled.

Ellen "loves LEADS" because it calls upon each of us, whatever our station in life, to see our role as a change leader. Imagine the possibilities if we spent just 10% of our time focused on the future, demonstrating LEADS capabilities and behaviour in support of improvement, reform, adaptation, advancement: whatever term you want to use for change. People need to see themselves as integral cogs in a smoothly functioning series of gears, all pulling in the same direction [8].

LEADS helps to level the playing field, Ellen says, because the LEADS approach to change recognizes that everyone in health care—including patients and families—have a role in leading change; and it outlines the capabilities needed to do so. From an organizational perspective LEADS promotes leading from the middle or at least ensuring that the middle gear (that is, middle management) is connected both to the executive and front-line delivery gears in any health care system. And as Ivy's text boxes have reminded us in each of the domains, bridging the gaps in terms of equity, diversity and inclusivity is part of getting all the gears aligned, with each doing their part to ensure that changes go smoothly.

Balancing the Tension Between Change Leadership and Change Management

Chapter 9 reminded us that leading change in the health sector involves dealing with a big, complex and often non-adaptive system. As Braithwaite et al observe, it is hard to change health care systems because they are so big, so political and so institutionalized, with so many vested interests.

> Construing health care as a complex adaptive system implies that getting evidence into routine practice through a step-by-step model is not feasible. Complexity science forces us to consider the dynamic properties of systems and the varying characteristics that are deeply enmeshed in social practices, whilst indicating that multiple forces, variables, and influences must be factored into any change process, and that unpredictability and uncertainty are normal properties of multi-part, intricate systems [11].

To be effective as a change agent in today's complex health care systems requires leaders to move beyond a step-by-step, evidence-based paradigm of change. Linear, reductionist or Cartesian approaches to leadership in the health sector limit our flexibility to respond to the peripatetic and reoccurring challenges of change.

Linear thinking builds on the adage that the shortest distance between two points is a straight line. It reflects how we have been taught to think, how we are taught to put everything in sequence; in order. One problem solved; move on to the next: however, in real change, a problem solved at one point might well reoccur at any time in the process of change. As Bill, one of your authors and building on his policy experience observed: "You never really solve serious health policy problems; you substitute one set of problems for another hoping the new set will be more manageable than the old set."

Indeed, we too have argued that alignment of effort is needed if visions are to be achieved and change to be realized (Chap. 7). It's true our best efforts are needed to create as much alignment as possible, in a system that is inherently misaligned. To approach change assuming that a cause-and-effect model of it, predicated purely on logic and reason—and typically associated with the construct of change management—can re-order human behaviour and sustain it, while moving on to the next step in the change process, is naïve. Even though alignment can be created in one moment, in one situation, new events and circumstances may well put it askew, requiring a return to an earlier stage of the change process. Other approaches to change, built around the principles of organic systems thinking, recognize this challenge. There are no straight lines, no simple answers or solutions to help human beings get from the current, unsustainable state to a preferred future state.

Complexity science is characterized by nonlinearity [12]. According to Miles, complex systems and problems require more than simplistic linear thinking [13]. With a complexity science perspective, there is an appreciation of the complex, dynamic and interconnected relationships occurring within a complex system or problem. And, as Dumas and Beinecke remind us: "Change leaders must encourage their organizations to learn, innovate, experiment, and question, preparing their organizations for change by constantly seeking new perspectives, and encouraging participation throughout the organization." [14]

We suggest the need for a fundamental change of our mindsets about change management and change leadership, along the lines suggested by one of the gurus of change management. Here's what John Kotter has had to say about the fundamental difference between change management and change leadership in complex, dynamic systems:

> There is a difference that is very fundamental and it's very big between what is known today as change management and what we have been calling for some time change leadership. Change management tends to be more associated, at least when it works well, with smaller changes. If you look at all the [management] tools, they're trying to push things along; trying to minimize disruptions or keep things under control. It's trying to make sure change is done efficiently. Change leadership is just fundamentally different. It's an engine. It's more about urgency. It's more about masses of people who want to make something happen. It's more about big visions. It's more about empowering lots and lots of people.
>
> Change leadership has the potential to get things a little bit out of control. You don't have the same degree of making sure that everything happens in a way you want and at a time you want when you have the 1000 hp engine. What you want to do of course is have a highly skilled driver and a heck of a car, which will make sure that your risks are at a minimum. But it is fundamentally different.
>
> The world we all know right now talks about, thinks about and does change management. The world we all know right now doesn't do much change leadership since change leadership is associated with the bigger leaps that we have to make, associated with the windows of opportunities that are coming at us faster, and staying open less time; bigger hazards and bullets are coming at us faster. So, you really have to make a larger leap at a faster speed.

Change leadership is going to be the big challenge in the future. And the fact that almost nobody is really very good at is, obviously, a big deal [15].

As Kotter suggests, getting behind the wheel of a race car is not for the faint of heart. Kotter understands the need for better management and enlightened leadership to come together for success. Managing and leading change can be seen as opposite sides of a piece of paper: they seem like two sides of a coin. But if you twist the paper and join the two ends, you have a Mobius strip; when the two sides no longer appear as opposites, but feed into one another. Change leadership and change management are those two sides.

We are reminded that while people may be forced to change via circumstance or environmental forces beyond their control, leaders need to ensure they and others have some freedom to choose *how* to change and *how much* effort and commitment they want to put into it. All the LEADS domains and many of the capabilities and the variety of ways that they can be put to work embrace the notion of making a choice of how to think about change, how to respond to forces we can't change, and whether or not we wish to be preemptive in shaping the society that will result from those forces.

To illustrate this point, let's look at a change many of us have gone through: renovating a house. "Personally, I hate change, but I love renovating my house," says Rosabeth Moss Kanter, author of the book *Evolve!* [16] Her point: nobody likes change when it's done to them. But change we choose is different; that's the kind of change we're willing to embrace. We own what we help create.

But getting an array of different people to work together to co-create anything is fraught with human foibles. Here's a variation on renovating the house of health care from our colleague Hugh MacLeod in his recent *book Humanizing Leadership*: [17].

Although all trade people are certified to perform their job, we observed that not all individuals perform their job to the same level of care and attention. Perhaps it was their individual work ethic that determines outcome; maybe it was the program, apprenticeship, or company they worked for that hinders their ability. Maybe they were wrapped up in personal problems outside of work, unable to separate their personal life from their business life. Or maybe it was fatigue; they have worked too many consecutive days, and the long hours are leading to burn out.

Extending beyond the individual worker, maybe the trade person has a personal conflict with their boss, or general contractor. Maybe it is the incompetence of the general contractor and their inability to orchestrate the project. Maybe the tools had an effect on outcome or the new techniques and technologies they have yet to master. Maybe some individuals on the project were working towards professional advancement, while others were complacent with where they are. Maybe some contractors looked for shortcuts, while others were consumed by perfectionism.

Ultimately, we learned that we have little control over execution, attitude, behaviours, skills, pride, deadlines, and completion timelines. We witnessed firsthand that trade apprenticeship development programs resulting in trade certifications did not guarantee quality, attitude, pride, and customer service. On sequencing and hand offs between framing, plumbing, electrical, drywall, finishing, and painting, we witnessed how one profession could hold others up and professional rivalry, pettiness, and blaming occurs. We learned that not all these individuals possessed the ability to articulate the problems and solutions and progress with absolute clarity and conviction.

> *The truth is that all the answers can be found in the hearts and minds of people. Every individual has the capacity to contribute to organizational growth. Individuals carry the seeds of success: skills, talents, potentialities, and enthusiasm. Unfortunately, for many those same seeds contain too many intellectual, emotional, and systemic barriers. Liberating the "bottoms" and integrating the "middles" is how learning organizations succeed.*

Does this resonate with you? The challenges of renovating the health care system are unrelenting and often the locus of control is outside your purview. This renovation metaphor reinforces the key takeaways from Ellen's story about ensuring that all the gears, or sub trades as a general contractor, are lined up; but it also states that to assume that people will act accordingly, and do so with the quality that is envisaged, is misguided. Yes, we must trust people to do their absolute best; but not blind trust. Our job is also to monitor people's efforts and provide supports for their work; and to make the adjustments to the process that are needed. As a recent report from the Health Leadership Academy and McMaster University on scenario planning points out: "Modern health care systems are complex. They continue to evolve under shifting and interacting external forces in difficult-to-predict ways" [18].

The good news is that LEADS, especially when used in concert with other change models, can help to build the case for and help sustain transformational change in the health care system [4]. Change leadership requires we consider (metaphorically speaking) taking a speed-reading course, where we don't read in sequence but in jumps and where we continue to practice, to get better ever faster. As we found in Chap. 9, system thinking and systems leadership is required to transform systems.

Given these limits of reductionist linearity, how can we put LEADS to work as a change leadership model to address the volatility, uncertainty, complexity and ambiguity (VUCA) of health systems change? We explore in the reminder of this chapter the challenges of getting beyond simply managing change [8]. This is the essence of distributed leadership and the power of LEADS as a change leadership tool. Let us explain how to put LEADS to work as a robust change leadership model in the dynamic context of leading change in today's health care system.

LEADS as a Model to Guide Change

> *Everybody likes progress. It's the changes they don't like!*
>
> Will Rogers

The first step in putting LEADS to work as a change model is for you as a leader to acknowledge and be able to clearly articulate why the *status quo* is not tenable or sustainable. This can be for any number of reasons. As we have seen from several vignettes already, the imperative for change is often created externally perhaps by new legislation, by a task force, by a court ruling, by a tragic bus accident or by the vagaries of democratic processes (changes in governments).

But change can also come from within, as this chapter encourages you to think about. Through the *power of one*, leveraging up your personal locus of influence and power or though the power of working as one as part of an internal team, or an external coalition, you can create or orchestrate the need for transformational change. Regardless of where the impetus for change comes from, it is important that you know why you are championing it and why it is important for you to lead it.

By personally accepting that the current state is not sustainable and then clearly articulating a clear and compelling vision for that better future state, you define a gap between the two that we call the *territory of change*. The size, seriousness or significance of the gap evokes comparison to the first step of John Kotter's [19] change model, creating a *sense of urgency*, often referred to as a burning platform [20]. Let's look now at how the five domains can be reconfigured as a change leadership model.

Five Domains of LEADS as a Change Model

The model reassembles or reframes the five domains as an interactive and iterative unit or operating system. This is depicted in Fig. 10.1.

As Fig. 10.1 below shows, the LEADS domains and capabilities are not just a list, but an integrated whole interacting with one another, in an ongoing series of cycles to move toward the preferred future. The model suggests leadership happens at an operational (or personal and interpersonal) level (left hand side) and at the strategic (organizational or systems) level: (the right side of Fig. 10.1). Activities associated with both are interrelated and interdependent. The gap between the current and future states defines the territory of change: the short vertical black line.

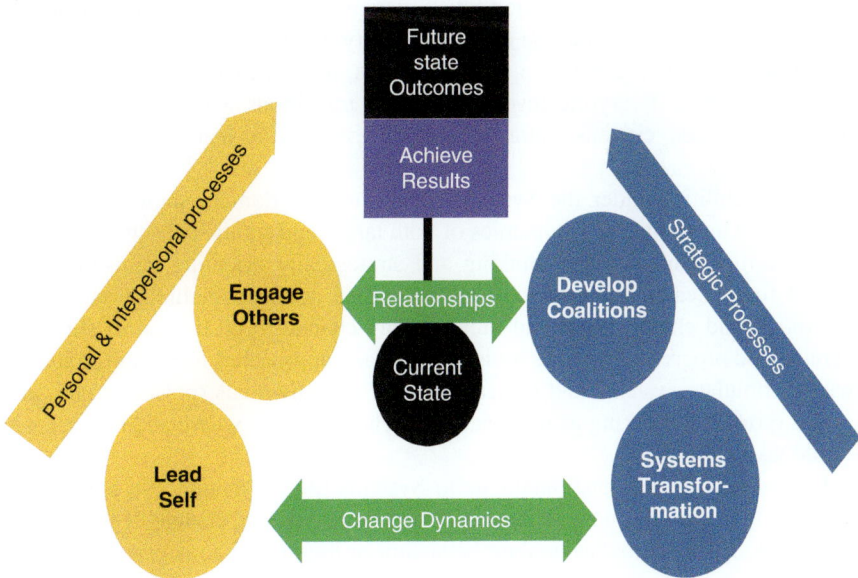

Fig. 10.1 LEADS as a model for change

Assessing the scope and breadth needed for change (context for change) is the first step of your change process. Once you have determined your locus of influence, you need to focus on the Set direction and Assess and evaluate capabilities of the Achieve results domain (featured at the top of the change pyramid) to establish a change destination. Vision, values and desired results help to define the preferred future. The model suggests you determine where the individual, organization or system is relative to the preferred future state. When expressed in measurable terms, the difference between current performance and desired performance shows the breadth and extent of the change you're undertaking. It also suggests short-term measurements (what Kotter called short term wins [21]) that can help guide course corrections along the way.

The other two capabilities of Achieve results (Align decisions with vision, values and evidence, and Take action to implement decisions) suggest ways leaders can align activities to ensure the journey stays on track. As change progresses, the Achieve results domain interacts with the capabilities of the other domains to keep change happening, to continue to achieve alignment of effort, and to help the corrective actions needed as you encounter those rocks in the field described in Chap. 7.

The second component of LEADS as a model of change highlights the need for leaders to have a sophisticated understanding of the human landscape of change and a high level of comfort with ambiguity and action learning. This component is represented by the horizontal green arrow linking the Lead self and Systems transformation domains. To achieve the desired results, you need to be attentive to the ever-changing external environment and need to understand what goes on psychologically when people—you and others—experience change. Individuals need support to transition from getting over the past to get to neutral before they can embrace the future [22]. To achieve a desired future, you and others will also have to change mindsets, behaviour, distribution of responsibility and resources, and the structure and culture of your organization. LEADS' tools, instruments and approaches can help you do that. Everyone involved in both transitions and change—whether they're employees, citizens, patients, or families—need to learn how to embrace change.

The capabilities under the Systems transformation domain show that leaders must clearly understand the dynamics of both large- and small-scale change. These include critical and systems thinking and strategically orienting yourself to the desired future, capabilities which let you outline actions—including supporting innovation and championing and orchestrating change—you'll need to stimulate learning and progress. All of the tools, models, and approaches in Systems transformation stimulate systems and critical thinking so individuals (power of one) and groups (power of working as one) can make choices about where and how change should take place.

Lead self is the personal analogue to Systems transformation. No meaningful change, big or small, can avoid the responsibility of personal change. If we as leaders are asking others to change their behaviour or their mindset as part of a change project, it is incumbent upon us as leaders to model the changes ourselves. The four capabilities comprising this domain—self-awareness, self-management, develop self and demonstrate character—recognize leaders themselves must change. Some of the changes are psychological, making demands on your emotional intelligence, or testing your resolve; others require you to acquire or unlearn knowledge and skills and others put demands on your integrity and character. Leaders who can't meet those demands have diminished ability to champion change. Above all, you need be authentic when you model those capabilities, or your credibility as a leader suffers.

A third component of the model emphasizes the power of relationships to lead change (the short green horizontal arrow in the diagram). Relationship-building comes ahead of tasks in the process of change and both Engage others and Develop coalitions focus on it—Engage others in the operational or inter-personal context and Develop coalitions strategically, within, or between organizations.

Collectively and interactively, the five domains of LEADS address the actions leaders need to take in order to accomplish small or large system change. Consider reviewing the five domains of LEADS as a territory to be traversed; not a linear sequence of actions to be slavishly adhered to. You may wish to revisit certain places because they need your presence, or because they are necessary for you to replenish your own needs.

Simple Rules and Change: A LEADS Approach

Systems thinking gives rise to a phenomenon called simple rules, which are broad principles of change that leaders can use in many different contexts. Simple rules operationalize the concept of concerted action implicit in the practice of distributed leadership [23]. Allan Best and colleagues, in an article called Large-System Transformation in Health Care: A Realist Review, describe studying transformation initiatives to inform change processes in Saskatchewan [24]. They identified simple rules of large-systems transformation they thought were likely to increase the success of the initiatives.

In adapting these findings, and to assist us in distilling the lessons learned so far from putting LEADS to work as a change model, we propose three simple rules of change which, when interpreted and applied according to LEADS, can help leaders determine what to do and how to do it. The three simple rules are shown in Fig. 10.2.

In keeping with the systems construct of interdependency, the three rules interact with each other on an ongoing, fluctuating basis to lead change. These rules work whether you're attempting to change yourself, your unit, your organization, or system. The diagram shows the context at the centre, as practices associated with each of the three rules interact with and are conditioned by context; and the model itself is placed in a broader environment that also interacts with each component of the model. As the first rule of Fig. 10.2 indicates, you must constantly focus your efforts on improving results. You must always come back to two key questions: what results do we need to achieve? How do we align our actions with desired results?

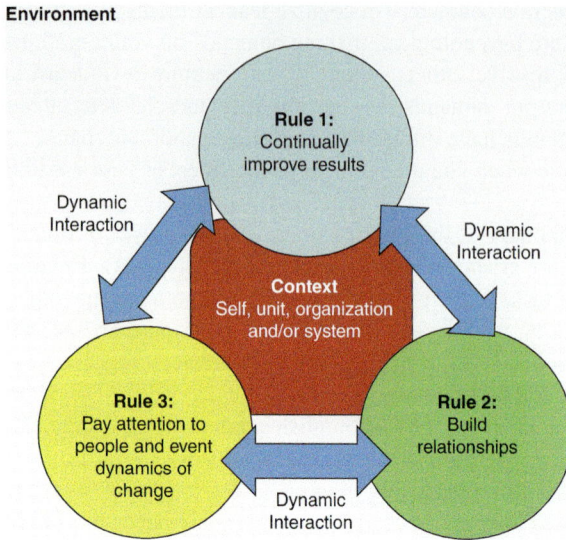

Fig. 10.2 Simple rules for leading change

The second rule is to build trusted relationships. It is through relationships that things get done. The LEADS domains of Engage others (interpersonal relationships) and Develop coalitions (inter-organizational relationships) outline the leadership actions necessary to build those relationships.

The third rule is to pay attention to the people and event dynamics of change. That's because dynamic interplay in a change is always a function of how people react and respond to events, in the larger world or in your change process. These can morph into new and unexpected challenges (Peter's wild cards from Chap. 7), either changing the desired result; or suggesting course corrections to the action plan on how to get there from where you are.

These LEADS change models are custom made by health, for health methods for thinking through and implementing system-wide change: we encourage you to use one of them to make change work. LEADS also provides a set of expectations by which to judge the quality of the change processes, and which could be used to set curriculum for aspiring health leaders. When applied by health care leaders, LEADS guides decision making, policy development and implementation at multiple levels in the system from patient care to system transformation.

Learning Moment
Picture your own workplace or locus of influence. Think about one practice you would like to change, on behalf of patients, families, or the community. Choosing either the five-domain LEADS change model, or the three simple rules approach, outline steps you would take to plan the change (your project).

Consider the following questions:
1. Is your project primarily operational or strategic?
2. In that context, clarify the change gap: the difference between the desired results and the current state of your project. How big a change is it?
3. What systems change implications does the project have? Consequently, what change challenges (unit, department, organization, coalition, system) will you face moving from where you are now to where you want to be?
4. Based on your understanding of the scope and breadth of those external changes, what internal personal challenges will you have to face?
5. Based on how big the change is, who will you need to build relationships with, and why? How will you do it? Are there approaches discussed in the Chap. 6 of this book (Engage others) that would help you build those relationships?

Putting LEADS to Work as a Change Leadership Model: Three Case Studies

Three success stories showcase how LEADS can and is being used by health leaders to lead change, not just react to what the health system is delivering in terms of challenges. Rather than follow either one of the two LEADS models of change directly, each leader has adapted them to context and improved them through their own thinking.

Nadine's Story: Context Is King

Our first case study comes to us from the Canadian province of Newfoundland and Labrador. The context is that in 2006 the government of the day decided to merge eight separate health care organizations into one to form Eastern Health. This regional authority serves the capital city of St. John's and the surrounding rural areas on the Avalon Peninsula. It also provides tertiary care services for the province.

After two years working on the consolidation of management and "back office" functions, the attention of the CEO and the senior team turned to a multi-pronged leadership development strategy. Nadine Whelan, initially as a member of the Organizational Development team and later as the head of the Leadership Development team, identified early on the need to build the strategy around a common framework which eventually turned out to be the LEADS framework. Here's her story.

As Nadine quickly found out, the most difficult obstacle to overcome in any post-merger integration process is the clash of cultures. And, as with any successful leadership development strategy, sponsorship from the top was key. Nadine also recognized that the pace of change and level of complexity in a large forming organization presented challenges to everyone's leadership, including her own. Nadine reflected on her own commitment from a Lead Self *perspective: This is going to be a long journey…what is my vision for this work?*

Nadine also recognized that she had her own values and beliefs about leadership and change and was still working through her own transition to the new organization. She turned to her colleague, Joseé, who was working on an employee engagement and culture strategy. Being strategic systems thinkers, they both saw this work as interconnected and recognized that engaging others and building leadership capacity were critical to success. They also knew that certain results articulated in the organization's strategic and operational plans needed to be achieved and enriched by a broader systems perspective. These results revolved around the triple aim objectives of better health, better care and a better bottom line for the people of Newfoundland and Labrador. "What if, we use LEADS to help us?" Nadine asked.

Against conventional wisdom in change leadership, they took a "middle out approach," believing that's where the leverage was. A core group of 17 people participated in an internal LEADS facilitator certification program. Using LEADS as a change leadership tool, Nadine and this cross-functional, multi-level "volunteer army" [20] formed a Leadership Network. They used the LEADS model to scaffold their learning, conversations and shared work; they lived LEADS.

Together, they designed a two-day LEADS learning program with the lofty goal of building leadership capacity through connecting formal leaders and doing workshops on the organization's new strategic plan with the entire team of 650 managers. To support this action learning, Nadine designed a set of "LEADS Change Planning" adaptive leadership questions under each domain to be used by the facilitators to help leaders frame and reframe their change challenges. Workshop by workshop over a two-year period, they fostered a leadership community dedicated to co-creating positive change in the health system.

Throughout this process of change, Eastern Health experienced a series of unforeseen external shocks or crises. There was a crisis over botched breast cancer screening, followed not long after by another public review involving child welfare services which led to leadership changes, but the experiment with LEADS-based change continued. While the new CEO and senior leadership team were occupied with operational issues and rebuilding trust and confidence, Nadine and the growing informal LEADS change team continued the process of engagement in an organic way, working through and with "mavens" or key influencers throughout Eastern Health and, importantly, at every level of the system.

Nadine reflected with Joseé upon the journey and lessons in change leadership. They agreed that in many ways, the change process resembled the diffusion of innovation theory [25], with early adopters being essential for testing the concept and engaging others. They recalled how the leadership network was essential in bridging formal and informal change approaches, each member playing an important role in helping people understand LEADS and putting it to work in nuanced contexts. One member, Cathy, was critical at first but eventually became an artful practitioner of Systems Transformation and key to helping leaders integrate LEADS with Lean and other improvement science methods.

"Building relationships and aligning with organizational directions is critical to success in shifting contexts," Nadine said. "You really need to have the contextual agility to identify the change levers, agents and partners. When a new CEO came in with an engagement platform, we had matured our LEADS-based practices and integrated to a point that we were able to step into a new place and meet emergent leadership challenges. Developing coalitions internally provided a solid foundation for advanced leadership and organizational development and, eventually, building a strategic alliance in growing leadership capacity across the province."

Reflecting on the broader lessons in Nadine's story, we see LEADS's three simple rules at play. The expected results were clear: merge eight organizations into one, do it seamlessly from a patients' perspective, guided by IHI's triple aim. Leveraging up existing trusted relationships (Josee) and building new ones (Cathy) became key to delivering on the desired results despite several wild cards (the cancer screening crisis and the new CEO). Nadine and the Eastern Health team made unanticipated adjustments along the way to keep the change process relevant and embedded the management deliverables the CEO and board were looking for in the LEADS change process. The story also underscores the need to balance change leadership with change management, as Kotter has suggested, which often means ensuring that the urgent (management issues such as dealing with the cancer screening crisis) don't crowd out the important (strategic issues around the merger, for example). One of the biggest lessons from Nadine's story is that "culture is king." When applying the LEADS pyramid of change, we need to remind ourselves of the adage: "culture eats strategy for breakfast."

Nadine's story testifies to the resiliency of both the LEADS model of change and of Nadine and her leadership team. She worked to establish a critical mass for change (her leadership network) and built momentum for the LEADS approach to change. Nadine has since moved on from Eastern Health. Like Collin's flywheel, however, LEADS is now embedded in Eastern Health as a vehicle for leadership development and systems change. This case study also supports the general observation that before you can effectively embrace LEADS as a change model, key team leaders must internalize the LEADS framework.

Finally, out of this process Nadine and her team also developed a change guide that continues to guide them through ongoing system and structural change (see Fig. 10.3).

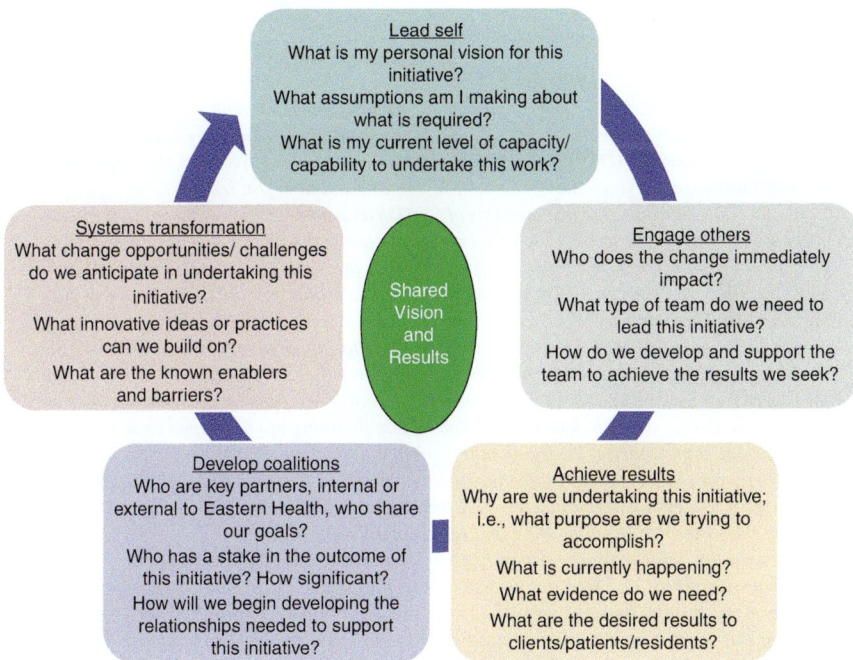

Fig. 10.3 Eastern Health's leadership of change framework as adapted from the LEADS model by Nadine Whelan (with permission)

The Eastern Health model provides leaders with questions to answer as they engage in change, a classic systems approach to change.

You are invited by Nadine—and us—to consider other questions that might populate the LEADS change planning approach used by Nadine and her team.

Hamilton Health Sciences Centre: The Drip Method of Leading Change

Our second case study on putting LEADS to work as a change leadership model is from Hamilton Health Sciences (HHS). HHS is a large academic health science centre in Southern Ontario, with over 15,000 staff, physicians, volunteers and researchers in 10 locations. It's affiliated with one of Canada's 17 medical schools, at McMaster University.

Hamilton Health Sciences was an early adopter of the LEADS framework dating back to 2009, initially sparked by a succession planning imperative. Early on, the two architects of the LEADS journey at Hamilton Health Sciences—Sandra Ramelli and Kathryn Adams—recognized that system change does not come through an orchestrated, top-down plan. In their words: "There are no big bang solutions. Our approach is more like a dripping tap that accumulates a significant amount of water over time: what we call, the 'Drip Method' of leading change." Here is their story of putting LEADS to work as a change model by the installment plan.

LEADS as a change model was not intuitive for Sandra and Kathryn in the beginning. In retrospect, however, LEADS did help guide them as a change leadership tool. Sandra's aha! moment came when she realized: We are the instruments of our success as leaders. As one learns more about LEADS, the framework becomes more intuitive and the capabilities become hard wired in you—they become who you are and how you lead.

While HHS didn't use the five domains of LEADS as a holistic change model in the beginning, our approach was to engage in incremental change using the LEADS domains as a guide. For example, LEADS as a philosophy preaches that who you are gets expressed in the way you behave as a leader. That gave us the confidence that we could lead our way. Also, the distributed leadership philosophy helped us to realize we can't create change without our people being engaged and empowered to actually lead the change with us. The Lead self domain was also an inspiration for us as it underscores that we are the instruments of our own success as leaders and, if we are committed to change, we can enhance and advance our ability to lead. Our work in developing a succession planning model helped us to recognize the value and importance of engaging others when leading change. Once we saw the advantages there, we saw the potential of engaging our people to help build an organization-wide program for leadership development with LEADS as the foundation. Gradually, drip by drip by drip, the water was accumulating and LEADS took hold.

We used the Achieve results capabilities to focus and clarify the results we were looking for. What was our vision? Why are we wanting to shift leadership? Part of the vision was to transform the system. Because we were an organization that was changing--we were transforming our system to a people-centred care model—we needed to change our culture, reaching beyond our walls. Leaders inside and outside our organization became the change agents. We realized we couldn't do this alone. How are we going to build the relationships that we need both internally and externally? Here's where we drew on the Develop coali-

tions capabilities. We realized that if LEADS was our foundation, we had to lead using it and we had to get others to lead, using it, with us.

One of the changes that came from this work was the creation of a Centre for People Development that opened in 2015. It now has oversubscribed programs to develop leaders. The guiding principle is that there is a "leader in every chair." Anyone in the organization who aspires to be a leader can learn what they need to create the change we agree we are collectively pursuing. Now, from a Systems transformation perspective, we see the Centre for People Development as just one important piece in the larger picture of transformation at HHS. We have since coupled overall strategy with leadership; it is part of our success formula. We are showing the value of developing better leaders in terms of achieving our organization's strategic priorities. This is one of the reasons that our CEO champions this work. Developing a LEADS based culture is our true north: you have to live LEADS. When it becomes internalized, we will have changed HHS together. This story can be told in a myriad of ways. We are living LEADS. We now embody it. It's inside us. You don't change who you are at 5 p.m.

We found so many aspects of this story, and the way in which it was told by Sandra and Kathryn, inspiring. While they didn't use the five domains of LEADS in the beginning, their "drip by drip" approach has been successful. In terms of conducting an after-action review against the three simple rules, while the initial impetus for change came from a succession planning imperative, over time it evolved. And, as it evolved, Sandra and Kathryn were successful in building relationships within Hamilton Health Sciences and within the broader health care community.

What was critically important to their success was engaging physician leaders. It started with engaging individual physicians. What started as a trickle, drop by drop, has now translated into physicians being passionate about LEADS and has translated into significant physician participation in leadership development programs offered by the Centre for People Development.

Advancing Psychological Health in the Workplace

For a third case study in putting LEADS to work as a change leadership model we turn to what is being done across Canada to advance psychological safety in the workplace. As adults, we spend more waking hours on average at work than at home or anywhere else [26]. About 30% of all short and long-term disability claims are now for mental health problems and illnesses. Taking a mental health day has gone from being a last-minute day off work to a serious and growing reality of the workplace. The health care sector is anything but immune from this growing challenge. "Staff working in the health care sector are more likely to miss work due to mental illness or disability than people in all other sectors. They face higher rates of burnout, compassion fatigue and sleep deprivation that can affect their psychological health and safety and the safety of their patients" [27].

To address this challenge the Mental Health Commission of Canada developed the National Standard for Psychological Health in the Workplace (the Standard) [28]. The Standard, which is the first in the world, is built around 13 psychosocial factors that can affect the mental health of employees and patients in the workplace.

Building on a strong track record of working together to advance the mental health agenda in Canada more generally, the CEO of the Mental Health Commission and the former CEO of HealthCare*CAN* (one of your co-authors representing Canadian hospitals and regional authorities) shared a common concern about the slow uptake of the Standard in health care workplaces. They agreed to form an issue-specific, time-limited alliance called the "By Health, For Health Collaborative" to help speed it up. They turned to the LEADS framework and one of your two co-authors to help frame a joint action plan.

Here's how LEADS was put to work as a change model to develop a seven-step change management process for accelerating implementation of the Standard in Canadian health care workplaces. The first step in the process was to map the 20 capabilities that comprise the LEADS framework against the 13 action-oriented, psychosocial factors that make up the Standard.

It became clear the factors that make up the Standard aligned very well with the LEADS capabilities, perhaps not surprising, given the emphasis LEADS puts on healthy workplaces and the acknowledgement in the Standard of the importance of leadership. For example, the Centre for Addiction and Mental Health in Toronto used LEADS and the Standard to develop a 360-assessment tool for their leaders that marries LEADS and the Standard to generate the 360 questionnaire [29].

After the mapping exercise, LEADS was used to develop a seven-step process to help health care and other organizations adopt the Standard (*see* Fig. 10.4).

As in the case of the two previous case studies, step one in applying LEADS as a model of change is to develop a clear consensus on what success looks like: in this case creating psychologically safe workplaces (vision and desired results: how will you measure success?) The second step is to assess the current state to determine the leadership gap, using meaningful metrics for the desired result and for monitoring progress. Step three is to ask those leading the change to look in the mirror to ensure they are modelling behaviour consistent with the Standard: can you lead the project if you yourself are psychologically unhealthy? Step four is essentially to put together your guiding team. Step five is ensuring that you are backing up the plan with the resources necessary to execute it. Step six reflects the reality that no organization is an island and the need therefore to work with community organizations, the regional authority or local networks to reinforce adherence to the Standard. And, finally, step seven is to recognize that the Standard is just one, albeit important part of creating a psychologically safe work environment. Laws, regulations, policies, practice and protocols can either help or hinder implementation of the Standard. This is where systems thinking is integral to success in achieving desired results.

In keeping with the Eastern Health model presented earlier, each of the seven steps of this model has a set of guiding questions for the leader. An astute leader will also note—contrary to our earlier statement that linear change models are not the best—this approach is expressed as a seven-step approach, suggesting linearity. However, once initiated, leaders will find themselves moving from one step to another not necessarily in a straight line, but iteratively relative to the needs of the change process. The seven steps are more an intellectual planning approach to help conceptualize the various challenges and see the journey holistically. Once embarked on the journey, you may have to revisit different steps to address new situations, new people, and unexpected events.

Create Vision & Results

What does a psychologically healthy environment look like for your organization? Work with staff at all levels to determine the desired vision.

Assess Current State

You've determined where your organization wants to go, but where are you now? Establishing benchmarks will help to measure progress throughout your journey to implement The Standard.

Prepare Leaders to *Lead Self* through Change

Leader-managers need the opportunity to *'ground'* themselves in the attitudes, beliefs, values and skills needed to be *'authentic'* change agents of psychological health and safety.

Engage Others in Change

Healthy, psychologically safe, and productive interpersonal relationships between workplace colleagues are critical to implementing The Standard.

Use a Systems Approach

Health care is complex in terms of the politics, professions and organizations involved. A broad, systems approach to organizational change is required to appreciate an organization's role within this complex environment.

Engage Stakeholders

Psychological safety and wellness goes beyond individual organization borders—because patients do! Ensuring a psychologically safe work environment ensures that patients receive equal quality care no matter which institution they visit.

Focus on Results

Aligning the limited budget, people resources, and technical expertise in support of efforts to create psychologically healthy workplaces can enhance efficiency and improve productivity.

STEP 1 ↔ STEP 2 · STEP 3 · STEP 4 · STEP 5 · STEP 6 · STEP 7

Using LEADS to create psychologically healthy workplaces.

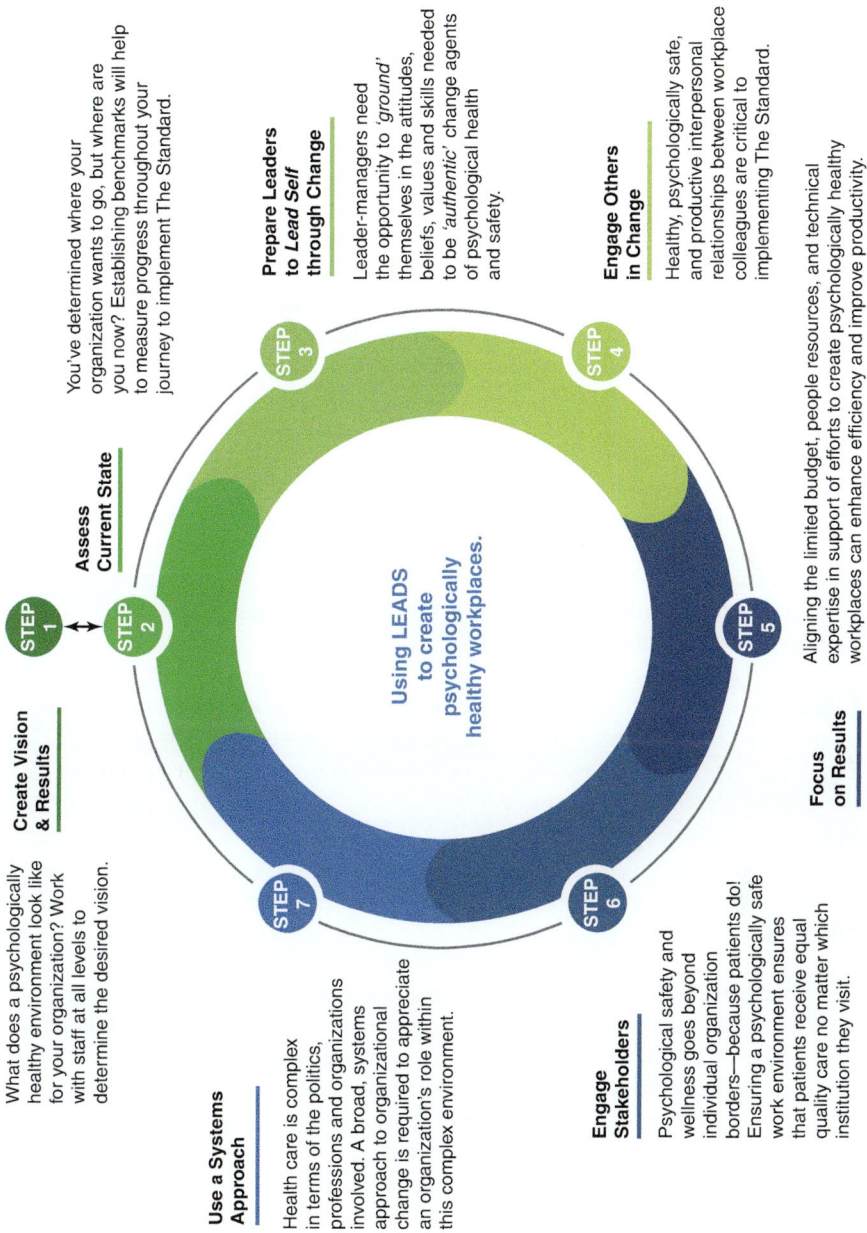

Fig. 10.4 LEADS model to implement psychological health and wellness standards in an organizational context

Three Case Studies: Key Takeaways

Each of these quite different case studies or stories show how the LEADS framework can double as a change model when your put all five domains to work in a holistic, interactive way. LEADS has been used with intention, as in the case of accelerating the uptake of the Standard and Nadine's story. Or, it can be adopted by the installment plan and introduced 'drip by drip' as it was at Hamilton Health Sciences. Don't go into the change process believing that you need to have it all figured out. If you employ LEADS methods, you can learn as you go, relying on others to co-create the desired change with you.

However you choose to use LEADS, either on its own or with other change models, remember the three simple rules of change: be clear about the results you are hoping to achieve; build and sustain relationships with other players; and pay attention to the change dynamics created by events and people you work with. Learn as you go, because nobody has all the answers.

Learning Moment: Healthy Workplaces
Reflect on your own workplace.

1. What evidence do you have, or do you need to have, to assess your organization's efforts to create and sustain a psychologically healthy workplace?
2. Based on that evidence, how healthy is it?

Using one of the change approaches in this chapter, where will you put your efforts to sustain what is working, or to improve what is not?
If not, take the LEADS-base change tool described here and see how you can use it to put the Standard in your workplace.

Summary

To be a good leader is to be good at leading not just managing change. The exercises and stories in this chapter highlight how to use the LEADS framework for that purpose and how important it is for you to see the interdependency of the leadership capabilities in that process. Change is a constant in all health care systems and LEADS can support you as you work with it, by outlining how you need to think and act differently to be a successful change leader.

This chapter describes how change management and change leadership are different. The difference is not determined by the order of magnitude or scale of the change being contemplated, rather by the number of people involved and the complexity of the change. We have reviewed the available literature around complex (non) adaptive systems like health care and how linear or reductionist approaches to change are ill-equipped to address current health care challenges. We see LEADS as a robust change leadership tool because it's intuitive, because it is a by health, for health framework and because it is built on the foundations of good leadership itself. Finally, this chapter features three live case studies of putting LEADS to work as a change leadership model, showing that like any change model, either using it on its own or in combination with other models, it must be adapted by leaders to each unique context for it to be successful.

References

 1. Drucker PF. Managing in turbulent times. London: Routledge; 2015.
 2. Dickson G, Lindstrom R, Black C, Van der Gucht D. Evidence-informed change management in Canadian healthcare organizations. Ottawa, ON: Canadian Health Services Research Foundation; 2012. http://www.cfhi-fcass.ca/Libraries/Commissioned_Research_Reports/Dickson-EN.sflb.ashx. Accessed 20 Jul 2019.
 3. Rosenbaum D, More E, Stane P. Planned organisational change management: forward to the past? an exploratory literature review. J Organ Change Manag. 2018;31(2):286–303.
 4. Al-Haddad S, Kotnour T. Integrating the organizational change literature: a model for successful change. J Organ Change Manag. 2015;28(2):234–62.
 5. Antwi M, Kale M. Change management in healthcare: literature review. Kingston: The Monieson Centre, Queens School of Business; 2014.
 6. Khaira M. Best practice leadership competencies for effective change management in Island Health. National health leaders conference [unpublished paper]. Toronto, ON: Island Health Authority; 2019. p. 41.
 7. Salem-Schatz S, Ordin D, Mittman B. Guide to after action review. Version 1.1: Center for Evidence Based Management; 2010. https://www.cebma.org/wp-content/uploads/Guide-to-the-after_action_review.pdf. Accessed 28 Aug 2019.
 8. Mintzberg H. Simply managing. San Francisco, CA: Barrett-Koehler; 2014.
 9. Dickson G. Health reform in Canada: enabling perspectives for health leadership. Healthc Manage Forum. 2016;2016:1–6.
10. Collins J. Turning the flywheel: a monograph to accompany good to great. New York, NY: Harper Business; 2019.
11. Braithwaite J, Churruca K, Long J, Ellis LA, Herkes J. When complexity science meets implementation science: a theoretical and empirical analysis of systems change. BMC Med. 2018;16:63.
12. University of Victoria. Complexity science in brief. Victoria, BC: University of Victoria; 2012. https://www.uvic.ca/research/groups/cphfri/assets/docs/Complexity_Science_in_Brief.pdf. Accessed 19 Aug 2019.
13. Miles A. Complexity in medicine and healthcare: people and systems, theory and practice. J Eval Clin Pract. 2019;15(3):409–10.
14. Dumas C, Beinecke RH. Change leadership in the 21st century. J Organ Change Manag. 2018;31(4):867–76.
15. Kotter J. Change management vs change leadership – what's the difference. 2012. Place unknown Video: 5 min, 4 sec. https://www.youtube.com/watch?v=2ssUnbrhf_U. Accessed 28 Aug 2019.
16. Kanter RM. Evolve!: succeeding in the digital culture of tomorrow. Boston, MA: Harvard Business Press; 2001.
17. MacLeod H. Humanizing leadership. Vancouver: Friesen Press; 2019.
18. DeGroote MG. Health Leadership Academy. Preparing for the alternative futures for health: why navigating the disruptive forces of healthcare require transformational leadership. Hamilton, ON: McMaster University; 2019. https://healthleadershipacademy.ca/files/2019/04/Alternative-Futures-of-Health.pdf. Accessed 29 Aug 2019.
19. Kotter JP. A sense of urgency. Boston, MA: Harvard Business Press; 2008.

20. Galloppin L. The giant misunderstanding on burning platforms. Online magazine for organizational change practitioners. 2011. http://www.reply-mc.com/2011/01/17/the-giant-misunderstanding-on-burning-platforms/. Accessed 19 Jul 2013.
21. Kotter J. Leading change: why transformation efforts fail. Harv Bus Rev. 1995;1995:59–67.
22. Bridges W. Bridges transition model. London: MindTools; 2019. https://www.mindtools.com/pages/article/bridges-transition-model.htm. Accessed 29 Aug 2019.
23. Currie G, Lockett A. Distributing leadership in health and social care: concertive, conjoint or collective? Int J Manag Rev. 2011;13:286–300.
24. Best A, Greenhalgh T, Lewis S, Saul J, Carroll S, Bitz J. Large-system transformation in health care: a realist review. Milbank Q. 2012;90(3):421–56.
25. Lidblad J. A review and critique of Rogers' diffusion of innovation theory as it applies to organizations. Org Dev J. 2003;21(4):50–64.
26. Mental Health Commission of Canada. What's the issue? Ottawa, ON: Mental Health Commission of Canada; 2019. https://www.mentalhealthcommission.ca/English/what-we-do/workplace. Accessed 23 Aug 2019.
27. Dickson G. Transforming healthcare organizations. Healthier workers. Healthier leaders. Healthier organizations. Ottawa, ON: Mental Health Commission of Canada; 2018. https://www.mentalhealthcommission.ca/sites/default/files/2018-11healthcare_crosswalk_eng.pdf. Accessed 23 Aug 2019.
28. Canadian Standards Association (CSA) in Association with the Mental Health Commission of Canada. Psychological health and safety in the workplace—prevention, promotion, and guidance to staged implementation. Ottawa, ON: Canadian Standards Association (CSA) in Association with the Mental Health Commission of Canada; 2013. https://www.csagroup.org/documents/codes-and-standards/publications/CAN_CSA-Z1003-13_BNQ_9700-803_2013_EN.pdf. Accessed 20 Jan 2019.
29. Dickson G. Mapping the national standard for psychological health and safety in the workplace to the LEADS in a Caring Environment capabilities framework [unpublished commissioned report]. Mental Health Commission of Canada: Ottawa, ON; 2018. https://www.mentalhealthcommission.ca/sites/default/files/2018-11/healthcare_crosswalk_eng.pdf.

Putting LEADS to Work in Canada and Abroad

11

Graham Dickson, Donald J. Philippon, Kelly Grimes, and Brenda Lammi

> *To us, LEADS means learning by example. The framework provides opportunities to heighten teamwork and, most importantly, cultivate collaborative partnerships with patients, families, and communities.*

Michelle Gilchrist[1]

Introduction

How leadership is understood and practised and how LEADS is put to work depends on context. To understand how LEADS is used and its potential for growth in Canada, we decided to examine both its evolution in the Canadian context and in

---

[1] Personal Communication, Gilchrist, M. Sun Country Health Region, Saskatchewan, 2017.

Don Philippon, Ph.D., is a former deputy minister of health and founding co-chair of Canadian Health Leadership Network; Kelly Grimes is its executive director of Canadian Health Leadership Network; and Brenda Lammi is vice-president, professional and leadership development, with responsibility for LEADS Canada, at the Canadian College of Health Leaders.

G. Dickson
Royal Roads University, Victoria, BC, Canada
e-mail: graham.dickson@royalroads.ca

D. J. Philippon
University of Alberta, Parkland County, AB, Canada
e-mail: don.philippon@ualberta.ca

K. Grimes (✉)
Canadian Health Leadership Network, Ottawa, ON, Canada
e-mail: kgrimes@chlnet.ca

B. Lammi
Canadian College of Health Leaders, Ottawa, ON, Canada
e-mail: blammi@cchl-ccls.ca

© Springer Nature Switzerland AG 2020
G. Dickson, B. Tholl (eds.), *Bringing Leadership to Life in Health: LEADS in a Caring Environment*, https://doi.org/10.1007/978-3-030-38536-1_11

four countries with which Canada shares a similar system of government: Australia, England, Scotland and New Zealand. Our comparator countries also have universal health care, but how it's administered differs in each one, resulting in different approaches to adopting and using health leadership frameworks. This analysis offers lessons for Canada and comparator countries.

This chapter has three sections. In the first section "What Happened: Putting LEADS to work nationally in Canada," we look at the efforts to catalyze leadership development and talent management nationally since 2014. The second section, "Lessons for Canada from Comparator Countries," starts with a description of efforts to implement leadership development and talent management—using national frameworks or not—in Australia, England, Scotland and New Zealand. We then distill some lessons for Canada from their efforts. In the third section, "Next Steps: Where to from Here," we outline where we think Canada's national efforts should head. This includes further deepening and broadening our understanding of spread processes implicit in the Systems transformation domain of LEADS.

What Happened: Putting LEADS to Work Nationally in Canada

Since the first edition of this book was published in 2014, significant efforts have been made across Canada to further embed leadership development, practice, and talent management across the country—primarily through the LEADS framework (see Chap. 3). We have not defined leadership talent management before: Talent management goes beyond our primary focus, leadership development, to include activities aimed at improving overall leadership capacity, such as succession planning, hiring practices and performance assessment.

Efforts to catalyze a national leadership development and talent management initiative in Canada have been spearheaded by coalitions of health organizations working together to improve leadership capacity, stewarded by two organizations: the Canadian Health Leadership Network (CHLNet) and the Canadian College of Health Leaders (CCHL). Since 2014 the two organizations have been working together through the LEADS Collaborative, a loose national coalition aimed at engaging their individual organizational members in a national strategy to develop health leadership talent management based on LEADS. It is important to know the role and function of the co-sponsors to better understand how LEADS has taken root across Canada.

The Canadian Health Leadership Network (CHLNet)

Let's first look at CHLNet's role. As an informal network of national and provincial organizations, CHLNet has taken on a catalytic leadership role [1]. Health workforce issues pertaining to health care leaders and managers laid the foundation for CHLNet, which was officially established in 2009·[2, 3]. Its mission is: "Working together to create value and grow leadership capacity across Canada" [4].

From the outset the work of CHLNet has been guided by two key principles: to be a coalition of the willing, meaning there is no compulsion to join; and leadership without ownership, which means the partners recognize no one organization owns leadership development, and the partners agree to share their efforts. These principles generated interest among a broad range of organizations and the membership began to grow. To be a part of this value network, partners must agree to embrace LEADS or a LEADS-compatible framework as a leadership platform for their own organization and promote the framework. Trust and reciprocity remain the twin pillars of its success.

Sustaining early momentum in the network was an ongoing challenge [5] and continues to be. With a minimal administrative budget, the executive director—working with an engaged secretariat drawn from the membership (similar to a working board)—has developed an action-oriented, inclusive agenda involving many leaders from across Canada. Almost 10 years later, 12 founding organizations have expanded to over 40 network partners. The vision for CHLNet remains the same: "*Better Leadership, Better Health—Together*" [6]. Members include governments, academic institutions, health associations, regional health authorities, patients' organizations, and health disciplines groups from many jurisdictions [6].

CHLNet's work has built and continues to evolve around three value streams: one, connecting people through dialogue and engagement; two, advancing health leadership research, knowledge and evaluation; and three, accelerating leadership practices and capabilities. Its value streams and many deliverables in the work plan use LEADS (or LEADS-compatible frameworks) as their foundation (see Table 11.1) to encourage use of a common leadership vocabulary across the country. CHLNet initiatives have evolved through a series of working groups, made up of decision makers and academics, who oversee specific projects to enhance leadership capacity for health reform. For example, a 2014 CHLNet's Benchmarking Group report [7] provided a window into health leadership across the county and identified a significant skills deficit, which formed the basis of the *Canadian Health Leadership Action Plan* [8]. This study is being updated for release in early 2020 (see below). The strategic plan, aimed at improving health system performance, reflected an innovative and collaborative approach to change leadership, consisting of five pillars:

- Create a collective vision.
- Establish a common leadership platform (such as LEADS).
- Gather more evidence on innovations and leading practices.
- Enhance capacity and capabilities.
- Measure and evaluate success.

Table 11.1 CHLNet value streams and primary deliverables

Value stream	Deliverables
1. Connecting People through Dialogue and Engagement	• Semi-annual network partner roundtables and leadership dialogues • Leadership top ten reading lists • Eblasts and webinars on leadership topics
2. Advancing Health Leadership Research, Knowledge and Evaluation	• Research and evaluation working group; Leadership Development Impact Toolkit • Toolkit on wise practices for leadership development • Partner on research grants such as: Status of Women empowering women leaders • Benchmarking study to examine extent of health leadership gap in Canada • Plain language briefs
3. Accelerating Leadership Practices and Capabilities	• Canadian Health Leadership Action Plan • LEADS as a common leadership platform • LEADS Collaborative structure to represent the needs of network partners and refresh the evidence and content of the LEADS framework • Health leadership exchange and acceleration working group in which members share leadership talent management needs, best practices, and innovations.

In 2019, benchmarking data was gathered to gauge progress in building leaders. Some of the survey data is organized according to LEADS capabilities. (Some early results are presented later in this chapter.)

Another significant CHLNet project is the Leadership Development Impact Toolkit. CHLNet member organizations placed a priority on assessing the impact of leadership development because it came up in many discussions with governments and other organizations. The toolkit, launched in 2019, was based on a systematic review of the literature [9] and designed by a steering group of experts (the Return on Investment Steering Group that included academics, advisors, and a representative from Return on Investment Canada). Engaged partners provided funding for a pilot study of three organizations [10]. The toolkit's systematic approach uses a four-step process: laying the foundation, assessing outcomes, evaluating impact and determining the rate of return on investment. The intention is to create a registry of shared impact measures across the country.

Canadian College of Health Leaders and LEADS Canada

The Canadian College of Health Leaders' vision is "Advancing leadership, shaping health systems" and its mission is "To develop, promote, advance and recognize excellence in health leadership." It is a not-for-profit organization with a voluntary membership of individual health leaders, as well as corporate members. It is stewarded by a CEO reporting to an elected board of directors. In 2012, the Canadian College of Health Leaders (CCHL) purchased a majority share of the intellectual property rights to the LEADS framework [11]. Its role in the LEADS Collaborative is to encourage the use of the LEADS framework as a common vocabulary for national leadership development, and to provide a certification process to recognize individual leaders who are proficient in LEADS.

In 2013 CCHL established a not-for-profit business arm, LEADS Canada, to help protect the integrity of the LEADS framework and to provide support to health organizations across the country who were interested in using the framework as a foundation for their own leadership talent management efforts. LEADS Canada's function is to market the framework, develop tools, control licensing and deliver related educational and developmental services through accredited facilitators, consultants and coaches. Working in a non-profit, sole-source model, LEADS Canada's approach to leadership talent management has been to contract or partner with health organizations to co-create LEADS-based leadership development programs and other talent management tools. The intent of LEADS Canada's suite of business lines is to work with health organizations to increase individual leadership and organizational capacity by utilizing practices such as: LEADS-based succession planning, generating positive cultural change, and taking organizations from dysfunctional or compliant cultures to sustainable, generative cultures in which distributed leadership and staff engagement flourish.

Another component of the Canadian College of Health Leaders' national strategy is to offer individuals who have demonstrated health leadership capability the Certified Health Executive (CHE) credential. In 2019, the credential was overhauled to reflect the uptake and distribution of LEADS across Canada. The revised version, called CHE Select [12], increased its standards by requiring people pursuing the credential to have formal LEADS-based leadership development learning, a LEADS 360 assessment, and a debriefing with an executive coach, in addition to a leadership development plan and LEADS in Action project. As LEADS is fully incorporated in the content and requirements for completing the Certified Health Executive credential, it will contribute to building a common leadership language across health systems in Canada. The Canadian Society of Physician Leaders also offers a LEADS-based credential for physician leaders, called the Canadian Certified Physician Executive (CCPE) (more on this in Chap. 15).

These approaches reflect the original approach to building a LEADS-based talent management system that began in British Columbia in 2006 and continues today.

Putting LEADS to Work in British Columbia

British Columbia's health authorities have used LEADS since its inception in 2006. Indeed, without their support, there would not have been a LEADS framework to be chosen as the leadership talent management framework by multiple organizations in BC and across Canada.

The BC health authorities' LEADS talent management is guided by the BC Health Authority Leadership Development Collaborative and individual organizational development practitioners in each authority. Administrative and strategic support for the BC Collaborative is provided by the Provincial Health Services Authority.

The BC Collaborative comprises development practitioners from each of the six health authorities in BC, who meet regularly to determine how to use LEADS for common programming—though each retains the ability to use it in their own way locally to respond to needs in their authority.

Leadership LINX was developed by Provincial Health Services Authority for the Development Collaborative. Leadership LINX is a portal designed to connect leaders across all health authorities in BC.

Leadership LINX offers three provincial programs based on LEADS:

- *Core LINX: A comprehensive leadership and management development program.*
- *Experience LINX: A powerful, experiential leadership development program designed for health care leaders recognized as influential in their organization.*
- *Transforming LINX: A comprehensive seven-month project-based leadership development experience designed specifically for senior health care leaders* [13].

BC's efforts contributed to the creation of the LEADS Collaborative and the transfer of the LEADS intellectual property to the Canadian College of Health Leaders.

The Canadian Health Leadership Network and the Canadian College of Health Leaders continue to endorse the founding principle of "leadership without ownership" and encourage organizations to work together for mutual benefit. "By working with others in the spirit of leadership without ownership, CHLNet has helped coalesce a groundswell of support for a growing set of practical, By Health, For Health leadership tools, all under the banner of the LEADS in a Caring Environment capabilities framework" [14].

For example, LEADS Canada's online Community of Practice, its LEADS Exchange Days (co-sponsored by CHLNet), and CHLNet's sub-committees (Research and Evaluation; Health Leadership Exchange and Acceleration Working Group, see Table 11.2) engage champions from across the country. LEADS Canada, on behalf of the LEADS Collaborative, has made the LEADS framework available to not-for-profit

Table 11.2 LEADS across Canada

	Licensed organizations	LEADS integrated organizations[a]	Ongoing LEADS services	Select LEADS services	Total users
National organizations	4	2	3	2	11
British Columbia		8		3	11
Alberta	3	3	2	2	10
Saskatchewan	1 (provincial)				1
Manitoba	1 (provincial)	9			10
Ontario	6	4	25	13	48
Quebec				4	4
New Brunswick			1		1
Prince Edward Island		1 (provincial)			1
Nova Scotia	1 (provincial)		1		2
Newfoundland & Labrador				4	4
Total	16	27	32	28	103

[a]These organizations are the early adopters of LEADS (e.g., health authorities in BC) which don't have licences or are negotiating one

health organizations in a variety of different ways, as outlined in Table 11.2. In addition, many people in the health system refer to and use the framework in a variety of ways without accessing any specialized services from LEADS Canada.

LeaderShift in Ontario

The LeaderShift [15] project is a cross-sector initiative funded by the Ontario Ministry of Health and Long-Term Care from 2018 to 2020. Its aim is to give leaders in the primary and community care sectors an opportunity to develop their leadership talent, ignite cross-sector collaboration, and play a stronger role in shaping the future of Ontario's health care system. The initiative is being coordinated by the Ontario Community Support Association on behalf of its five member associations comprising Community Health Ontario (a voluntary coalition) and covering three subsectors in the community health: home and community support, addictions and mental health and team and community based primary care.

The project was designed to involve 575 leaders over the two-year period. The Ontario Community Support Association partnered with LEADS Canada to develop a leadership capacity building program based on the LEADS framework. The learning opportunities include a five-day face-to-face learning series focused on LEADS, a moderated community of practice, leadership focused webinars, YouTube videos and an online series of webinars to introduce LEADS. At total of 23 cohorts have been involved so far, averaging around 27 persons each.

In addition to providing direct services, LEADS Canada licenses the use of LEADS and certifies individuals within organizations to build capacity for the sustainability of LEADS without creating dependency on external service providers. The purpose of licensing and certification is to ensure integrity of the application and integration of LEADS [16]. (An example of a licensing agreement is outlined below in a vignette provided by HealthCare*CAN*).

Putting LEADS to Work: CHA Learning

HealthCareCAN is the national voice of health care organizations and hospitals across Canada. Its goal is to improve the health of Canadians through an evidence-based and innovative health care system. An example of the power of LEADS Canada partnering, is CHA Learning (a division of HealthCareCAN) [17].

In 2014 CHA Learning negotiated a licence from LEADS Canada to use the framework and has been integrating elements of LEADS into its online learning programs, where it uses LEADS as its leadership language and as the framework on which to build the competencies it develops.

For example, in 2016, CHA Learning published Leading from the Boardroom: Bringing "LEADS in a Caring Environment" to Canadian Healthcare Boards [18]. In 2017, it launched an innovative course called Change Leadership Certificate, built on LEADS.

The partnership between LEADS Canada and CHA Learning shows the framework can work for both individuals and organizations.

The Impact of LEADS

What impact is LEADS having across Canada? Measuring the impact of leadership development on the actual behaviour of leaders or on culture and system performance is a complex task. The King's Fund distinguishes between impact on leader development and on leadership development: the former is focused on individuals and the latter on the health system [19].

We have the benefit of three studies providing some insights into the impact of LEADS 1. A pan-Canadian qualitative study looking at the impact of LEADS on an organization, referred to here as the LEADS Impact study [20], 2. The evaluation of the LeaderShift program in Ontario [21], and 3. preliminary results from the 2019 CHLNet Benchmarking study.

LEADS Impact Study

The LEADS Impact Study 2014-2016, funded by Mitacs (a network linking industry and post-secondary institutions) and CCHL, was conducted by a team of researchers and gathered information from five organizations across Canada [20]. The study provides insights and conclusions on the impact of LEADS at the individual level, on organizational functioning and on health systems achievement.

Its key findings:

- At the individual level, the LEADS framework was empowering and enabling by helping to address challenges and priorities, providing a common language that facilitates multidisciplinary collaboration, offering a framework teams can use to work together to address specific tasks and strategic goals, increasing communication effectiveness, and enabling professional development and succession planning.
- At the organizational level, the study found the LEADS framework helps build trust by encouraging reflection and collaboration; assists managers in engaging and guiding their teams, supports succession planning and provides motivation to build positive feedback systems to enable systems change.
- At the systems level, the study found LEADS provides a flexible framework to achieve change, fosters innovation by enabling individuals to link their ideas to strategic objectives, helps achieve strategic health priorities by linking each individual's tasks to priorities through personal professional planning, performance assessments, and reporting and provides a language for senior leaders to connect with all staff.

Evaluation of the LeaderShift Project

The LeaderShift Project in Ontario described in the previous section—using LEADS as the foundation for the curriculum—was extensively evaluated for its impact. The evaluation included individual self-assessments and follow-up interviews with organizations and participants six months later. The self-assessment ratings on how confident participants feel about their own capabilities in each of the LEADS domains before and after the five-day learning session show clear gains on all five LEADS domains, but particularly with Lead self and Engage others domains (Fig. 11.1).

Preliminary findings from the follow-up interviews with employers of LeaderShift graduates indicate they are seeing positive changes in behaviour from people in the course, who appear more confident and strategic. This has had positive spillover effects in their organizations, inspiring others to be more strategic as well. Employers said LeaderShift graduates work more collaboratively and are taking on larger or more complex projects compared to before the training [21].

CHLNet Benchmarking Study (2014–2019)

At the time of writing, only preliminary results are available for CHLNet's 2019 Leadership Benchmark study. Results are mixed, with the use of LEADS increasing on the one hand but significant gaps remaining in terms of the current state of leadership capabilities. The 2019 Benchmarking study builds on a 2014 baseline survey [22], using tracking questions on the use of a leadership framework and to what extent the one being used was LEADS. Early results show 81% of the respondents were using a leadership framework in 2019 as compared to 47% in 2014, and two-thirds in 2019 were using LEADS (see Fig. 11.2). For up-to-date results see: www.chlnet.ca.

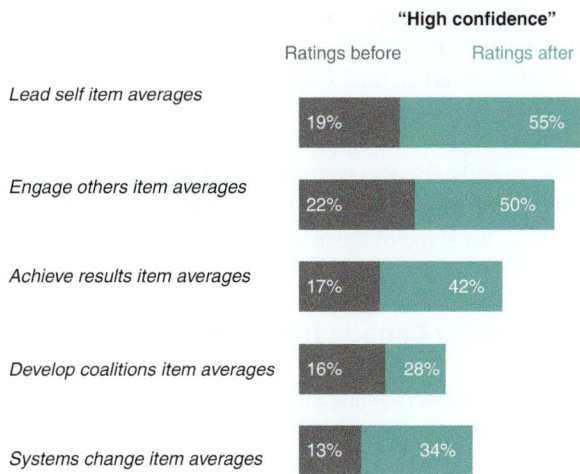

Fig. 11.1 LEADS Capabilities

"High confidence"

Ratings before   Ratings after

Lead self item averages — 19% / 55%

Engage others item averages — 22% / 50%

Achieve results item averages — 17% / 42%

Develop coalitions item averages — 16% / 28%

Systems change item averages — 13% / 34%

Data source: Post-training survey data up to Jan 25, 2019

What is being done?

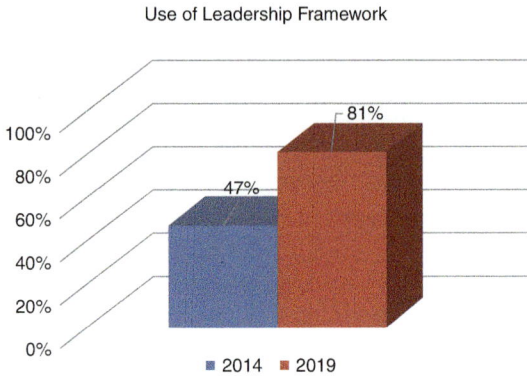

Use of Leadership Framework

Note: 2/3 are using LEADS

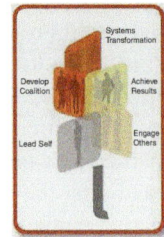

Fig. 11.2 CHLNet benchmarking study: are you using a leadership framework?

In 2019, the three capabilities leaders demonstrate most are: modelling honesty, integrity, resilience, and confidence (from Lead self), contributing to the creation of a healthy organizational culture (from Engage others) and demonstrating a commitment to customers and service (people-centred care) (Develop coalitions). The three capabilities least in evidence were fostering the development of others (Engage others), encouraging and supporting innovation, including the use and of new technology and demonstrating systems and critical thinking (both from Systems transformation) [22].

Taken together, the LEADS Impact Study, the LeaderShift Evaluation Study, and the CHLNet Benchmarking Study attest to how effectively LEADS can be put to work to improve local, provincial, and national leadership. But what else might be done to truly create a national leadership talent management initiative, available to all Canadian health leaders? We explore what is happening in other national jurisdictions for some of those answers.

Lessons for Canada from Comparator Countries [23]

Universal publicly funded health systems, it has been argued, have a particular interest in leadership because they are accountable to the public through their elected leaders to show they are optimizing scarce resources [24]. Accordingly, we thought it would be appropriate to look at other countries with universal, mostly publicly funded systems to compare approaches to improving leadership. We'll discuss what we learned in two stages: first, by outlining their approaches to leadership talent management and second, by suggesting lessons for Canada from these countries.

National Approaches to Leadership Talent Management

Health leadership frameworks fall into two categories. Australia is the only one of the four countries we looked at that uses an analogue of LEADS—Health LEADS Australia—to catalyze a national approach to leadership talent management. New Zealand, NHS England and NHS Scotland each have adopted national approaches to leadership talent management; some with a national framework, some without. Regardless, the emphasis in those jurisdictions in on stimulating leadership development and talent management at the local level.

Australia
The situation in Australia is of special interest to Canada because of its similar large remote and rural areas. A government agency (since dissolved), Health Workforce Australia, signed a licensing agreement to use the Canadian framework to inform the development of Health LEADS Australia. As an agency of government, Health Workforce Australia had resources to implement the framework across the country and the work was endorsed by the Australia Health Minister's Advisory Council—the peak health advisory body in the country. The intent was to follow this up with LEADS based tools and a leadership network similar to CHLNet (Dr. Neale Fong, Personal communication, 2019 Jun 12). However, a major change in political leadership led to Health Workforce Australia being dismantled in 2014 and follow-up work on Health LEADS Australia lost momentum.

The Australasian College of Health Service Management continued support for Health LEADS Australia by endorsing the framework as its leadership capability guide, using it to revamp the College's Master Health Service Management Competency framework. This framework underpins College activities including accrediting health management qualifications in 11 universities across Australia (and one pending in New Zealand), the Health Management Internship Program with over 65 interns at any given point, the Fellowship Program which is offered in Australia, Hong Kong, and New Zealand and in continuing professional development programs. The College is also promoting the LEADS Australia framework in work it's doing with other countries in southeast Asia including delivering programs in leadership, management and governance for hospitals in China, delivering a Health Leadership Program for the Vanuatu Ministry of Health, agreements being developed with Thailand, India, the Philippines and in discussions with the Indonesian College for Healthcare Executives.

Health LEADS Australia is used by organizations across Australia in a variety of ways, but it is not nationally endorsed and is only used extensively by two states: Queensland and South Australia. The Queensland Department of Health developed a 360-degree feedback tool aligned with Health LEADS Australia to use in its clinician leadership programs. The framework is also used by the universities of Melbourne and Tasmania and the National Mental Health Commission.

NHS England and NHS Scotland

The United Kingdom consists of four countries: England, Scotland, Wales and Northern Ireland. Each has its own version of the National Health Service (NHS). We looked only at England and Scotland for this book, because each has its own approach to leadership talent management.

NHS England began building a Leadership Qualities Framework in 2001 with significant work done with several groups of health system leaders, particularly physicians. However, when the government changed in 2010, the Leadership Qualities Framework was replaced with the Healthcare Leadership Model (see Chap. 3). The centralized approach faded away, leaving some of its aspects in place in the NHS Leadership Academy but with a much-reduced mandate.

In England in 2013 the Francis Inquiry report made numerous recommendations to resolve issues of poor care and high death rates revealed by the Stafford Hospital scandal where an investigation by the Healthcare Commission in 2008 found poor care at the hospital between 2005 and 2008 led to as many as 1,200 more patients dying than would have been expected.

One of the Francis report's key recommendation was to improve "support for compassionate caring and committed care and stronger healthcare leadership" [25]. Yet by 2015 little progress seemed to be made in terms of addressing the leadership problems described in the report [26]. Issues of pace-setting leadership (see Chap. 6), an overriding focus on targets and performance, and a preference for top-down management with a command-and-control style, created a feeling among staff "that they were working in an environment that was described overall as 'demotivating'" [26].

In 2016, this led to a resurgence of interest in a national leadership strategy, but with a focus on organizational culture development. While the NHS Leadership Academy still uses the nine-dimension Healthcare Leadership Model to develop leadership in the health care system in England, the current approach allows variation in leadership competency frameworks so they can be in line with the needs of particular groups (Stephen Hart Personal Telephone interview, 2019 April 1). The Academy offers a significant array of programs, both person-to-person and online, to support leadership talent management including National and Local Leadership Academies, coaching and mentoring, board development, and supports for emerging student leaders [27].

Leadership talent management in NHS England also is supported by Health Education England and NHS Improvement. "Health Education England exists for one reason only: to support the delivery of excellent health care and health improvement to the patients and public of England by ensuring the workforce of today and tomorrow has the right numbers, skills, values and behaviours, at the right time and in the right place" [28]. Its most recent mandate statement (2018–2019) says one major focus is to "grow the workforce rapidly, including consideration of additional staff and skills required, build a supportive working culture in the NHS and ensure first rate leadership for NHS staff" [29].

Health Education England works with the NHS Leadership Academy and NHS Improvement to support leadership talent management. NHS Improvement emphasizes the importance of leadership at all levels to champion culture change and clinical improvement [30]. The NHS Leadership Academy will become part of it in 2019–2020 to "create a systematic and considered approach to talent management and development for all staff" [29]. From the perspective of the leadership capabilities needed to create transformational large-scale change, NHS Horizons, a small, specialist team within the Strategy and Innovation Directorate of NHS England, is dedicated to developing the skills and capabilities leaders need [31].

NHS Scotland has more recently developed a national leadership initiative called Project Lift [32]. The program has significant ongoing funding and political support from government and has two unique features. First, it's customizable to individual leader needs, allowing individuals to select areas of leadership to develop. In addition the project's role is to provide tools to complement local and regional Health and Social Care approaches, but not to replace them. The government's role is to provide commonly needed supports only affordable when developed system-wide.

The second unique feature is that it's offered and mediated online through a sophisticated interactive website, rather than through person-to-person programming. The online project's approach to leadership development "is all about fostering and enabling learning *in* practice and *from* practice. It is informed by the concept of 'vertical development,' i.e., helping you to understand and make sense of your context as you develop your capacity to think and act differently" [33]. Interested individuals are linked with an online leadership assessment, and to a suite of multi-professional development opportunities.

Project Lift focuses on six elements of leadership talent management: staff engagement, value-based recruitment, talent management, performance appraisal and leadership development. It starts with a self-assessment and numerous follow-up activities are made available to those who are seen to have leadership potential. Its leadership profile has eight elements: two each under the titles of Ability, Ambition, Values and Insight. These are high level descriptors of the desirable qualities of leadership in NHS Scotland.

New Zealand
New Zealand has had a national health care workforce agency called Health Workforce New Zealand, since 2009. Early in its development a commitment was made to create a national leadership institute, however in the decade since only a centre at the University of Auckland has opened, falling short of the plan to develop a national institute. Health Workforce NZ has steered away from a central framework, choosing instead to focus on culture to bring about organizational change. Its rationale is that a single competency framework could divert attention from critical issues facing a particular group or organization.

International Hospital Federation
In this discussion of international perspectives, it's fitting to note work being done by the International Hospital Federation on the Global Competencies Directory. The Canadian College of Health Leaders and Australasian College of Health Service Management participated in the work, so LEADS and Health LEADS Australia

were among the frameworks shaping the directory [34]. With over 80 capabilities
and more than 20 domains, the directory was intended to advance the professionalization of health care delivery managers anywhere in the world [35]. However, it is
a directory and because of its size and complexity, not something easily supplanting
context-driven national frameworks. Broader talent-management strategies are left
to each individual country.

Lessons from International Comparisons

In all the jurisdictions we looked at, efforts to build the leadership modern health
care demands were the stimuli for developing leadership frameworks and talent
management strategies. We've drawn five lessons from our international comparisons about how to get the most from national leadership frameworks and related
talent management strategies.

1. *Don't rest on your laurels: Deliberately evolve your leadership frameworks and
   related talent management approaches to maintain relevance and impact.*

   Every country's leadership framework was designed to enhance leadership
   skills and abilities to meet the demands of complex, rapidly changing health
   systems. However, awareness of the scope and breadth of the challenge of
   improving leadership to meet those obligations has only recently become clear.
   The three important functions of health leadership—integration of service for
   patients and families; the creation of healthy and productive workplaces so people can deliver optimal service; and successfully implementing desired health
   reform policies and practices that we introduced in Chap. 1– help to define both
   the content of national frameworks and how they are used.

   Originally, one of the motivations for the use by NHS England, Canada and
   Australia of a capabilities framework was to facilitate successful implementation
   of government policy. In the past seven years the reality is that such policy
   changes demand service integration and the creation of healthy workplace cultures to implement them. This circumstance emphasizes the need for distributed
   leadership. For example, the Francis report on the Stafford Hospital scandal in
   the UK identified leadership as a primary factor contributing to the unhealthy
   workplace culture that caused poor patient care. NHS England then developed a
   new version of the NHS framework and how it is to be used. In Canada and
   Australia the imperative to create healthy workplaces and service integration has
   become a priority and different organizations are adapting their talent management strategies accordingly. National frameworks and how they are used must
   therefore continually evolve as our own understanding of the role they and leadership can play in future system development.

   The kind of evolution we're talking about can be seen in how Canada has
   worked to use LEADS in efforts to create psychologically healthy workplaces,
   in how LEADS has been re-interpreted to reflect the values of Indigenous peoples and to address the challenges of offering person-centred care. The national
   health services of both England and Scotland are also engaged in modifying their
   leadership frameworks and their talent management strategies to help shape

healthy workplace cultures. In both instances, processes to engage local leaders in making sense of how the frameworks can help them improve their leadership, and to provide the opportunities to do so, should be co-created with them if grass roots change is to happen.

2. *Frameworks and talent management programs should be designed so grassroots organizations and individuals can feel ownership in them.*

The ultimate goal of a national framework is changing behaviour. If leaders don't change what they do and how they do it, then services don't get integrated, workplaces don't become healthier and new policies aren't implemented. But it's important to note formal leaders can only direct and model behaviour change; the actual change must be created by people much closer to, or actually on, the front lines. That's why leadership frameworks can't just be directed at senior executives; they must also focus on formal and informal leaders at the frontlines of service delivery. If grassroots leaders cannot see what behaviour ought to be changed or believe in the need for change, they are unlikely to change what they do. We call this combination of awareness, belief and willingness to act "ownership." National frameworks and talent management approaches that don't inspire a sense of ownership are a waste of money and effort.

Our knowledge of Canada's LEADS efforts and study of leadership frameworks in the comparator countries shows a sense of ownership can be promoted several ways. The most important thing is to ensure the framework is valid—that it's based on good evidence and makes sense to the organizations and individuals using it. Then work should be done to help the people who use the framework make sense of it, by dedicating the time and effort it takes for them to see its direct relevance to their day-to-day practice. Leadership development programs based on the framework are essential—but they must be understood by organizations and the individuals who participate to be valuable. Use of what people learn in those programs should be promoted by making knowledge transfer an integral part of their design. Finally, talent management approaches, such as succession planning, hiring and performance management should be based on the leadership qualities your framework seeks to instill.

3. *Leadership frameworks must be adapted to the unique national context, but all countries can and should learn from each other.*

Canada, England, Scotland and Australia have developed national strategies for leadership talent management that reflect their political, constitutional, geographic and situational context. For example, the way Canada's constitution divides power over health care has meant there is no broad governmental drive or willingness to build leadership capacity, so grassroots organizations have sprung up to promote leadership development. In Australia, the loss of government support (after initial interest) has undermined efforts to implement Health LEADS Australia nationally. In England and Scotland, central government stewardship of health care has encouraged each country's NHS to develop centralized programs and supports for leadership talent management.

Those variations do not mean the jurisdictions have nothing to learn from each other about maximizing the benefits of leadership development and talent management. Indeed, mobilizing knowledge—one of the capabilities of the LEADS Develop coalitions domain—will stimulate innovation and spread. Canada should reach out to NHS England and Scotland to learn about gaining government support. Australia is already learning about building grass roots support from Canada—and Canada's future work on it, in turn, will likely be influenced by how Australia applies what it learns. England and Scotland could probably learn about how to adapt and adjust national frameworks for local use from Canada and Australia.

4. *Government involvement must be carefully constructed and artfully led.*

Another lesson from our country comparisons is that government stewardship of leadership talent management must be carefully constructed and artfully led. Carefully constructed so it provides resources to support a broad effort and is not seen as a top-down, imposed requirement. Artfully led so the ownership of effort remains in the hands of local leaders.

England's efforts to devolve greater ownership of leadership development to local authorities suggests that its own acknowledged failures in changing leadership behaviour may have been because of a top-down approach. Scotland's online learning strategy, built centrally, but employed locally, appears to have great promise. But withdrawal of government support can also mitigate success: LEADS foundered in Australia when government pulled the plug on funding.

In Canada, governments (national and provincial) played only a limited role with a one-time grant in 2006 providing the initial incentive for organizations in BC to come together [36] and generate action learning strategies for using LEADS, creating early momentum to build support across the country. Since then, government has only provided limited project funding (e.g. to support benchmarking studies Canada's coalition-led approach to leadership talent management—the LEADS Collaborative—has been successful in creating commitment to a common framework, but struggles to maintain funding and support, which the other countries get from government. This weakens Canada's ability to ensure leadership in talent management and development are offered nationwide, minimizes the breadth of what's available and leads to duplicated effort.

5. *Canada should develop more online talent management supports to reach more leaders*

Modern online learning technology and support systems like those in England and Scotland are not fully developed in Canada (due to limited resources). LEADS Canada, HealthCareCAN and CHLNet have online support systems for leadership talent management, but they don't match the level of investment of the sophisticated websites pf NHS England's Leadership Academy, NHS Improvement, Horizons, and Health Education England. Scotland's online material combines the ability to overcome the challenges of reaching people in rural and remote areas with customization that tailors to the needs of each individual.

Using the newest technology could reach more leaders than person-to-person programs. Programs that blend in-person learning with online work may have even more impact. Also, online programs of self-directed learning can reach a national audience, reinforcing shared values and the common vocabulary that LEADS offers.

We believe these five lessons drawn from our international comparisons can accelerate national efforts for system-wide change everywhere.

Next Steps: Where to from Here

There are many important actions for the LEADS Collaborative and its coalition partners to take as they work to strengthen their cross-country initiative to support leadership capacity development and related talent management approaches:

1. *Ensure the LEADS framework and related talent management strategies are refreshed through evidence-based continuous improvement cycles.* The LEADS framework has gone a long way toward creating a common approach for Canadian organizations working to improve leadership. However, it cannot be allowed to grow stale or out of date. The LEADS Collaborative and its partners should use quality-improvement principles to keep LEADS a vibrant model of ideal leadership practice, and maintain efforts to increase its spread and acceptance through the coalition of the willing.
2. *Redouble efforts to get federal government funding and support for LEADS programs and evidence building.* The LEADS Collaborative has made numerous appeals to the federal government and some of the provinces for financial support. Some provincial and territorial governments have stepped up with support for health leadership development. The advantage to federal government action, however, is that providing national supports would move Canada away from local efforts to re-invent leadership and drive the country toward a national, evidence-based leadership development program. In keeping with our earlier lesson from international comparisons, how that support is structured and utilized must continue to facilitate local ownership and action for leadership development and talent management approaches.
3. *Create an international network of experts and resources.* Health Education England has called for an international network of experts and resources to support their health-workforce, leadership development and talent management efforts. An international network would encourage countries to share emerging practices and new knowledge. Canada has begun this effort working through and with the International Leadership Association to build a health leadership community of practice. But a more formal approach to learning and sharing from other national jurisdictions (in research, knowledge mobilization, programming, and online

learning, among other areas) should be pursued. In particular, Canada should explore in greater detail the approaches currently being used in NHS Scotland.

4. *Improve health care through greater leadership support for healthy work-places and engaged workforces.* The LEADS framework encourages leader-ship behaviour that creates healthy, productive workplaces and an engaged workforce (including leaders). This goal is common to all comparator coun-tries because reforming health care systems is a demanding process requiring healthy, committed workers. More efforts to support leaders, clinicians and employees are essential for successful efforts to improve health care.

5. *Begin work to create an integrated national centre for health leadership development.*

One of the most challenging attributes of coalitions is they are hard to sustain over time (see Chap. 8). They either evolve or disappear. The Canadian coali-tion—the LEADS Collaborative and its coalition partners—which is currently stewarding the use of LEADS and providing LEADS supports, needs to consider formalizing its arrangement. Creating a co-funded hub, such as a health leader-ship institute designed to support building leadership capacity across the country, could be a natural evolution for the Collaborative (CHLNet and CCHL). And as we will see in Chap. 16, the foundations for a more professional approach to health leadership is possible.

Summary

As we've seen, while many countries have recognized the importance of improving the quality of leadership in their health care systems, there are many different approaches to achieving that goal. Canada has had good success with LEADS, and can certainly continue on that path, but that's because LEADS was designed to suit the context of a federal system of government that gives much of the power over health care to its provinces and territories. Context also dictates England's central-government support, offered through National Health Service and the variations we've discussed in Scotland, Australia and New Zealand.

That is not to say, however, that LEADS has nothing to offer other countries. Indeed, Australia has based some of its leadership work on LEADS. For example, the relationship between the Canadian Health Leadership Network with its organi-zational membership, and the Canadian College of Health Leaders, which offers credentials to individual leaders, has been fundamental to establishing wide acep-tance of LEADS. Now, the Australasian College of Health Service Management is trying a similar approach, according to its chair, Dr. Neale Fong. Early assessments indicate it's making a difference, particularly in elevating the confidence of leaders to tackle major changes to improve the performance of the system to achieve better health outcomes.

The point is, every country working on developing better health care leaders can learn from others, and efforts to do so should be formalized and jointly supported among nations.

References

1. Tsuchiya K, Caldwell CH, Feudenberg N, Silver M, Wedepohl S, Lachance L. Catalytic leadership in food & fitness community partnerships. Health Promot Pract. 2018;19(1):458–548.
2. Romilly L. Development of a comprehensive situational analysis of human resources and skill needs of Canada's health executive/management sector. Ottawa, ON: Canadian College of Health Service Executives in partnership with the Academy of Canadian Executive Nurses, Canadian Society of Physician Executives, and Human Resources Skills Development Canada; 2005. https://www.cchl-ccls.ca/document/1585/HRD_HumanResourcesSkillNeeds_LornaRomilly_EN.pdf.
3. Da Prat C. Health care leaders and managers in Canada: analysis of the human resource issues and information gaps. Discussion report. Ottawa, ON: Canadian College of Health Service Executives; 2006. https://www.cchl-ccls.ca/document/1583/HRD_HealthCareLeadersCanada_ChristineDaPrat_EN.pdf. Accessed 22 Aug 2019.
4. Canadian Health Leadership Network. Vision and mission. Ottawa, ON: Canadian Health Leadership Network; 2019. https://chlnet.ca/about-us/about-us-vision-mission. Accessed 31 Jul 2019.
5. DAunno T, Hearld L, Alexander JA. Sustaining multistakeholder alliances. Health Care Manage Rev. 2019;44(2):183–94.
6. Canadian Health Leadership Network. Network partners. https://chlnet.ca/about-us/current-network-partners. Accessed 20 Jun 2019.
7. Canadian Health Leadership Network. Canadian health leadership benchmarking report: CHL-Bench. Ottawa, ON: Canadian Health Leadership Network; 2014. http://chlnet.ca/wp-content/uploads/CHLNet-Leadership-Benchmarking-Study-Final-Report.pdf. Accessed 20 Jul 2019.
8. Canadian Health Leadership Network. Closing the gap: a Canadian health leadership action plan. Ottawa, ON: Canadian Health Leadership Network; 2014. https://chlnet.ca/wpcontent/uploads/Canadian-Health-Leadership-Action-Plan.pdf. Accessed 29 Sep 2019.
9. Jeyaraman M, Qadar SMZ, Wierzbowski A, Farshidfar F, Lys J, Dickson G, et al. Return on investment in healthcare leadership development programs. Leadersh Health Serv (Bradf Engl). 2018;31(1):77–97. https://doi.org/10.1108/LHS-02-2017-0005.
10. Canadian Health Leadership Network. Pilot test of the leadership development impact assessment toolkit: final report. Ottawa, ON: Canadian Health Leadership Network; 2019. http://chlnet.ca/login. with authorized username and password. Accessed 20 Aug 2019.
11. Dr. Graham Dickson, the Principal Investigator for the research that created LEADS, owns 25% of the IP and CCHL 75%.
12. Certified Health Executive (CHE) Select Program. Ottawa, ON: Canadian College of Health Leaders; 2019. https://www.cchl-ccls.ca/site/cert_che. Accessed 20 Aug 2019.
13. Leadership LINX Help. Supporting your leadership development. Vancouver: BC: Health Authority Leadership Development Collaborative; 2019. http://help.leadershiplinx.ca/. Accessed 22 Aug 2019.
14. O'Rourke B, Bryden B. CHLNet annual report. Ottawa, ON: Canadian Health Leadership Network; 2011.
15. LeaderShift. The future of health care leadership is here. Toronto, ON: LeaderShift; 2019. https://www.leadershiftproject.ca/. Accessed 19 Aug 2019.
16. LEADS organizational license. LEADS Canada, Canadian College of Health Leaders; 2019. https://leadscanada.net/site/license. Accessed 20 Aug 2019.
17. HealthCareCAN. Ottawa, ON: HealthCareCAN; 2019. http://www.healthcarecan.ca/. Accessed 22 Aug 2019.
18. Dickson G, Waite G. Leading from the boardroom. HealthCareCAN: Ottawa, ON; 2016. http://www.healthcarecan.ca/wp.
19. West M, Armit K, Loewenthal L, Eckert R, West T, Lee A. Leadership and leadership development in health care: the evidence base. London: The King's Fund and the Center for Creative Leadership; 2015. https://www.kingsfund.org.uk/sites/default/files/field/field_publication_file/leadership-leadership-development-health-care-feb-2015.pdf. Accessed 20 Aug 2019.

20. Vilches S, Fenwick S, Harris B, Lammi B, Racette R. Changing health organizations with the LEADS leadership framework: report of the 2014–2016 LEADS impact study. Ottawa, ON: Fenwick Leadership Explorations, the Canadian College of Health Leaders, & the Centre for Health Leadership and Research, Royal Roads University; 2016. https://leadscanada.net/document/1788/LEADS_Impact_Report_2017_FINAL.pdf. Accessed 1 May 2019.
21. Cathexis Consulting Inc. Interim report: how LeaderShift is making a difference. Cathexis Consulting 17 September 2018. https://www.leadershiftproject.ca/blog/interim-report-how-leadershift-is-making-a-difference. Accessed 20 Aug 2019.
22. Canadian Health Leadership Network Breakfast Session. Does Canada have the leadership capacity to innovate? Benchmark 2.0. Toronto, ON: National Health Leadership Conference; 2019. http://chlnet.ca/wp-content/uploads/NHLC-CHLNet-Breakfast-Session-2019-V02.pdf. Accessed 20 Aug 2019
23. Key informants from Australia were Dr. Elizabeth Shannon, who was part of the Health LEADS Australia consultation team and who has subsequently utilized Health LEADS Australia in a number of different projects across the country; and Dr. Neale Fong, President of the Australasian Health Leadership and Management Association, and also a senior executive with Health Workforce Australia during the Health LEADS Australia project. The key informant from England was Stephen Hart, national director for leadership development at Health Education England (HEE); from Scotland, Ms. Carolyn MacLeod, Leadership and Talent Management Division, Directorate of Health Workforce Leadership & Service Reform; and from New Zealand, Desmond Gorman, Medical Professor at Auckland University and former Executive Chair of Health Workforce New Zealand.
24. Philippon DJ. The leadership imperative in publicly funded universal health systems with a particular focus on the development of the Canadian Health Leadership Network (CHLNet). A project submitted a partial fulfillment of the requirements for the Fellowship Program. Canadian College of Health Leaders: Ottawa, ON; 2011. https://cchl.in1touch.org/document/1548/DonPhilippon_FellowshipProject.pdf. Accessed 21 Aug 2019.
25. The Health Foundation. About the Francis inquiry. London: The Health Foundation; 2019. https://www.health.org.uk/about-the-francis-inquiry. Accessed 8 Aug 2019.
26. Lynas K. The leadership response to the Francis report. Fut Hosp J. 2015;2(3):203–8.
27. Resources. NHS Leadership Academy; 2019. https://www.leadershipacademy.nhs.uk/resources/. Accessed 21 Aug 2019.
28. NHS Health Education England. Transforming maternity services; 2019. https://www.hee.nhs.uk/. Accessed 2 Aug 2019.
29. Department of Health & Social Care. DHSC mandate to Health Education England March 2018 to April 2019; 2019. https://assets.publishing.service.gov.uk/government/uploads/system/uploads/attachment_data/file/781757/DHSC_mandate_to_Health_Education_England_-_April_2018_to_March_2019.pdf. Accessed 2 Aug 2019.
30. Leadership. NHS improvement; 2019. https://improvement.nhs.uk/resources/valued-care-leadership/. Accessed 21 Aug 2019.
31. About us: The Horizons Team. Horizons; 2019; http://horizonsnhs.com/about/. Accessed 22 Aug 2019.
32. Project Lift. NHS Scotland. https://www.projectlift.scot/. Accessed 31 Jul 2019.
33. Talent Management. Project Lift: NHS Scotland. https://www.projectlift.scot/our-elements/talent-management/. Accessed 31 Jul 2019.
34. International Hospital Federation. Leadership competencies for healthcare services. Geneva: International Hospital Federation; 2015. https://www.ihf-fih.org/resources/pdf/Leadership_Competencies_for_Healthcare_Services_Managers.pdf. Accessed 31 Jul 2019.
35. International Hospital Federation Special Interest Groups. Healthcare management SIG. Geneva: International Hospital Federation 2015. https://www.ihf-fih.org/activities?type=sig&section=healthcare-management. Accessed 10 Jun 2019
36. Dickson G. Genesis of the leaders for life framework. Victoria, BC: LeadersforLife; 2008.

Putting LEADS to Work in Provincial Health Regions

12

Stevie Colvin and Sharon Bishop

The greatest danger in times of turbulence is not the turbulence; it is to act with yesterday's logic.

Peter Drucker [1]

Introduction

Meeting the challenges of twenty-first century health care requires strengthening leadership skills. Integrating LEADS into organizational processes and daily work is crucial to moving the system forward. This chapter focuses on how the *LEADS in Caring Environment Capabilities Framework* (LEADS) has been put to work in leadership and leadership development in Canadian and Australian health regions. To do that we reviewed academic and grey literature on regionalization and spoke with health organization leaders in both countries. Case studies of leadership development efforts in three jurisdictions—Alberta and Saskatchewan in Canada and New South Wales in Australia—are included. Regionalization is an established feature of health care in both countries and in each the scope and breadth of leadership development is province- or state-wide.

We view leadership as a strategic enabler of organizational and system performance, therefore our focus in this chapter is to offer a pragmatic approach for adopting and leveraging LEADS. We also highlight critical points in the employee lifecycle where LEADS can be embedded in talent management programs. We

S. Colvin
Alberta Health Services, Edmonton, AB, Canada
e-mail: steviecolvin@shaw.ca

S. Bishop (✉)
Saskatchewan Health Authority, Regina, SK, Canada
e-mail: sharon.bishop@saskhealthauthority.ca

© Springer Nature Switzerland AG 2020
G. Dickson, B. Tholl (eds.), *Bringing Leadership to Life in Health: LEADS in a Caring Environment*, https://doi.org/10.1007/978-3-030-38536-1_12

believe the approach we're recommending can be adapted to different governance structures and both small and large organizations.

A Brief Overview of Regionalization in Canada

Regional health authorities were created by provincial or state governments to be responsible for the administration and delivery of health services in specific geographical areas [2, 3]. Many of Canada's provinces have introduced regional health authorities, beginning in the early 1990s, to address problems with their health care systems during a fiscal crisis. Considered the most important policy shift since Medicare was introduced [4], regionalization was seen "as a promising space to assemble capacities and commitments to achieve health system transformation and improvement" [5].

The main goals of regionalization are integrating and coordinating health care organizations and services (vertical integration), consolidating and rationalizing hospital services (horizontal integration), decreasing variation in care and improving quality through evidence-based practices and decentralizing decision-making and resources to better meet population needs [4, 6, 7]. Essentially, regionalization strives for the right balance between decentralization and centralization of authorities and accountabilities. While regionalization has been part of the Canadian health care landscape for three decades, the consensus is that regional health authorities have not fully met their objectives [4, 6, 8].

Regardless, decision-makers continue to consolidate health systems as a solution to fiscal and fragmentation issues in health care. In the last 10 years in Canada there has been a trend to greater centralization, with provincial ministries of health consolidating and reducing the number of regions. Most recently, in 2019, the government of Ontario decided to merge 20 agencies, which employ more than 10,000 people, into one big agency to be called Ontario Health [9].

Alberta and Saskatchewan have single provincial health authorities responsible for coordinating all acute and continuing care and these two provinces are our main focus; as one of us works in Alberta and the other in Saskatchewan. The provinces of Nova Scotia, Prince Edward Island and Manitoba as well as the Northwest Territories have also gone from having several regions to operating a single authority. We also discuss experiences in New South Wales (Australia) and the provinces of British Columbia and Newfoundland and Labrador (Canada), which are all taking multi-organizational collaborative approaches to health care.

Leadership: Strategic Enabler of Health System Innovation and Performance

The need for transformational change in Canadian health care is widely recognized, although achieving and sustaining improved performance has proven difficult. The "wicked problems"[1] [10] facing provincial health systems has increased pressure on

---

[1] Wicked problems are ones that are complex, ill formulated, confusing, full of unsolvable dilemmas. They require multi-party collaboration to address. In the words of Chap. 9, they are people driven change problems.

stakeholders to work together. Consequently, collective, distributed leadership has become important for enabling innovation and improving health system performance [11–13].

As was described in Chap. 9, the challenge of creating large-scale change requires more sophisticated levels of strategic and systems thinking, relationship development and self-leadership than many formal leaders, including physicians, are capable of [14–16]. Leaders from across the system need to be engaged in collaborative teamwork and collective decision-making to achieve large system change. As a result, considerable investment is required to develop leadership capacity, both administrative and clinical, at all levels of the system [17].

The Wisdom and Lived Experience of Those in the System

We interviewed several LEADS-certified practitioners including Julie Sullivan from Eastern Health in Newfoundland; Sheila Betker from Winnipeg Regional Health Authority in Manitoba; Brad Dorohoy from Alberta Health Services; Peter Martin from Northern Health in British Columbia; Peter Vaughn in Nova Scotia, and David Sweeney from the Health Education and Training Institute, New South Wales, Australia (see Chap. 3 for a description of the leadership framework used in New South Wales: it is an analogue of LEADS). Content from some informal conversations is also included in this chapter.

Our key informants are advocates for learning and development as an effective mechanism for introducing LEADS to individuals and organizations. It was also obvious that they believed everyone in their organizations needs to be familiar with LEADS. Learners told them that familiarization with LEADS had taught them how to leverage their own sphere of influence effectively (Sullivan J. Key Informant, Eastern Health, Newfoundland; 2019 May 12). These ideas and practices are supported in the literature published by the Centre of Creative Leadership and the National Health Service in England, where they make a strong and persuasive case for distributed and collective leadership [18]. This thinking and approach contrasts dramatically with traditional approaches focused on developing individual capability in leaders.

However, learning and development initiatives are only a small part of the work of our key informants. Most of our interviewees are also concerned with the entire talent management continuum (pre-hire to retire). For this chapter we have adopted the definition of talent management offered by Silzer and Dowell [19] who describe it as: "an integrated set of processes, programs, and cultural norms in an organization designed and implemented to attract, develop, deploy, and retain talent to achieve strategic objectives and meet future business needs."

People we interviewed supported integrating LEADS into talent management. Nova Scotia's Peter Vaughn said to us, "As deputy minister I very much supported LEADS as a modus operandi" (personal communication, 2019 Aug 15). We heard that to be effective, learning and development must be part of an integrated suite of practices that align with and fuel the organization's overarching strategy. The Centre for Creative Leadership reinforces this idea: "When setting strategies that call for changes in the direction or capabilities of the organization, the leadership gap must be considered. One of the first questions to ask is: *Do we have the leadership we need for the strategy we've set?"* [20].

Our interviews provided evidence that the LEADS framework is elastic enough to be used at any point along the talent management continuum, which means it could be used to deal with urgent needs at the same time work is going on to embed it organization-wide. Practitioners told us they got buy in and commitment for LEADS by working on the most evident leadership gap. Once its credibility was established it gave them more latitude to work on embedding LEADS elsewhere in the organization.

The leader's story in the following case study from Alberta Health Services tells us how important credibility is. Leaders working in the health care system have many pressing demands, which can make it difficult to pause long enough to consider the validity of LEADS, or how it can be used to ease their challenges. Her story validates the practitioners' proof of effectiveness helps them move LEADS deeper into the system.

Case Study, Alberta: Building Leadership Capability on the Fly

Alberta Health Services (AHS) was Canada's first province-wide, fully integrated health system. Its formation in 2009 brought together 12 organizations, nine regional and three province-wide health authorities. The consolidation was one of Canada's largest health mergers, forming an organization that now has more than 110,000 employees and a total annual budget of about $21 billion. With little lead time between the government's announcement and the actual merger much of the restructuring work occurred after the fact.

Moving to the new AHS posed many challenges for leaders. Forming and leading a province-wide health service demanded significantly different capabilities than their past roles, but leadership development was the last thing anyone had time for. As the organization's thousands of formal leaders worked to ensure the merger did not take away from safe patient care, their own experiences were both challenging and largely unattended to.

Dr. Stephen Duckett, the original CEO of AHS, when asked what he wished he had done more of, said he wished he had paid much more attention to the leadership and management needs of leaders at all levels throughout the organization (G. Dickson, personal communication, 2019 May 12).

Consolidating and collapsing multiple systems into one caused turmoil. Across the system, leaders' portfolios grew, and their responsibilities mounted. Public confidence and workforce engagement had dropped, as leaders faced new challenges and tried to develop processes to resolve problems. This was the environment a newly formed Talent Management Strategies team needed to navigate in order to support the leadership team.

In 2010, the talent management team adopted the LEADS in a Caring Environment leadership framework. They chose LEADS because it offered a common vocabulary of leadership, and we hoped it would help unify Alberta's health leaders in the practice of leadership. The framework was new to everyone. In addition, the idea of a national framework with a vocabulary that could connect health care leaders across the country was appealing, offering the possibility of connecting AHS leaders to each other and their peers nation-wide.

The intent was to embed LEADS into AHS' leadership language and practice by building it into the learning continuum. The plan was to construct a system of programs and services that would sustain leaders in their development from individual assessment, through planning and learning, to practicing the leadership capabilities defined in the LEADS framework (see Fig. 12.1).

In this framework the LEADS self-assessment and LEADS 360 feedback tool were the foundation for individual assessment. The LEADS model anchored learning plans and learning reports. All courses and programs were constructed with the purpose of helping leaders build their LEADS capabilities.

One of the serious consequences of the turmoil the merger caused was lost relationships and broken connections. We hypothesized that putting learners in cross-functional cohorts (made up of people with different expertise, at different levels and from different program areas) would help rebuild connections and break down silos.

We started with a residential executive education program that had two core purposes: building leadership capabilities and creating networks among our senior leaders. All components of the program were aligned with all five domains of the LEADS framework. The program included 360 assessment, executive sponsored action learning projects, one-to-one coaching, LEADS-based learning plans, and reports to support a learner's ability to practice; to make sense of and apply what they learned. The time and energy required was and remains challenging for program participants, but many said they would recommend the program to others and our evaluations indicate the program's objectives are being met.

Reflecting on the decade of putting LEADS to work in Alberta Health Services' leadership development efforts—where we've been, and where we are—provides opportunity for celebration and begs the question "how might LEADS be leveraged even more broadly in our work?" Certainly, our greatest success has been in the creation of leadership development programs and services. We have achieved wide recognition of the LEADS framework and hear leaders' stories of how the framework is informing their personal practice. Here's what one program graduate, Stephanie T. Donaldson, said of her experience (Personal interview 2019 Apr 5):

> LEADS rolled out at a time that was incredibly busy for operations. Programs and services were coming together across the organization and non-stop pressures were facing leaders including the introduction of organizational best practices, public health emergencies, natural disasters and the day to day business of caring for the people we serve. As a leader it felt like one more initiative being rolled out. I felt I didn't have adequate time to understand and determine its application in my team let alone from a personal perspective. I

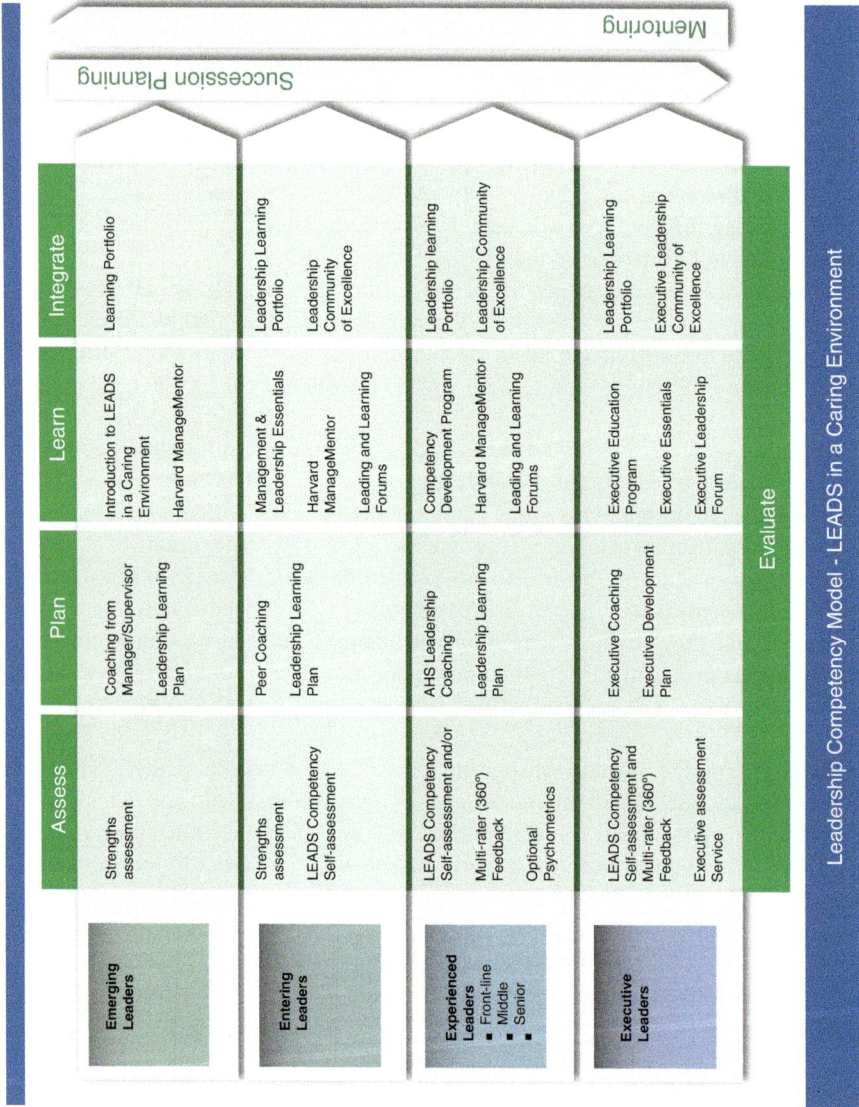

Mentoring

Succession Planning

	Assess	Plan	Learn	Integrate
Emerging Leaders	Strengths assessment	Coaching from Manager/Supervisor Leadership Learning Plan	Introduction to LEADS in a Caring Environment Harvard ManageMentor	Learning Portfolio
Entering Leaders	Strengths assessment LEADS Competency Self-assessment	Peer Coaching Leadership Learning Plan	Management & Leadership Essentials Harvard ManageMentor Leading and Learning Forums	Leadership Learning Portfolio Leadership Community of Excellence
Experienced Leaders ■ Front-line ■ Middle ■ Senior	LEADS Competency Self-assessment and/or Multi-rater (360°) Feedback Optional Psychometrics	AHS Leadership Coaching Leadership Learning Plan	Competency Development Program Harvard ManageMentor Leading and Learning Forums	Leadership learning Portfolio Leadership Community of Excellence
Executive Leaders	LEADS Competency Self-assessment and Multi-rater (360°) Feedback Executive assessment Service	Executive Coaching Executive Development Plan	Executive Education Program Executive Essentials Executive Leadership Forum	Leadership Learning Portfolio Executive Leadership Community of Excellence

Evaluate

Leadership Competency Model - LEADS in a Caring Environment

Fig. 12.1 The now-retired leadership development framework from AHS

certainly didn't understand it was a tool used globally with significant efficacy behind it. Somewhere in the day-to-day life I missed that in translation.

It wasn't until I had the gift of participating in our executive education program that I had the time and space to really dig into the LEADS framework. I could reflect on what the potential of LEADS—peeling back the onion to further understand myself as a leader and how I choose to show up. Additionally, I had time to reflect on how I could use it in my team to more effectively develop my staff and achieve the outcomes at a system level.

My view and understanding of the framework quickly moved to a much deeper appreciation of how robust it could be. I began to see the benefits it could afford to me personally as a leader and bringing it forward to my leadership table for shared learning and development. I could see how it could support teams and the goals we wanted to achieve in engaging with one another, transforming the health care system in Alberta in our communities and our teams who serve them and achieving the results that we were accountable for and that Albertans expected of us.

Utilizing the LEADS framework sometimes took me to places I didn't want to go in understanding myself as a leader and the teams that I lead. Ultimately as we embraced it, our staff and our leadership team were strengthened, and we have been able to make tangible and measurable steps towards transforming our health care system for the people we serve. And THAT is why we are all here!

As AHS moves forward, our goal is to continue to develop a shared, collective and extended leadership practice that builds capacity for change and improvement throughout the system. We're taking steps to embed LEADS in other talent management practices such as recruitment, performance, recognition and succession planning. At the same time, we are examining the creation of a refreshed leadership strategy and anticipate LEADS will play an even bigger role across the talent management continuum from attraction, through recruitment, on-boarding and socialization as well as development and retention, while bilaterally meeting leader and organizational needs.

The Alberta Health Services case study demonstrates the possibility of parallel and complementary purposes: using LEADS to develop leaders (focusing on the individual) and strengthening relationships across the system (focusing on organizational needs). Collective leadership is about good individual leaders but is also inherently about the quality of relationships amongst them. Organizational success is dependent on how leaders work together. Collective leadership "means everyone taking responsibility for the success of the organization as a whole—not just for their own jobs or work area [18]." Peter Vaughn, from Nova Scotia, one of our interviewees, acknowledges that collective leadership was crucial to their regionalization:

In terms of engaging leaders from across the province, we put out an expression of interest to help us design the new authority. It was widely seen as time for a transformational change and the response was overwhelming. Despite maybe not having a job after the changes, people stood up with great enthusiasm. Engagement was key...You co-own what you co-create...and you cannot understate the importance of physician engagement in that process (Personal interview 2019 Aug 15).

Our key informants also had unique stories about why, when and how to begin working with LEADS in their organizations. The common message was "start where the organization is most likely to benefit by integrating the framework's underpinning tenets." We heard once early needs are addressed, appreciation for the framework will deepen and other opportunities to use it will become evident (Brad Dorohoy, Alberta Health Services, Personal Interview, May 12).

Without exception, our key informants spoke about how important linkages are across the talent management continuum. In support of their view the NeuroLeadership Institute states that "coherence is a special kind of relationship between systems of concepts, in which each set of ideas and their relationships, reinforce and help explain the other" [21]. By coherence they mean that each piece needs to fit with the whole: coherence in messaging, policy, process and in all that individuals, teams and the organization interact with. Daily work must also be aligned and integrated. It is through coherence that each element of learning and strategic initiative can contribute to the creation of a leadership culture defined by LEADS. As Julie Sutherland from Eastern Health stated: "Everything needs to be connected. People need to see how it fits with our strategic priorities" (Personal interview, 2019 Mar 25).

Our case study on the creation of the Saskatchewan Health Authority offers insight into how an organization can make pragmatic decisions to ensure strategic positioning of LEADS and leadership development.

Case Study, Saskatchewan: Develop Better Leadership, Deliver Better Care

In August 2016, the Government of Saskatchewan announced the appointment of an Advisory Panel on Health System Structure tasked with providing advice on the future structure of the health system. The most prescriptive element of their mandate was to provide a recommendation of a future health system with fewer regional health authorities [22]. The primary goal of consolidation was to achieve improvements to patient care while finding administrative efficiencies [23].

The provincial government endorsed the Advisory Panel's recommendations. In particular the panel supported consolidating the 12 health authorities into a single provincial one, to create a system focused on meeting patient needs through seamless, integrated, team-based care. On December 4, 2017 it became official: the Saskatchewan Health Authority was announced as a legal entity [24]. Even though wholesale system-wide change was expected, and a lot of transitional preparation had already occurred, the move to one provincial region came as a surprise and shock to many. Although optimistic, senior leaders across Saskatchewan have acknowledged they don't have all the answers and have openly expressed (in keeping with the Lead self domain of LEADS) feelings of vulnerability.

In the initial stages of the merger, a Transition Team of senior leaders from the former regions was established. The Transition Team researched leading practice and reached out to other provinces—such as Alberta, PEI, and Nova Scotia, which had already merged their regional authorities into province-wide ones—to learn from their experiences. The emphasis was—and is at the time of writing—to encourage and support innovation: take what is working well and to adopt, scale and spread leading practices provincially. When reflecting on the first year as the SHA, Scott Livingstone CEO of the new province-wide authority, said: "December 4, 2017 is not the day we amalgamated, it is the day we came together to combine our strengths" (SHA News Release, December 4, 2018).

While there is a lot of trepidation, there is also a lot of enthusiasm. Across the health authority, we've become fond of the expression "we are building the plane as we are flying it," acknowledging the messiness of trying to stabilize during transition at the same time as innovating. We need to ensure service continuity for the people of Saskatchewan, and design for transformational change. We view leadership development as a strategic vehicle for this transformation.

"Leadership development is essential if we are to succeed in our new health authority… As we change from 12 regions to one it's so important that we speak and act as one and resist falling back into old safe ways. Change is hard but leadership is imperative as we move forward." (Client- and family-centred care advisor, Saskatoon, March 28, 2018).

Our leadership challenge is to channel the healthy excitement and motivation to proceed with building our desired future-state system. Leadership, in the current context, is constantly presenting challenges to leaders and their capabilities. Many leaders and managers, for example, have been conditioned to think about regionalization from the viewpoint of mechanical systems, rather than adopting perspectives suited to the complex adaptive system health care is (see Chap. 9).

Restructuring tests people and relationships (in keeping with the Engage others and Develop coalitions domains of LEADS) with the major leadership challenges lying in the interconnections—the interfaces and relationships among people, teams, functions and different stakeholder needs. Collaboration within and between portfolios is essential to ensure they are aligned, and roles and responsibilities clear. In the Saskatchewan Health Authority and across the system, there is a growing appreciation that a more collective, distributed leadership approach is needed to transform the health system.

"As we grow into our new role as one health authority the importance of leadership to guide us and sustain us becomes paramount. All we ask of our new leadership is that you be mindful of the trust we place in you" (Client- and family-centred care advisor, Swift Current, SK 2018 March 28).

In this complex and dynamic environment, we need new ways of thinking, doing and being, as well as organizational structures and processes to support them. For example, the Saskatchewan Health Authority's leadership structure places physician executives and vice presidents for all clinical portfolios in dyad partnerships—sharing the authority to make decisions on budgets, quality, safety and clinical practice standards. We have also focused on organizational design and establishing reporting relationships. Implementing new ways of thinking, doing and being requires the right talent, therefore retaining top performers is critical; at the same time, we've taken a phased approach to recruiting for leadership positions. The amalgamation presented an opportunity to standardize job titles and descriptions to ensure we have people with the right capabilities for positions. Although many have been patient through the transition, talent has been lost to early retirement, other provinces, and industry.

Over the first year (and in keeping with the Achieve results domain of LEADS), the most critical focus for the authority's board and executive, beyond building a senior leadership team, has been on developing a mission, vision, values and strategic plan. It has also emphasized establishing clear lines and structures for communication.

Well in advance of the official announcement of the amalgamation, a group of individuals who considered leadership the single most important enabler of organizational and system-level innovation and health-system performance [25, 26] established the Leadership Development Coalition. Orienting themselves strategically to the future, and challenging the status quo, this motivated group sought to proactively leverage the knowledge and best ideas that currently exist for leadership development. This collaborative effort, inclusive of patient and family advisors and external partners, was anchored in the LEADS in a Caring Environment Framework.

"Trained leaders are essential to maintaining the high standards Saskatchewan has established in health care. Leadership development programs allow continuous staff education and maintain a high level of interest in improving our system" (Client- and family-centred care advisor, Regina 2018 March 28).

The aim of the coalition was to "develop and demonstrate individual and collective leadership behaviours at all levels that support a healthy workplace and the delivery of high quality, safe, compassionate patient and family-centred care," an adaptation of the definition of leadership presented and discussed in this book. The proposal integrated leadership with management processes in the Saskatchewan Health Management System with a patient- and family-centred care approach (see Chap. 13). To do that, the coalition built additional partnerships, and engaged others in a coordinated networked effort—successfully navigating the socio-political environment, mobilizing knowledge and influencing collective action to achieve results (Develop coalitions domain of LEADS).

Even though Saskatchewan's flagship of health leadership development, the Saskatchewan Leadership Program, had been in place since 2014, efforts to mobilize knowledge and leading practices for leadership development had mostly been ad hoc. Across the province considerable variation existed in access to leadership development for all levels of leaders. In addition, there was limited internal capacity to plan, deliver and support licensed LEADS-aligned programming and integration in a systematic way.

The timing was right; and with senior level sponsorship secured, there was considerable strategic value in applying a systems perspective to leadership, leadership development and talent management. Executive leadership also recognized that leadership and improvement capabilities would have to keep growing to meet the needs of the ever-changing health care environment and advance transformation of the system in Saskatchewan. Equally important was to align leadership development with other culture strengthening activities including improving team-based care in community, supporting continuous improvement, strengthening cultural

Table 12.1 Leadership Development Coalition's proposal for action submitted to the Saskatchewan Health Authority executive

Leadership Development Coalition—Proposal for Action
1. **Formally adopt the LEADS in a Caring Environment Framework**
2. **Reaffirm SHA commitment to leadership development**
3. **Deeper dive into understanding needs/capabilities at the system-level**
4. **Co-create 'learning pathways,' for leaders at all levels, that develop both individual and collective leadership capabilities, consider key leadership transitions, and the succession planning pipeline**
5. **Leverage and build LEADS capacity by certifying internal organizational facilitators**
6. **Focus future leadership development action planning on the five identified Critical Development Elements:** emotional intelligence; leader presence; communication skill; cross-functional teamwork; and the discipline to deliver
7. **Develop a robust evaluation strategy (people, process, results)**
8. **Functionally integrate the LEADS framework into provincial talent management, organizational strategies, and daily work**
9. **Strengthen cross-functional partnerships with SHA leaders to ensure alignment and integrated action:** In particular, executive directors and directors responsible for oversight of Patient and Client Experience, Safety and Quality, First Nations and Métis Health, Strategy & Innovation, as well as with physician leaders will be important partners in advancing a leadership culture in the SHA
10. **Build and strengthen mutually beneficial relationships with external partners:** Building and strengthening relationships with external partners (i.e. CHLNet; LEADS Canada; CCHL; HealthcareCAN; ICF-Coaching) will enable the SHA to contribute to and learn from provincial and national leadership development action. Potentially leveraging internal capacity and providing momentum to move leadership development strategy forward more rapidly

awareness and responsiveness and increasing patient and staff safety. The coalition's proposal for action appears in Table 12.1.

Although LEADS was previously endorsed by the Provincial Leadership Team in 2013, uptake across the former regional authorities had been inconsistent at best. After amalgamation, and aligned with Accreditation Canada's Leadership Standards, the opportunity arose to make the LEADS framework the foundation of a more coherent and collaborative leadership development effort, as well as integrating it into the talent management strategy.

The first step was to partner with LEADS Canada, sign the licensing agreement and formally adopt LEADS as the Saskatchewan Health Authority's leadership capabilities framework. To align with the focus on designing an organization that supports the mission and vision, LEADS has been integrated into the job descriptions and interview guides at all management levels. Doing this raised awareness of the LEADS framework across the system and also encouraged the hiring of leaders whose capabilities aligned with strategic and operational requirements.

Efforts are underway to embed LEADS into elements of the SHA People Strategy, particularly in organization-wide strategic initiatives such as orientation and onboarding, leadership learning pathways, performance management, succession planning, team building and change leadership.

We are also working to raise awareness and knowledge of the LEADS framework and build capacity more broadly. Strengthening cross-functional networks, with physician leaders and colleagues in quality, safety and strategy, is crucial for identifying leadership development champions, integrating LEADS more fully, and achieving results over the long term. Partnerships are being established with physician leaders and cross-functional colleagues to create experience-based leadership development opportunities. Over time, the goal is to make leadership development accessible at all levels—a substantial culture shift from what was done in the past.

We made a point of discussing cross-boundary collaboration on leadership development with key informants from other provinces. Manitoba, British Columbia and Newfoundland have all tried it. In BC, the idea was to be "centrally designed, locally delivered." In Newfoundland and Manitoba, the collaborations are structured more loosely, with peers co-developing leadership development resources with options to adopt and adapt. Each of these working collaboratives faced challenges. One key informant, Peter Martin from Northern Health in BC, said, "the process of collaboration was messy" (Personal communication, 2019 May 12). The success of a collaboration can be affected by different needs, desired outcomes and the pace and focus of work. Nevertheless, key informants said inter-organizational collaborative practices are worth the time and energy.

Our third case study of putting LEADS to work in a regionalized system comes from New South Wales in Australia.

LEADS in New South Wales: The Health Education and Training Institute

Unlike in Alberta and Saskatchewan, leadership education in New South Wales (NSW) is a responsibility of the regional health system but is provided by the Health Education Training Institute (the Institute), which is a discrete part of the health system. The independent agency has a performance agreement with NSW Health.

The Institute's performance agreement says: "The primary role of the Institute is to provide leadership to Local Health Districts, Networks and other NSW public health organizations and training providers on the development and delivery of education and training across the NSW Public Health System." HETI ensures education and training across the system:

1. Supports safe, high quality, multi-disciplinary team based, patient-centred care.
2. Meets service delivery needs and operational requirements.
3. Enhances workforce skills, flexibility and productivity [27].

The Institute describes its purpose as "Working with health partners to develop contemporary and responsive health education and training to enable a world-class workforce" [28]. This includes the responsibility to "design, commission, conduct, coordinate, support and evaluate management, leadership and professional development programs" for the health system in NSW.

Since 2012, the Institute has used its own LEADS-related framework (see Chap. 3) as the foundation for leadership talent management, to assist NSW health executives and clinician leaders to support excellence in organization and patient outcomes. Philosophically speaking, they share with LEADS Canada a belief in leadership as distinct from management; a greater focus on leadership than individual leaders; believing that leadership is a collective distributed phenomenon; and ascribing to the ideology of the power of learning leadership in an organizational setting [29]. The NSW Health Leadership Framework has been critical in framing the curriculum design of their leadership programs which also draws heavily from the adaptive, collective and relational leadership literature [30–32].

There are several categories of leadership programs at the Institute—Leadership Quarter events designed to provoke thought, a 10-month inter-professional leadership and organizational development program delivered locally in partnership with NSW health organizations, a two year development program for the next generation of leaders, intensive senior executive development to support new senior managers and chief executives and people- and financial-management courses. The whole array of courses is shown in Fig. 12.2.

The Institute also uses CORE Chat for Managers' workshops to assist NSW staff to understand how to use NSW Health core values as tools for everyday action. To prepare for those, there are Values in Action workshops, where participants learn about effective team cultures and high performing teams, and how they can use specific techniques to improve their own teams' performance. While the NSW approach is unique it was constructed to address specific organizational challenges and reinforces the importance of constructing programs with clear objectives.

In the next section we discuss embedding LEADS across the talent management continuum and synthesize Saskatchewan's process with the best advice from the other case studies and interviews to create a pragmatic approach for integrating LEADS in large health authorities, or in collaborations among smaller ones.

LEADS and Leadership Development in Health Regions

Earlier on we introduced the importance of integrating LEADS into the talent management continuum and explored it in each of the case studies. While this was not a direct focus of our key informant interviews, we were told "as you work with it [LEADS] you see more and more opportunities for how to use it" (Betker S. Key Informant, Winnipeg Regional Health Authority, Manitoba, 2019 May 12). Considering the full employee life cycle (pre-hire to retire) helps talent managers design learning and development interventions that meet both organizational goals and individual's needs, while recognizing the capabilities needed to sustain organizations and ensure leaders integrate effective leadership behaviour into

Leadership and Management development pathway

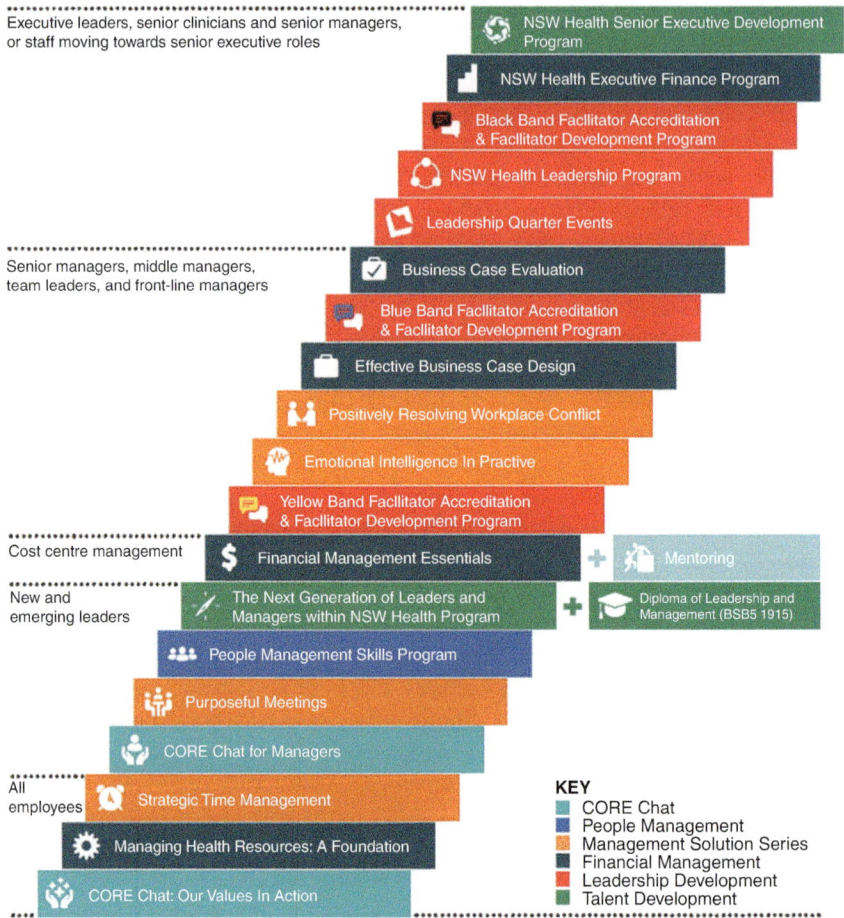

Executive leaders, senior clinicians and senior managers, or staff moving towards senior executive roles
- NSW Health Senior Executive Development Program
- NSW Health Executive Finance Program
- Black Band Facilitator Accreditation & Facilitator Development Program
- NSW Health Leadership Program
- Leadership Quarter Events

Senior managers, middle managers, team leaders, and front-line managers
- Business Case Evaluation
- Blue Band Facilitator Accreditation & Facilitator Development Program
- Effective Business Case Design
- Positively Resolving Workplace Conflict
- Emotional Intelligence In Practive
- Yellow Band Facilitator Accreditation & Facilitator Development Program

Cost centre management
- $ Financial Management Essentials   + Mentoring

New and emerging leaders
- The Next Generation of Leaders and Managers within NSW Health Program   + Diploma of Leadership and Management (BSB5 1915)
- People Management Skills Program
- Purposeful Meetings
- CORE Chat for Managers

All employees
- Strategic Time Management
- Managing Health Resources: A Foundation
- CORE Chat: Our Values In Action

KEY
- CORE Chat
- People Management
- Management Solution Series
- Financial Management
- Leadership Development
- Talent Development

Fig. 12.2 Health education training institute leadership and management development pathway [33]

practice throughout their careers. Figure 12.3 introduces four dimensions of talent management to consider when "weaving LEADS through related collateral" (Dorohoy B. key informant, Alberta Health Services, Alberta; 2019 May 25).

We advocate an integrated and coherent practice otherwise there is a risk of focusing on developing leadership capability one person at a time [34]. A one-at-a-time approach is a concern because it assumes individuals will stay with the organization long term, resulting in sustained transfer of learning rather than creating a culture of leadership practice (discussed at length in Chap. 4). Similarly, developing individual leaders assumes an individual can exercise leadership in any environment and neither culture or context play a role in their success or failure. Research, however, suggests the opposite: "the effectiveness of training programs, development experiences, and self-help activities depends in part on organizational conditions that facilitate or inhibit learning of leadership skills and the application of this learning" [35]. Taking a collective and integrated approach shifts leadership development efforts away from individuals towards the concept of shared accountability and emphasizes the need for a culture that empowers leaders to act.

Based on what we learned from our three case studies, Table 12.2 suggests how to maximize the value of leadership development in talent management efforts.

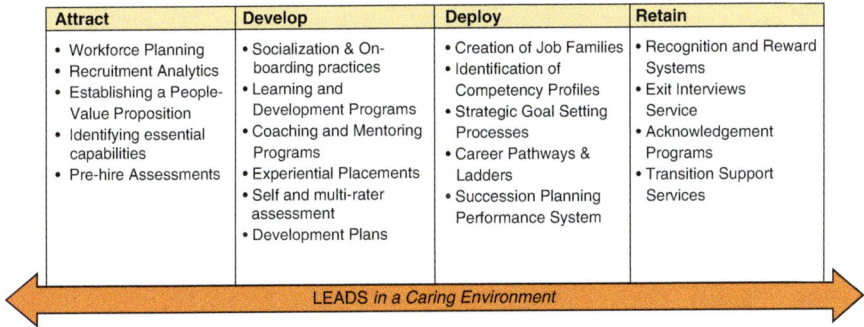

Attract	Develop	Deploy	Retain
• Workforce Planning • Recruitment Analytics • Establishing a People-Value Proposition • Identifying essential capabilities • Pre-hire Assessments	• Socialization & On-boarding practices • Learning and Development Programs • Coaching and Mentoring Programs • Experiential Placements • Self and multi-rater assessment • Development Plans	• Creation of Job Families • Identification of Competency Profiles • Strategic Goal Setting Processes • Career Pathways & Ladders • Succession Planning Performance System	• Recognition and Reward Systems • Exit Interviews Service • Acknowledgement Programs • Transition Support Services

LEADS *in a Caring Environment*

Fig. 12.3 Weaving LEADS through four dimensions of talent management

Table 12.2 Maximize value of leadership development in talent management efforts

1.	**Formally adopt the LEADS in a Caring Environment Framework**
	The decisions here are: *How will you determine the best leadership framework for your organization? What criteria will you use in making that assessment?*
	Some of the essential considerations for every practitioner in determining framework fit are validity and usability. In this book you will find all the information you need to assess the LEADS framework. "Behind the apparent simplicity of the LEADS framework lies a six-year process of research, dialogue, discussion and use of LEADS…" [36, 37]
	Questions to consider Is there value for us in having a common vocabulary and expected behaviour for leaders in the organization? If there is value, what would it be? What need or gap would LEADS fill for us? What outcomes are we expecting from the adoption of LEADS? How does the adoption of LEADS align with current processes, products, programs and policies?
	Key informant wisdom: Key informants shared thoughts on this matter. They spoke about how LEADS is:
	Evidence-based: "Through our international search for a leadership framework we landed on LEADS as the most robust, evidenced based framework available." (David Sweeney) **Accurate**: "From what I have seen and experienced it [LEADS] is as good and robust a model as there is, and it seems to have hit the mark." (Brad Dorohoy) **Accessible**: "LEADS was ready made, came in a package." (Peter Martin) **Usable**: "It's simple, it's easy to use, it just makes sense." (Julie Sutherland) **Powerful**: "The network supports each other's work. We also share our products with each other" (Sheila Betker)

(continued)

Table 12.2 (continued)

2.	**Reaffirm organizational commitment to leadership development**

The decisions here are: *Will we, as an organization, make a long-term commitment to leadership development? Can we get a formal commitment from our senior leadership to support leadership development?*

There is a strong argument that all members of the workforce need to engage in ongoing learning and development. This need is often linked to the pace of change [37] and the increasing complexity of work [38]. Leaders in health care are faced with unique challenges that shift with technological advances, population demographics and medical advances [38] which are exacerbated by public health emergencies and natural disasters. These leadership challenges also support the need for ongoing learning.

Questions to consider
- How does leadership development fit in with and support the organization's strategic direction?
- Are the organization's senior leaders committed to leadership development?
- How does LEADS support our organization's leadership needs for now and in the future?
- Who needs to sponsor, advocate and advance the adoption of LEADS for a successful investment of leadership development in the organization? What will their roles be? How must they be engaged in this work?

Key informant wisdom: Our interview participants shared their thoughts on the value and impact of investing in leadership development and the unique benefits of internally designed and delivered programs that 'fit' organizational context. Julie Sullivan describes the benefits in her experience: *"You can feel it [LEADS] in the organization. When you feel that energy and support, and you see the cascading supportive system that's there. When you see people pausing and asking where is my role in this, understanding that it's ok [to pause] ... it's shifted the culture from do, do, do, do, do to...[a culture of]... doing what is valuable"*

3.	**Dive into understanding needs/capabilities at the system-level**

The decisions here are: *How will we work with LEADS to leverage its full potential?* If an organization is going to benefit from its leadership development programs, they need to fulfill a relevant and practical need. "Needs assessment is a process for figuring out how to close a learning or performance gap" [39]. Therefore, the questions each organization needs to ask and answer will be unique.

Questions to consider
- What do we need to learn in our needs assessment/gap analysis for now and into the future?
- How will we collect the information we are seeking?
- With whom and how will we share what we learn?
- What will we use the information to achieve?

Key Informant Wisdom: The driver for investing in LEADS for Newfoundland's Eastern Health was a need for leadership sustainability: *"We came to a point when many of our leaders were set to retire, and no one was applying. People were intimidated by ...[leadership roles] ...and didn't think they had the skills to do the jobs. They were thinking 'How can I step into that?' We realized we needed to skill up our own people, and support them to take on the leadership roles."* (Julie Sullivan)

Table 12.2 (continued)

4.	**Co-create learning strategy and framework that aims to develop both individual and collective leadership capabilities** **The decision here is:** *Who needs to be involved in the development and/or refresh of our organization's learning strategy?* The benefits of thinking big picture in leadership development are exponential. Not only do individuals grow their leadership capabilities, but teams and the organization benefit in ways that are measurably significant. The National Health Service in the UK has invested in leadership research and works through the King's Fund in partnership with the Centre for Creative Research. Two articles that discuss collective leadership may be of interest as you consider how you want to construct your programs: "Developing Collective Leadership for Healthcare" [18], and "Delivering a Collective Leadership Strategy for Health care" [34]. These articles make a case for the importance of thinking beyond the development of individuals and designing programs that ensure leadership becomes encultured in the organization. NOTE: The Canadian Health Leadership Network (CHLNet—see Chap. 11) has a working group dedicated to learning strategy and another to research in health leadership. Connecting with the CHLNet coalition may be to your advantage. **Questions to consider** • Where are there sensitivities about leaders and leadership philosophies and practices in your organization? • How will you navigate any differences in definition, philosophy and/or practice? • How do individual capabilities link to collective capabilities? What is the relationship between the two? **Key Informant Wisdom:** David Sweeney describes the benefits of building collective leadership: *"the other evidence for us ... now, after four years, people are drawn to our program because it is helping the organization deliver its strategy, deliver its strategic intent."*
5.	**Consider leveraging and building LEADS capacity by certifying internal organizational facilitators** **The decision here is:** *Should the organization invest in having internal practitioners with deep knowledge of the LEADS framework?* There are multiple options available to organizations who wish to adopt LEADS. Either way LEADS Canada is the gateway to the framework, for understanding the options surrounding adoption and for connecting into the community. **Questions to consider** • What could certification of internal organizational facilitators offer your organization? • What are the risks and benefits of certifying facilitators in your organization? • What would certified internal organizational facilitator's roles entail? **Key informant wisdom:** Manitoba reports experiencing unforetold benefits through internal certification. Sheila Betker's experience indicates internal certification offers the opportunity for innovation because it increases the number of people involved in the use of the framework. *"Through certification we have undertaken projects and as a result we have seen [LEADS] integrated in a variety of ways. Examples include using it in job descriptions, in interviews, in engagement, leadership development, meeting structures, different people are using it in other ways."*

(continued)

Table 12.2 (continued)

6.	**Focus future leadership development action planning on the critical development elements**

The decision here is: *How will our organization focus on building a solid foundation of a few critical core capabilities required of everyone at every level?*

Organizations need to ensure that all staff know their roles, and are empowered to take individual and collective responsibility for delivering care. A solid foundation for that is identifying a few critical core capabilities required of everyone at every level. Core capabilities describe the essential knowledge, skills and attitudes necessary for all members of the workforce. They are the basic building blocks of development programs and encourage desired behaviour. They also support recruiting, developing and retaining the workforce [40, 41].

Questions to consider
What is the purpose of identifying core capabilities ?
How can and will we distill which behaviour is core to the entire organization?
Can we distinguish which capabilities are associated with progressive levels leadership in our organization? Does LEADS fulfill the role for us?

Key informant wisdom: The Saskatchewan Health Authority identified emotional intelligence, leader presence, communication, cross-functional teamwork and the discipline to deliver (using continuous improvement methodology) as the essential LEADS capabilities for leaders. The Leadership Development Coalition was guided by the organization's strategic needs and the capabilities essential for supporting a successful transition.

7.	**Develop a robust evaluation strategy (people, process, results)**

The decision here is: *What level of evaluation do we need to apply to each of our programs, products and services?*

Measurement is undertaken in levels: reaction, learning, application, impact and return on investment. True measures are derived from collecting the appropriate data before, during and after any initiative or intervention is undertaken. Decisions about what data to collect derive from the initial objectives for doing the work. Clear objectives connected directly to organizational impact measures provide the guideposts for evaluation [42].

Questions to consider
- How will this initiative help our organization? How is this initiative aligned with organizational goals?
- What are the critical things our organization will want to know about our initiative[s]?
- What are the objectives for this specific initiative? How can we measure for these things?

Key informant wisdom: David Sweeney shared his thoughts on the value of evaluation and what it can do as an embedded practice in leadership development: *"The notion of sustainability preoccupies me a lot...one thing that would be terrible is to do all this work and it to not be sustained or grown. Two things are important: (1) a commitment to good evaluation processes and techniques that need to be present right from the beginning and (2) how do you measure over time and what systems do you put in place to promote sustainability once [participation in] the [formal] program is over?"*

Table 12.2 (continued)

8.	**Functionally integrate the LEADS Framework into provincial talent management, organizational strategies and daily work**
	The decision here is: *Where does this project—the integration and embedding of LEADS—fit in the other activities and priorities in the organization right now?*
	Organizations need to take a long-range approach to leadership development considering not only leadership development programming and its myriad of activities but the whole span of employment from pre-recruitment to retirement [43]. This means really considering the ongoing relationship between the individual and the organization, and creating a robust talent management strategy that includes excellent leadership development programming but goes beyond it.
	Questions to consider • How would the integration of LEADS support program, portfolio and organizational strategies? • What is the scope of this work? What kind of resources will this require? • What are the timelines?
	Key informant wisdom: Brad Dorohoy spoke about how important it is to be realistic about engaging in this work, to align with and be sensitive to everything else that is happening, and use that information to begin appropriately: *"You have to start somewhere, you have to put the flag in the ground and I think that enables the other pieces to be connected.... The flag enabled us to weave LEADS into the other product and processes when the time was right."*
9.	**Strengthen cross-functional partnerships with leaders to ensure alignment and integrated action**
	The decision here is: *What actions need to be taken to build appropriate partnerships to achieve your goals? How do we effectively integrate physician leadership into organizational leadership initiatives?*
	Patrick Lencioni [44] acknowledges leaders everywhere espouse a belief in teamwork, but laments those same leaders rarely manage to foster it. Rather they seem to build environments of competition, political in-fighting and silos.
	Questions to consider • How will we establish cross-functional partnerships to champion leadership and leadership development across the whole organization? • How will we build and strengthen the relationships needed to be successful in this endeavor? • What are the biggest barriers to building and sustaining the right relationships? Who can help you overcome any real or perceived barriers?
	Key informant wisdom: David Sweeney: *"We try to work with local health districts... to support their objectives... through working on cross-boundary issues, and building a sense of collaboration, working on something more than ourselves that will benefit the bigger system."*

(continued)

Table 12.2 (continued)

10.	**Build and strengthen mutually beneficial relationships with external partners**

The decision here is: *Are we willing to work and learn with others, identifying and keeping a shared purpose to guide our partnerships?*

Working to establish mutually beneficial relationships with external partners is another way of saying build relationships across boundaries, or develop coalitions: "Coalitions are a multidimensional construct and building them is both an art and a science. They create the need for many leaders to become 'boundary spanners,' individuals who are skilled at building relationships across boundaries rather than in them" [38]. This type of work requires strategic thinking and effective relationships and a multipronged approach.

Questions to consider
- What goals do you have in mind? How negotiable are they?
- What are the anticipated benefits for your organization and for proposed partners?
- What characteristics define a successful relationship like this?
- How will potential partners be identified and invited to connect?
- What structures, mechanisms or agreements need to be created?
- Who will negotiate the desired relationships and outcomes?
- What is the timeframe?
- What are the boundaries? How will these boundaries be clarified?

Key informant wisdom: There is no doubt the establishment and maintenance of a coalition is hard work. Words of wisdom from Peter Martin: *"The process of collaboration was messy, drawn out, and at times painful... when going into this type of collaboration talk about it at an executive level."*

Summary

A provincial health region, with its mix of centralized and decentralized features and unique culture, offers a unique context for leadership and leadership development. Increasingly it is acknowledged that to improve system performance we need to go beyond traditional approaches to leadership, which focused on developing individual capability. In the past, we underappreciated the need for developing collective capability as well as underemphasized the importance of designing the development of leaders for the context of the organization they work in.

The in-depth case studies in this chapter, the wisdom and lived experience of key informants, and the literature have important lessons for health regions. We have outlined how leadership development requires a different approach in highly centralized health regions. To organizations or health systems looking to adopt or leverage LEADS, we've offered a pragmatic ten step approach—relevant and adaptable to both province-wide and regional health systems as well as to small and large organizations. We have argued it is necessary to develop multipronged strategies for coherent, effective and forward-looking collective leadership as well as actively seek out opportunities to partner with others, across and beyond the organization, to successfully champion leadership and leadership development. We have also recommended functionally integrating LEADS across the talent management continuum and aligning and embedding it in organizational processes and daily work.

Our approach highlights how organizational development practitioners and system leaders need to orient themselves to the future and continue to challenge the status quo. Leadership for transformational change in provincial health regions requires continual adjustment and adaptation. In a dynamic health care environment, an ongoing and iterative assessment of the collective capabilities and intentional design of the leadership culture is required.

References

1. Drucker PF. Managing in turbulent times. London: Routledge; 2015.
2. Manitoba Centre for Health Policy. Definition: regional health authority; 2013. http://mchp-appserv.cpe.umanitoba.ca/viewDefinition.php?definitionID=103476. Accessed 2 Sep 2019.
3. Bergevin Y, Habib B, Elicksen K, Samis S, Rochon J, Adaime C. Towards the triple aim of better health, better care and better value for Canadians: transforming regions into high per forming health systems. Ottawa, ON: Canadian Foundation for Health care Improvement; 2016. https://www.cfhi-fcass.ca/sf-docs/default-source/on-call/oncall-regionalization-report-e.pdf?sfvrsn=2.
4. Marchildon GP. Regionalization in Canada: will Ontario become the new ground zero in health system reorganization? Inaugural Chair Lecture presented at Institute of Health Policy, Management & Evaluation, University of Toronto, 19 Nov 2015. http://ihpme.utoronto.ca/wp-content/uploads/2015/10/G.-Marchildon-Inaugural-Chair-Lecture-19-N-ov-2015.pdf.
5. Denis J-L. Is there a future for regionalization in Canada? Keynote presented at Canadian Association for Health Services and Policy Research, 28 May 2015. https://www.cahspr.ca/en/presentation/5574f6a537dee8b718501959.
6. Barker P, Church J. Revisiting health regionalization in Canada: more bark than bite? Int J Health Serv. 2017;7(2):333–51.
7. Lewis S. A system in name only – access, variation, and reform in Canada's provinces. N Engl J Med. 2015;372(6):497–500.
8. Van Aerde J. Has regionalization of the Canadian health system contributed to better health? Can J Phys Leadersh. 2016;2(3):6.
9. CBC News. What you need to know about Ontario's new model for health care, 1 Mar 2019. https://www.cbc.ca/news/canada/toronto/what-are-ontario-health-teams-doug-ford-government-1.5035750. Accessed 2 Aug 2019.
10. Sturmberg JP, Martin CM, editors. Handbook of systems and complexity in health. London: Springer; 2013.
11. Harrison MI, Kimani J. Building capacity for a transformation initiative: system redesign at Denver Health. Health Care Manage Rev. 2009;34(1):42–53.
12. Denis J-L, Langley A, Sergi V. Leadership in the plural. Acad Manag Ann. 2012;6(1):211–83.
13. Chreim S, MacNaughton K. Distributed leadership in health care teams: constellation role distribution and leadership practices. Health Care Manage Rev. 2015;41:200–12.
14. Marchildon GP, Fletcher AJ. Systems thinking and the leadership conundrum in health care. Evid. Policy. 2015. http://www.ingentaconnect.com/content/tpp/ep/pre-prints/content-EvP_070. Accessed 27 Feb 2019.
15. Merlino JI, Raman A. Health care service fanatics. Harv Bus Rev. 2013;91(5):108–16.
16. Duckett S. Getting the foundations right: Alberta's approach to healthcare reform. Healthc Policy. 2011;6(3):22–6.
17. Bishop S. Accelerating health system transformation in Saskatchewan. Lessons learned from the Saskatchewan surgical initiative (SkSI). Ottawa, ON: Canadian Foundation for Health Improvement; 2014. https://www.cfhi-fcass.ca/sf-docs/default-source/reports/sask-report.pdf?sfvrsn=2. Accessed 15 Aug 2019.

18. West M, Eckert R, Steward K, Pasmore B. Developing collective leadership for health care. The Kings' Fund & The Centre for Creative Leadership: London; 2014.
19. Silzer RF, Dowell BE, editors. Strategy-driven talent management: a leadership imperative. 1st ed. San Francisco, CA: Jossey-Bass; 2010.
20. Centre for Creative Leadership. How to create a strong leadership strategy; 2019. https://www.ccl.org/articles/leading-effectively-articles/got-a-strong-leadership-strategy/. Accessed 1 Mar 2019.
21. Chesebrough C, Davachi L, Rock D, Slaughter M, Grant H. Coherence: the architecture of efficient learning. NeuroLeadersh J. 2019;8:1–21.
22. Kendel D. Opinion: health system restructuring in Saskatchewan – reflections of an interim chief executive officer; 2018. https://hqc.sk.ca/news-events/hqc-news/health-system-restructuring-saskatchewan-ceo-reflections. Accessed 31 Mar 2019.
23. Abrametz B, Bragg T, Kendel, D Saskatchewan Advisory Panel on health system structure report.pdf; 2016. http://publications.gov.sk.ca/documents/13/105089-Saskatchewan-Advisory-Panel-on-Health-System-Structure-Report.pdf. Accessed 30 Jan 2019.
24. The Provincial Health Authority Act (Chapter P-30.3). Saskatchewan Statutes; 2017. https://www.canlii.org/en/sk/laws/stat/ss-2017-c-p-30.3/latest/ss-2017-c-p-30.3.html. Accessed 6 Jun 2019.
25. Unleashing innovation: excellent healthcare for Canada/report of the advisory panel on healthcare innovation. Ottawa, ON: Canada Advisory Panel on Healthcare Innovation. 2015. https://www.canada.ca/en/health-canada/services/publications/health-system-services/report-advisory-panel-healthcare-innovation.html. Accessed 22 Jul 2019.
26. Better health, better care, better value for all: refocussing health care reform in Canada. Ottawa, ON: Health Council of Canada Archive. 2013. https://healthcouncilcanada.ca/773/. Accessed 22 Jul 2019.
27. 2019–20 Performance Agreement. An agreement between: Secretary, NSW Health and the Health Education and Training Institute for the period 1 July 2019–30 June 2020. https://www.heti.nsw.gov.au/__data/assets/pdf_file/0003/436701/performance-greement.PDF. Accessed 2 Aug 2019.
28. Health Education and Training. Vision and purpose. https://www.heti.nsw.gov.au/about-heti/our-organisation/vision-purpose-mission. Accessed 2 Aug 2019.
29. Sweeney D. Beyond frameworks: developing leadership in health care. A presentation to the Canadian Health Leadership Network Knowledge Acceleration Working Group. Ottawa, ON: Canadian Health Leadership Network; 2018.
30. Heifetz R, Grashow A, Linsky M. The practice of adaptive leadership. Boston, MA: Harvard Business Press; 2009.
31. Dunoon D. In the leadership mode. Bloomington, IN: Trafford Publishing; 2008.
32. Brown A, editor. Developing collective leadership for healthcare. London: The King's Fund; 2014.
33. Health Education and Training Institute. Leadership and management. https://www.heti.nsw.gov.au/education-and-training/our-focus-areas/leadership-and-management. Accessed 2 Aug 2019.
34. Eckert R, West M, Altman D, Steward K, Pasmore B. Delivering a collective leadership strategy for health care. Ottawa, ON: Centre for Creative Leadership; 2014. https://www.ccl.org/wpcontent/uploads/2015/04/DeliveringCollectiveLeadership.pdf. Accessed 23 May 2019.
35. Yukl G. Leadership in organizations. 8th ed. Boston, MA: Pearson; 2013.
36. Dickson G, Tholl B. Bringing leadership to life in health: LEADS in a caring environment: a new perspective. Kindle edition. London: Springer; 2014.
37. Vilches S, Fenwick S, Harris B, Lammi B, Racette R. Changing health organizations with the LEADS leadership framework: report of the 2014-2016 LEADS impact study. Ottawa, ON: Fenwick Leadership Explorations, the Canadian College of Health Leaders, & the Centre for Health Leadership and Research, Royal Roads University; 2016. https://leadscanada.net/document/1788/LEADS_Impact_Report_2017_FINAL.pdf. Accessed 1 May 2019.

38. Snowden DJ, Boone ME. A leader's framework for decision-making. Harv Bus Rev. 2007;85(11):68–71.
39. Gupta K, Sleezer C, Russ-Eft DF. A practical guide to needs assessment. 2nd ed. San Francisco, CA: Pfeiffer/Wiley/ASTD; 2007.
40. Lucia AD, Lepsinger R. The art and science of competency models: pinpointing critical success factors in organizations. Jossey-Bass/Pfeiffer: San Francisco, CA; 1999.
41. Boyatzis RE. Competencies in the 21st century. J Manag Dev. 2008;27(1):5–12.
42. Phillips JJ, Phillips PP, Ray R. Measuring leadership development: quantify your program's impact and ROI on organizational performance. New York, NY: McGraw-Hill; 2012. http://www.books24x7.com/marc.asp?bookid=47650. Accessed 30 May 2019
43. Groves KS. Talent management best practices: How exemplary health care organizations create value in a down economy. Health Care Manag Rev. 2011;36(3):227–40.
44. Lencioni PM. The trouble with teamwork. Leader to leader. 2003;2003(29):35–40.

The LEADS in a Caring Environment Framework: Putting LEADS to Work in People-Centred Care

13

Cathy Cole, Heather Thiessen, and Brenda Andreas

Living LEADS means putting the needs of patients and families first.

Effective leadership requires a deep connection to the people that you work with and the people you serve. LEADS can guide health system leaders at all levels on how to connect, partner and co-design with patients, families, communities, and citizens. The *LEADS in a Caring Environment* framework is a foundational model for health system transformation and one of the most notable transformations in this era is the activation of patients, residents, clients and their families and communities as our partners.

Since 2014, when the first edition of this book was published, the field of patient and family engagement has grown tremendously. Patient engagement has become a cornerstone of quality care [1] and, while it originally focused on the direct relationship between patients and providers, it has grown to recognize users of health services have important contributions to make to the design and delivery of services—from grassroots to governance [2].

The motto of the LEADS framework is "in a caring environment," but what does creating a caring environment mean? And not just from the perspective of an organization's leadership and providers but to patients, their families and the community at large? Many organizations and leaders aspire to be people-centred, yet many leaders feel they are "faking it until they make it."

It's commonly thought being patient-centred is an essential part of improving patient safety, yet many organizational leaders struggle to create a culture to put it into practice [3, 4]. If used correctly, LEADS can effectively guide leaders to developing skills in people-centred care and improvements in patient safety (as well as other improvement goals). In this chapter, we're focusing on the need for leaders to

C. Cole (✉) · H. Thiessen · B. Andreas
Saskatchewan Health Authority, Saskatoon, SK, Canada
e-mail: cathy.cole@saskhealthauthority.ca

© Springer Nature Switzerland AG 2020
G. Dickson, B. Tholl (eds.), *Bringing Leadership to Life in Health: LEADS in a Caring Environment*, https://doi.org/10.1007/978-3-030-38536-1_13

operationalize people-centred care and how LEADS can be put to work to do that. We also offer examples of how health care organizations across the world are using LEADS to increase their people centredness.

The World Health Organization defines people-centred care as "an approach to care that consciously adopts individuals, carers, families and communities as participants in, and beneficiaries of, trusted health systems. People-centred care extends beyond care interactions as it focuses on health services to the role of communities and their role in shaping health policy and health services" [5].

There's a variety of terms for patient and family engagement, including patient and family-centred care, client and family-centred care, patient and family engaged care and people-centred care. We're using people-centred care because it expands the idea to include community, and is in line with the World Health Organization, Accreditation Canada, and the Canadian Health Standards Organization. However, we do use other terms when they are the words used by an organization we're writing about.

The Evidence-Based Case for People-Centred Care

The World Health Organization Framework on Integrated People-Centred Health Services says a people-centred approach is crucial to developing health systems that can respond to emerging and varied health challenges [6]. It identifies five strategies for doing that.

1. Empowering and engaging people and communities.
2. Strengthening governance and accountability.
3. Reorienting the model of care.
4. Coordinating services in and across sectors.
5. Creating an enabling environment.

Despite the increasing emphasis on people-centred care, many health systems remain focused on hospital-based, disease-focused, siloed care. Such health organizations likely offer limited accountability to the people they serve and have little incentive to provide care that actually responds to the needs of their users. Their patients may be unable to control or contribute to decisions about their care or the health of their communities.

Developing integrated people-centred care systems generates significant benefits, including improved access to care, improved health and clinical outcomes, better health literacy and self-care, increased satisfaction with care, improved job satisfaction for health workers, improved efficiency of services and reduced overall costs [7–10]. The 2017 Commonwealth Fund comparison of heath care system performance reveals striking variations in performance across its five domains—Care Process, Access, Administrative Efficiency, Equity, and Health Care Outcomes. No country ranked first across all domains or measures, suggesting all countries have room to improve. The U.S., France, and Canada scored lower than the 11-country average across most of the five domains [11]. Because people-centred care is understood to be a key contributor to patient safety and quality improvement, many countries are focused on integrating it into daily practice. In the Institute of Medicine's report *Crossing the Quality Chasm*, patient-centredness is identified as one of six dimensions of quality [12], driving health care leaders to value people-centred care and include patients in all aspects of care [13].

Policy makers are increasingly recognizing that patient preference and insights need to be integrated in professional knowledge and experience to produce better care [14]. But real change requires going beyond token involvement toward genuine collaboration such as co-production [15]. Recently in Canada, there have been legislative efforts putting greater emphasis on people-centred care, such as Ontario's Excellent Care for All Act (Bill 8 [16]) and Patients First Act [17]. All call on health care organizations to focus on a more holistic patient journey.

The Health Standards Organization in Canada and Accreditation Canada have played major roles in coordinating organizational efforts to boost people-centred care [18]. Accreditation Canada added people-centred care criteria to its standards in 2016; they include partnership and co-design with patients and families in all areas of program and service delivery and in governance and leadership. The criteria indicate high quality care is possible only through co-design and co-production [18].

Introducing people-centred care means every care interaction, every contract negotiation and every policy debate must include careful consideration of who gets a seat at the decision-making table. Another component of people-centred care is developing cultural safety, which is different from a culture of safety. The latter is risk management, while cultural safety is about ensuring our patients and their families feel safe and cared for—and staff do as well. Cultural safety also requires recognizing the inequities in engagement: we serve many diverse and vulnerable populations and it's important to ensure all patient voices have the chance to be heard in an ethical and caring way. Patient engagement moves health care from the traditional view of the patient as a passive recipient of service to an integral member of teams in redesigning care [19].

Family engagement is just as critical as patient engagement. Historically, families have been an untapped resource, viewed as visitors, not partners. But increasingly families and friends are taking on caregiver roles and supporting patients through their health care journeys. Families have a valuable role to play sharing information with the patient and care team, identifying safety issues and concerns, and supporting patients when they're not receiving direct care [20]. Family presence policies let patients designate family members or other loved ones whom they want to have unrestricted access to them during their care. Studies show unlimited access to family and loved ones reduces complications and stress for everyone involved and improves the overall experience of care and outcomes [21].

Many leading health systems around the world have begun implementing family presence policies [22], including in Canada. For example, the Canadian Foundation for Health Care Improvement's *Better Together: Partnering with Families* campaign, conducted in partnership with the Institute for Patient and Family-Centered Care is designed to help hospitals change from seeing families as visitors to recognizing them as partners in care, starting by easing restrictive visiting hours [23].

Continuum of engagement

Levels of engagement	Consultation	Involvement	Partnership and shared leadership
Direct care	Patients receive information about a diagnosis	Patients are asked about their preferences in treatment plan	Treatment decisions are made based on patients' preferences, medical evidence, and clinical judgment
Organizational design and governance	Organization surveys patients about their care experiences	Hospital involves patients as advisors or advisory council members	Patients co-lead hospital safety and quality improvement committees
Policy making	Public agency conducts focus groups with patients to ask opinions about a health care issue	Patients' recommendations about research priorities are used by public agency to make funding decisions	Patients have equal representation on agency committee that makes decisions about how to allocate resources to health programs

Factors influencing engagement:
- **Patient** (beliefs about patient role, health literacy, education)
- **Organization** (policies and practices, culture)
- **Society** (social norms, regulations, policy)

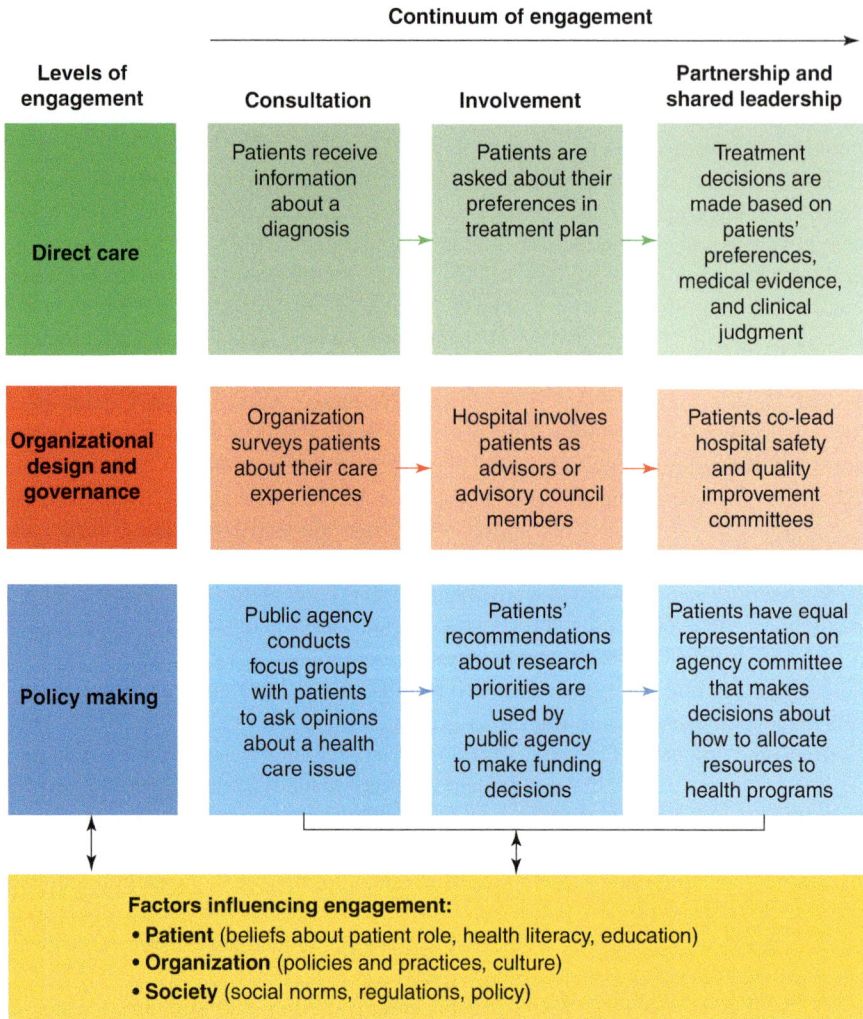

Fig. 13.1 Carmen framework to guide engagement of patients, families, and citizens [24]

In addition to high-level polices, there are several frameworks describing what's required to create people-centred care. One developed by Carmen and colleagues (see Fig. 13.1) describes various levels of engaging patients and families from consultation to partnership in three levels of the health system: direct care, organizational design and governance, and policy-making [24]. The authors say health care organizations must work on all three levels to succeed in achieving people-centred transformation.

The Patient and Family Engaged Care framework (see Fig. 13.2) developed by Frampton and colleagues [25] describes the organizational foundations, activities and structures needed to create patient and family-engaged care, which will result in

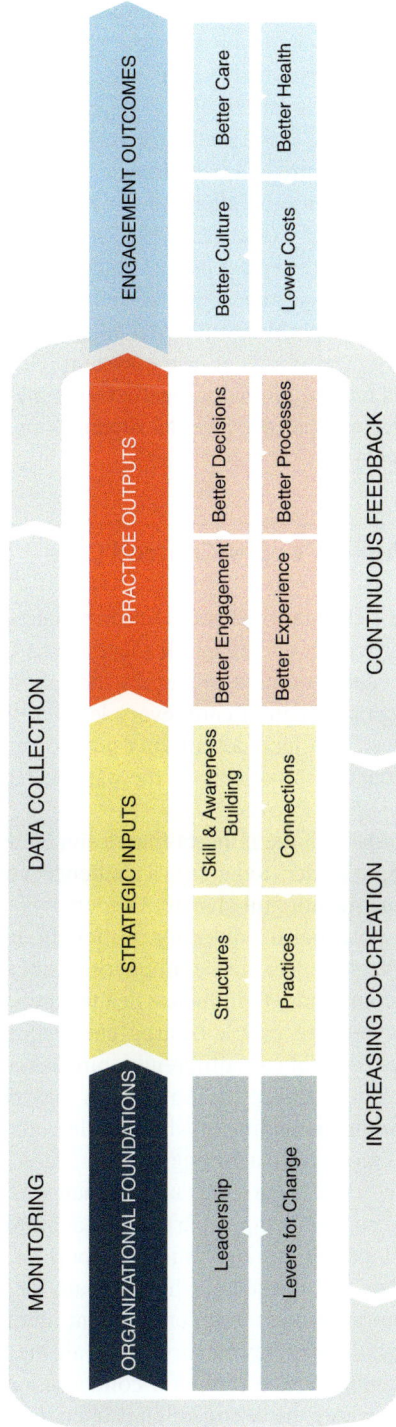

Fig. 13.2 Patient and family engaged care framework [23]

better engagement, decisions, experiences and processes. It envisions clients and families meaningfully and continually involved in decision-making at all levels (from the point of care, to organizational system-wide quality improvement and in developing policy). Informed by a variety of literature showing a clear intentional role for leaders in people-centred care, the framework demonstrates the need for organizations to make people-centred care a strategic priority, with the support of leaders whose behaviour, decisions and allocation of resources show they're committed to success and sustainability (i.e., LEADS). Organizations need to start by developing a clear vision of what effective patient engagement looks like and identifying the strategies and investments needed to make it happen [26].

We won't solve health care's problems until patients, families, residents, clients and communities are all engaged partners in the system. Health care leaders and teams must learn the skills required to work together with the people they serve to realize the benefits of patient partnerships at organizational and system-wide levels.

The Role of Leadership in People-Centred Care

Changing an organization's culture to be people centred takes some revolutionary adjustments to services, provision of care and leadership. As Chap. 7 said, results-oriented leadership is needed to create processes that align toward a common goal—and if the goal is people-centred care, every level of the organization will have to change its practices. That includes altering professional identities to leave behind their traditional concept of patients as the passive recipients of the work they do [27].

This is, of course, at odds with the mindset that designed many of the ways we go about improving health, so leaders today face a challenge: connecting people and changing mindsets to create meaningful change. Leaders who foster a wider set of relationships increase the potential for diversity of thought, experience and background. Bringing new, diverse voices into conversations about change empowers patients, families and the community to influence health care's evolution into being people-centred. However, because people-centred care requires leaders to think about patients and families' role in care differently, mindsets—depending on how set they are—must also change. Given those mindsets may differ from person to person, establishing a clear understanding of what people-centred care means to the organization is critical to successfully adopting it [28].

Effective leadership is essential to driving cultural change [29, 30] and also a key factor in successful patient engagement, which can't be achieved without high-level action such as policy development, but also official support for front-line and grass-roots innovation. Executives and managers who advocate for patient and community partnerships foster empowerment and commitment among patients, families and staff [1, 31, 32]. They are also key in supporting all the actions essential for major transformation in health care: meaningful collaboration, shared power, and learning are all more likely where the organization is open to co-designing changes.

The best leaders are arguably the ones who are continuously monitoring their external and internal people environments so they understand what needs to be changed and how they should go about it [33, 34]. Culture begins to shift when people in leadership roles throughout the organization believe in the value of patient experience, such as talking about patient experience in a way that shows it matters to them; talking about patient experience in discussions of daily tasks; modelling the behaviour they want to see in staff; guiding and coaching those they influence; and recognizing people who do the right things [1, 22]. As Bowers, Nolet, Roberts, and Esmond said, "Strong leadership is an important ingredient to any successful practice or organizational change. The more extensive the change, the more important leadership becomes. Taking on the role of change champion, leaders often make the difference between success and failure" [35].

LEADS can guide leaders through the challenging transition to truly people-centred care. The Develop coalitions capability, demonstrates a commitment to customers and service, says leaders "...facilitate collaboration, cooperation and coalitions among diverse groups and perspectives...to improve service." Strategies for doing that include emphasizing engagement in all aspects of people-centred care, overseeing thoughtful recruitment of patients and families for meaningful partnership roles and taking intentional leadership action to support and sustain change.

Chapter 5: Lead self will help leaders change their behaviour in the ways needed to run a people-centred organization or system. The capability of self-awareness is essential: leaders need awareness of their own assumptions, values and strengths to alter how they and their organizations function. Demonstrating character, another Lead self capability, through honesty, integrity, resilience and confidence, will be key in earning the trust of new partners and moving people-centred care from a goal to practice.

Informal leaders, such as patients and family members, who don't have a position of power in the formal system but do have influence through their networks and connections are also important in making the people-centred care culture shift. Best and colleagues identified five factors for creating large-system transformations, three of which involved working with informal leaders, including bringing them into a distributed leadership model and engaging patients and families and physicians [36]. Helen Bevan and colleagues in their recent white paper [37] argue there is an emerging movement of informal leaders who are committed to their organizations and want them to succeed. They are typically passionate people who support the people and patient-centred goals of their health care organizations. They are willing to take responsibility for change but question the way it's being done now. These radicals, many of them patient and family leaders, operate at the edge of current thinking and practice. The ePatient movement for example, is led by strong, highly motivated and connected patient leaders who push boundaries and paradigms [38].

The important message is to remember leadership is not reserved for CEOs: each of us, by the fact of our shared humanity, can show leadership. Global thought leaders in disruptive transformation such as Clayton Christensen [39] suggest that the most radical thinking about future possibilities is unlikely to come from the centre or top of organizations. Helen Bevan says [37] diverse groups of people consistently make better decisions than small groups of senior leaders or experts. By investing in informal leaders, we open up our decision-making processes to different kinds of conversations with people [40].

Putting LEADS to Work: Developing Informal Leaders

Holland Bloorview Kids Rehabilitation Hospital [16] *in Toronto, Canada, is a long-time leader in patient and family engagement. Among other examples, the hospital has a formal committee—the Family Leader Accreditation Group—that fully integrates 17 family and youth leaders into its accreditation preparation process. In the group, staff, clients and family leaders meet as equal partners to update quality and safety initiatives to prepare for accreditation.*

In another example from Hotel Dieu Grace Healthcare *in Windsor, Canada, front line employees can self-identify as emerging leaders and receive LEADS training to support their leadership development. The training includes the option to work on a leadership project to make improvements based on their own ideas to build confidence in leading change. This example shows how LEADS can be used to develop informal leaders to be effective in leading change.*

A shift to people-centred care requires a systems view, a massive shift in vision, and cultural adjustments, all of which demand leaders deft in change who have the skills and ability to inspire others to action. As the two examples above show, the LEADS framework is useful for both formal and informal leaders looking to acquire the skills they need to lead.

Case Studies: Putting LEADS to Work in People-Centred Care

Where organizations and leaders can get lost developing people-centred care is in the *how*. By using the LEADS framework to develop leaders, organizations can begin to move people-centred care from principles to behaviour and action at all levels, but it's important to remember context and culture matter, because leaders don't shift to people-centred care in isolation. This next segment gives several examples from Canada and around the globe of how LEADS has been used as a framework to improve people-centred care in different settings.

Case Study: Saskatchewan Health Authority—Engaging Patients in Transformation

In 2017, twelve health regions in Saskatchewan were amalgamated into one organization, the Saskatchewan Health Authority (see Chap. 12). Patient and family-centred care was at the forefront of planning to build the new organization.

Saskatchewan's journey toward patient and family-centred care started in 2009 with the Patient First Review [41], which called for major changes in how patients experience the health system, how health services are delivered and how the system is designed. The report's overarching conclusion was that the health system should make patient and family-centred care the foundation and principal aim of the province's health system, through a new policy framework to be adopted system wide. The Patient First Review said active engagement of patients is key to transformation and outlined how patients should be routinely involved in all planning exercises as well as in developing new accountability tools.

The creation of the Saskatchewan Health Authority in 2017 provided the opportunity to put the report's recommendations into practice. It did so by redesigning and aligning services for better care, and the LEADS framework was the leadership team's guide as it reimagined health care, including patient and family-centred care. Health system leaders drew on LEADS as they worked to link their own ideas to action aligned with the new health system's strategic objectives. They also used LEADS to support them as they worked through the disruption of reorganization, innovation and communication challenges. LEADS principles also shaped the vision of the culture shift into partnerships with patients and families, when executive leaders had to demonstrate how the strategic goal of people-centred care became standard practice.

Here are some examples of how LEADS was used to put the report's recommendations into practice:

Making patient and family-centred care the foundation of the Saskatchewan Health Authority's values, so all the Authority's activities are grounded in it. (The values were co-written with patients and families).

Embedding patient- and family-centred care as a distinct portfolio in the organizational structure (titled Patient and Client Experience). It has a dedicated executive director, directors, and staff. The portfolio also covers accreditation, creating strategic alignment and operational links to Accreditation Canada's people-centred care standards.

Developing patient and family partnerships at various levels of the organization, including:

- *Forming a Patient and Family Leadership Council, with a mandate to achieve a patient and family-centred culture. Its membership includes patient and family advisors representing the diversity of the people of Saskatchewan as well as executive leaders of the Saskatchewan Health Authority.*
- *Involving patients and families in the transition to a single health authority, through consultations and focus groups on organizational design and structure.*
- *Including patient and family advisors and knowledge keepers (an indigenous phrase signifying individuals [elders] who possess wisdom and carry teaching and practices to be preserved) on hiring committees for executive leadership positions. Their role included asking questions and participating in evaluating and choosing candidates.*
- *Teleconferencing monthly with different groups of members of the Advisor Partnership Forum, a community of 600 patients and family members to inform developers of a Patient Client Experience Portfolio. Because the health authority is growing rapidly, getting in touch on key issues ensures engagement with patients and families guides the work.*
- *Partnering with patients and families to design events such as the Accreditation Vision Day, the Patient and Client Experience Vision Day and strategic committees such as Provincial Policy Development, Patient Safety and Provincial Health Network; patients and family advisors also participated.*

The Saskatchewan Health Authority recognizes meaningful engagement with patients and families requires deliberate attention of leaders at all levels. The leadership team learned they must lead with their hearts, be willing to be vulnerable, and honour the lived experiences of patients and families by creating space for co-design.

Menno Place: Strengthening Leadership in Long-Term Care [42]

Menno Place, home to 700 long-term-care residents in Abbotsford, BC, wanted to shift from a medical model with an emphasis on task-focused acute care practice to a holistic, people-centred model with a home-like environment. It chose LEADS as the foundation of its effort to strengthen its leadership, a strategy dubbed "Living LEADS" by the CEO. Resident and family-centred care was introduced as its strategic framework in January 2015 and expanded in 2018.

Shifting Menno Place's culture from the traditional medical model of "provider knows best" to a resident and family-centred model required bold leadership and intentional support from the executive team. LEADS was used by the senior executives to develop an awareness of and common vocabulary for leadership and guided the transformation. In accordance with the Achieve results domain, for example, each leader developed a purpose statement and a personal goal related to resident- and family-centred care, which were then shared with one other.

As part of building leadership, Menno Place announced each leader would be accountable for identifying and submitting two departmental goals designed to shift culture. The goals had to be measurable and would be shared with the leadership team, so leaders could support each other. One proposed goal shared by the team was to improve the organization's ability to form partnerships, using the Develop coalitions capabilities as a guide. Menno Place had been relatively insular, and leaders were now encouraged to look outside of Menno to develop coalitions.

One project that emerged from this was school groups and family members being invited to discuss the redesign of the Menno Place Special Care Unit. Although this slowed the work down, trying out co-design on a real project helped leaders learn the process for partnering with families and others in future changes to Menno Place.

Menno Place executives have been coaching staff to think in new ways and step out of their comfort zones. Naturally some ideas have been met with resistance from staff. Menno Place leaders have learned that resistance often reflects a fear of the unknown or of loss of power. Consistent messaging and working together by all formal leaders to move the resistors forward is showing progress. Regular meetings with staff and face-to-face discussions have helped to make the new vision for care at Menno Place clearer. Empowering leaders, staff, residents and family members has reduced cultural barriers to change.

One of the most effective ways in which Menno Place leaders now show families the sincerity of their commitment to resident and family-centred care is to act on their suggestions. Demonstrating they're listening and genuinely want families to bring forward ideas is also an effective way to get buy-in for future initiatives.

Case Study: Strengthening Leadership Through LEADS for the Uganda Alliance of Patient Organizations

The Uganda Alliance of Patient Organizations (UAPO) was founded in 2011 by 10 nongovernmental organizations dedicated to advancing the interests of patient groups neglected by the over-burdened and underfunded health care system in Uganda. This example highlights the importance of contextual leadership in engaging multiple stakeholders in redesigning services.

UAPO's strategic priorities include promoting meaningful engagement of patients in their health care, providing a strong patient's voice on health care policy, and stimulating initiatives to advance patient-centred research and care. UAPO is a coalition that takes an integrated approach to problem solving, comes together to share expertise and provide a structured, united front for key health care stakeholders to advance patient-centred care.

In August of 2017 a program providing an overview of the five domains of LEADS was delivered to UAPO representatives. The audience comprised administrators, advocates and physicians from UAPO organizations and the workshops were intended to increase the personal and organizational leadership capacity of the participants so they could improve UAPO's ability to bring about positive change in the Ugandan health care system. The LEADS domains were applied in novel ways to both amplify the personal as well as organizational leadership capabilities. A focus in the Develop coalitions module was to highlight the role service has in transformational change, including a discussion of the service value chain and how a common focus on service in improving patient care can breed better engagement and outcomes for the organization.

A module on Daniel Kahneman's [43] research on unconscious biases, and how an awareness of strengths and weaknesses created a foundation for authentic leadership, helped participants uncover potential mental models that were undermining their leadership abilities, instincts and decision-making prowess. Feedback from participants included 100% of them reporting their leadership skills had improved, and they could apply those skills to improve patient care.

Facilitators later circled back to gauge if people followed through with efforts to bring positive change. Respondents said applying what they learned led to better engagement with patients and health care stakeholders, "greatly improved team cohesion and performance" and enhanced their personal abilities at all levels, including listening, personal confidence and improving relationships with clients. The workshops clearly provided them with skills and the belief they could use them in in the health system (Stewart Dickson, Personal interview 2019 Jul 10).

ViTA South: Using Health LEADS Australia in an Extended Care Home [44]

ViTA South is part of a not-for-profit organization called Aged Care and Housing, which has been supporting older South Australians since 1952. The organization offers a wide range of services including retirement and residential options, domestic, personal and nursing care in the home, respite choices and short-term transition services. ViTA South opened in Adelaide, South Australia in June 2014.

At ViTA a research project facilitated applying the concept of distributed leadership as described in Health LEADS Australia: the Australian health leadership framework, to generate conditions required to support sustained collaborative practice. The decision to try distributed leadership was based in the assumption it would enhance inter-professional teamwork, collaborative decision making and "whole resident" care.

Some of the goals identified by ViTA South were to showcase a culture that supports a rights-based approach to people-centred care; to deliver services which contribute to maximizing quality of life for older people; and to promote rehabilitation and restoration for older people in a flexible environment. Evidence from interviews with ViTA South's formal leaders confirmed distributed leadership did lead to more collaborative care by staff.

LEADS as a Framework for Developing a People-Centred Health System

The LEADS framework doesn't explicitly mention people-centred care or say effective health care leaders need to be proficient in it; however, the language of LEADS does not preclude the potential use of LEADS capabilities to engage patients and families better; nor does it exclude the use of LEADS by patients and families to support their leadership efforts. As the examples above show, LEADS capabilities can provide valuable support for the individual and organizational transformation needed to adopt and sustain people-centred care. For example, although the Engage others domain does not mention patients as partners, statements like "[Leaders]… support and challenge others to achieve professional and personal goals" could certainly refer to patients and clients, if leaders consider them part of the system.

In formal and informal health care leadership, patient partnerships are determined by where leaders put the boundary around their sphere of influence. People-centred care expands traditional provider boundaries to include a broader community and a broader understanding: working *with* patients and families, not simply doing *to* or *for* them.

There is a not-to-be-missed opportunity to give people-centred care special attention in LEADS, so individuals developing their leadership through it will emerge with a new way of thinking about and acting toward patients, families and the community. People-centred care on its own isn't enough to support leaders to lead but the five domains of the LEADS framework can be used to show leaders how to move people-centred care from a principle to actions, words, and behaviour that will contribute to changing culture. To help with that, we have developed the following guide to support leaders in people-centred care, shown in Table 13.1, below.

Table 13.1 LEADS in a people-centred care context

Lead self
- Leaders connect to, and are guided by the humanity of health care
- Leaders are committed to leading with patients, families and communities as partners
- Patients' and families' lived experience is valued and grounds the leaders' perspective
- Leaders are open and seek to understand the perspectives of those they serve
- Leaders develop a rigorous practice of hearing the voices of patients and families

Engage others
- Leaders engage patients, families, and communities as their partners at all levels, and act on ideas, concerns and co-created recommendations
- Leaders seek diversity to ensure voices that are often missed or underrepresented are heard
- Leaders model engagement with patients and families to others in the organization
- Patient, family and community engagement recognizes providers don't have all the answers and partnership should be daily practice

Achieve results
- Leaders are humble and curious and play a key role in connecting people and ideas
- Leaders ensure patient-centred care, engagement and partnership are expressly included in the organization's vision, values, strategic plans and training
- Leaders always integrate user perspectives and related evidence in decision-making
- Leaders align and ground their work in the broader patient experience
- Planning for projects, communications and quality improvement tools involves patients and families
- Improvement efforts begin with user and staff experiences and include patients and families as partners to guide meaningful change
- Patient and family involvement is measured, assessed and evaluated and the results used to guide future action

Table 13.1 (continued)

Develop coalitions
• Specific goals are established for community partnerships on health care improvement
• Leaders build relationships with community organizations and their representatives to improve client and patient care
• Leaders understand how to widen the circle of involvement and share power, knowledge and how to mobilize it
• Leaders facilitate collaboration at all levels and across organizations to improve care and service
System transformation
• Leaders consider the entire patient journey across systems when working to improve their organizations and the system overall
• Leaders see patients, residents, clients and family members as whole people
• Innovations are planned with patients and families; successful ones are shared across the system
• Leaders use patient experience data and input to determine emerging trends and make strategic adjustments
• Leaders at all levels champion patient and family partnerships to support a culture of continuous improvement and innovation across the system

What's Important to Patients and Families

When thinking about what patients and families want and need from leaders, the patient and family co-authors identified four themes that emerged from the examples featured in this chapter.

First, value for patients and families is created at the point of care. As a patient, it does me no good if the CEO gets it and my family doctor doesn't. The patient experience is created by interactions with front-line care providers. If organizations have their values, systems and processes focused on people-centred care and the care providers aren't included, then they have failed. The challenge for formal leaders is first, to create a culture for the authentic partnerships at all levels to thrive; and second, to focus the value of those partnerships at the point of care.

A second theme to achieve meaningful patient partnerships is that patients and their families will have to be given, and accept, much larger roles with frontline care teams, including identifying needs, proposing solutions, testing them out, and implementing them together [24]. A foundational role for the health provider is to engage patients as part of the care team and activate them in participating in their care including:

- Understand and respect me and my goals, and co-design together a care plan tailored to me.
- Understand and respect how my care connects to other providers and systems.
- Ensure continuity of my care and see me as a whole person including the context that I am living.

A third theme identified by our patient authors is that people-centred care is about humanity. It is achieved by developing trust, respect, and truth between patients and providers at all levels of the health system. As a patient I come to you in *trust* that you will engage with me on my healthcare journey. I expect you will *respect* both my expertise and my lived experience as I will respect your expertise and lived experience as a provider. And I expect *truth*, in that we can share, in a timely manner, in difficult conversations, information about unexpected or difficult outcomes. Improving processes, medications, treatments and technology is only part of the picture. The human dimension of care is likely one of the biggest contributions to how patients and families experience care and thus one of the biggest opportunities for transformation [45]. The transformation of human interactions happens at three levels:

- At the individual level (What care works for you and me?)
- At program level, unit, or organizational level (How should care be designed and delivered for all patients like you and me?)
- At a system level (What services should be available, for whom and in what way?)

A fourth theme is that patient engagement needs to be construed as a moral issue as well as an economic issue [46]. Money and cost are important; but engagement of patients and families often reduces costs while improving the quality and safety of care. Yet, many health care providers still believe professional knowledge trumps patient experience [47]. Leaders at all levels need to understand how to take people-centred care from a philosophy to behaviour that operationalizes trust, respect and truth at the point of care. In healthcare there are many comprehensive pieces that, while operating distinctly, each have value; yet unless brought together, are nowhere as powerful as when integrated. People-centred care is the catalyst for an exponential opportunity to impact healthcare [2].

> The case here in raising the imagery of a patchwork is to acknowledge both the chaos and beauty of healthcare, recognize the individuality of various efforts and their power in coming together and to make the case that under this umbrella of experience we can create powerful alignment and purposeful grounding for focused action in moving forward. The idea that experience is the soft stuff of healthcare must come to an end for as intricate and challenging as the science of healthcare is, there may be no more complex opportunity than that of tackling the human experience in healthcare overall [2].

If we frame this concept within the Systems transformation capabilities of the LEADS framework, all leaders must see the entire journey of the patient and how all parts of the system contribute to the patient experience. Mobilizing this idea requires leaders to give up some of the edges of their own turf. Leaders are required to be mindful of the ways systems are organized and how they may create boundaries that limit people-centred care. Concerns about the health system extend beyond traditional boundaries of the broader community in which the population is being served. Coalitions between communities, community-based organizations, systems beyond health such as education and justice all need to be built as they all contribute to an individual's overall health. How do we make people centred care everyone's role? How do we ensure lived experience is woven throughout leader's regular work?

Summary

The LEADS in a Caring Environment framework describes the capabilities needed to be an effective leader in health care. As noted in Chap. 5, to truly be effective, your behaviour must be consonant with who you are and embedded in the values that connect you to the human experience. Our additional message is that leading the health care challenges of today requires leaders to lead in a people-centred way.

Leaders need to shift their thinking towards partnerships with patients and families and communities as a necessary part of leadership in health care. The domains of LEADS provide an effective framework for formal and informal leaders to build the skills required for people-centred care, as the stories of health organizations in our examples show. But having an effective framework for leadership is insufficient unless people-centred care is the goal of all parts of the health care system.

References

1. Bombard Y, Baker GR, Orlando E, Fancott C, Bhatia P, Casalino S, et al. Engaging patients to improve quality of care: a systematic review. Implement Sci. 2018;13(1):98.
2. Wolf J. The patchwork perspective: a new view for patient experience. Patient Exp J. 2017;4(3):1–3.
3. Power C, Stevens P, Munter A, Hughes L. Patient safety culture "bundle" for CEO's/senior leaders. Toronto, ON: Presentation at the National Conference for Health Leadership; 2018. http://www.nhlc-cnls.ca/wp-content/uploads/2017/01/NHLC_Schierbeck.pdf. Accessed 23 Aug 2019.
4. Groene O, Suno R. Patient involvement in quality management: rationale and current status. J Health Organ Manag. 2015;29(5):556–69.
5. World Health Organization. Framework on integrated, people-centred health services. Geneva: World Health Organization; 2017. http://apps.who.int/gb/ebwha/pdf_files/WHA69/A69_39-en.pdf?ua=1&ua=1. Accessed 20 Jul 2019.
6. World Health Organization. People-centred and integrated health services: an overview of the evidence. Geneva: World Health Organization; 2015. http://www.who.int/servicedelivery-safety/areas/people-centred-care/evidence-overview/en/. Accessed 20 Jul 2019.
7. Simpson E, House A. Involving users of the delivery and evaluation of mental health services: systematic review. BMJ. 2002;325(7375):1265.
8. De Souza S, Galloway J, Simpson C, Chura R, Dobson J, Gullick NJ, et al. Patient involvement in rheumatology outpatient service design and delivery: a case study. Health Expect. 2017;20(3):503–18.
9. Herdam B, Boolsen MW. Patient involvement in own rehabilitation after early discharge. Scand J Caring Sci. 2017;31:859–66.
10. McKevitt C, Ramsay A, Perry C, Turner S, Boaden R, Wolfe C, et al. Patient, carer and public involvement in major system change in acute stroke services: the construction of value. Health Expect. 2018;21:685–92.

11. The Commonwealth Fund. Health care system performance rankings. New York, NY: The Commonwealth Fund; 2017. https://www.commonwealthfund.org/chart/2017/health-care-system-performance-rankings. Accessed 25 Jul 2019.
12. Institute of Medicine (US) Committee on Quality of Health Care in America. Crossing the quality chasm: a new health system for the 21st century. Washington DC: National Academy Press; 2001.
13. McCannon J, Berwick DM. A new frontier in patient safety. JAMA. 2011;305(21):2221–2.
14. Batalden M, Batalden PB, Margolis P, Seid M, Armstrong G, et al. Coproduction of healthcare service. BMJ Qual Saf. 2016;25(7):509–17.
15. Filipe A, Renedo A, Marston C. The co-production of what? Knowledge, values, and social relations in health care. PLoS Biol. 2017;15(5):e2001403.
16. Excellent Care for All Act, Bill 8. Ontario Law; 2010. https://www.ontario.ca/laws/statute/10e14. Accessed 18 Sep 2019.
17. Patients First Act, Bill 41. Ontario Law. 2016. https://www.ontario.ca/laws/statute/s16030. Accessed 18 Sep 2019.
18. Health Standards Organization. HSO 76000: integrated people-centred systems (IPCS) standard. 2018. https://healthstandards.org/ipcs/. Accessed 2 Aug 2019.
19. Bate R. Experience-based design: from redesigning the system around the patient to co-designing services with the patient. Qual Saf Health Care. 2006;15(5):307–10.
20. Canadian Foundation for Healthcare Improvement. Much more than just a visit: a review of visiting policies in select Canadian acute care hospitals. Ottawa, ON: Canadian Foundation for Healthcare Improvement; 2015. https://www.cfhi-fcass.ca/sf-docs/default-source/patient-engagement/better-together-baseline-report.pdf?sfvrsn=bb65d044_10. Accessed 26 Aug 2019.
21. Liu V, Read JL, Cheng E. Visitation policies and practices in US ICUs. Crit Care. 2013 Apr 16;17(2):R71. https://doi.org/10.1186/cc12677.
22. Belanger L, Bussieres S, Rainville F, Coulombe M, Desmartis M. Hospital visiting policies – impacts on patients, families and staff: a review of the literature to inform decision making. J Hosp Adm. 2017;6(6):51–62.
23. Canadian Foundation for Healthcare Improvement. Family presence and visiting hours. Ottawa, ON: Canadian Foundation for Healthcare Improvement; 2019. https://www.cfhi-fcass.ca/WhatWeDo/a-z-topics/family-presence. Accessed 26 Aug 2019.
24. Carman KL, Dardess P, Maurer M, Sofaer S, Adams K, Bechtel C, Sweeney J. Patient and family engagement: a framework for understanding the elements and developing interventions and policies. Health Aff (Millwood). 2013;32(2):223–31.
25. Frampton S, Guastello S, Hoy L, Naylor M, Sheridan S, Johnston-Fleece M. Harnessing evidence and experience to change culture: a guiding framework for patient and family engaged care. National Academy of Medicine discussion paper; 2017. https://nam.edu/wp-content/uploads/2017/01/Harnessing-Evidence-and-Experience-to-Change-Culture-A-Guiding-Framework-for-Patient-and-Family-Engaged-Care.pdf. Accessed 2 Aug 2019.
26. Baker GR, Judd M, Fancott C, Maika C. Creating engagement-capable environments in healthcare. In patient engagement: catalyzing improvement and innovation in healthcare. Toronto, ON: Longwoods Publishing; 2016.
27. Van Aerde J. Relationship-centred care: toward real health system reform. Can J Phys Lead. 2015;1(3):3–6.
28. Li J, Porock D. Resident outcomes of person-centred care in long-term care: a narrative review of interventional research. Int J Nurs Stud. 2014;51(10):1395–415. https://doi.org/10.1016/j.ijnurstu.2014.04.003.
29. Houmanfar RA, Mattaini MA. Leadership and cultural change. J Organ Behav Manage. 2015;35:1–3. https://doi.org/10.1080/01608061.2015.1036645.
30. Edwards M, Penlington C, Kalidasan V, Kelly T. Culture change, leadership and the grassroots workforce. Clin Med. 2014;14(4):342–4.
31. Pryor C, Holmes RM, Webb JW, Liguori EW. Top executive goal orientations' effects on environmental scanning and performance: differences between founders and nonfounders. J Manag. 2019;45(5):1958–86. https://doi.org/10.1177/0149206317737354.

32. Li C, Lin C, Tien Y. CEO transformational leadership and top manager ambidexterity. Leadership Org Dev. 2015;36(8):927–54. https://doi.org/10.1108/LODJ-03-2014-0054.
33. Tse H, Troth A, Ashkanasy N, Collins A. Affect and leader-member exchange in the new millennium: a state-of-art review and guiding framework. Leadersh Q. 2018;29(1):135–49. https://doi.org/10.1016/j.leaqua.2017.10.002.
34. Weiner AS, Ronch JL. Culture change in long-term care. Binghampton, NY: The Haworth Press; 2003.
35. Bowers B, Nolet K, Roberts T, Esmond S. Implementing change in long term care: a practical guide to transformation. The Commonwealth Fund: Washington, DC; 2009. https://www.commonwealthfund.org/publications/other-publication/2009/apr/implementing-change-long-term-care-practical-guide. Accessed 2 Aug 2019.
36. Best A, Greenhalgh T, Lewis S, Saul J, Carroll S, Bitz J. Large-system transformation in health care: a realist review. Milbank Q. 2003;90:421–56. https://doi.org/10.1111/j.1468-0009.2012.00670.x.
37. Bevan H, Fairman S. The new era of thinking and practice in change and transformation: Improving Quality NHS (white paper); 2017. doi:10.13140/RG.2.2.10237.77289.
38. deBronkart D. How the e-patient community helped save my life: an essay by Dave deBronkart. BMJ. 2013;346:f1990.
39. Christensen C, Bohmer R, Kenagy J. Will disruptive innovations cure health care? Harv Bus Rev. 2019. http://hbr.org/web/extras/insight-center/health-care/will-disruptive-innovations-cure-health-care.
40. The Change Foundation. Leadership is key, and other lessons learned from the UK's Helen Bevan. Toronto, ON: The Change Foundation. https://www.changefoundation.ca/leadership-is-key/. Accessed 17 Jul 2019.
41. Publications Saskatchewan. For patients' sake: patient first review commissioner's report to the Saskatchewan Minister of Health; 2009. https://pubsaskdev.blob.core.windows.net/pubsask-prod/108631/108631-Patient_First_Review_Commissioners_Report.pdf. Accessed 17 Jul 2019.
42. Baillie K. One organization's journey to develop leadership competencies related to culture change. [An Organizational Leadership Project to fulfill the requirements for the Fellowship Program, unpublished]. Canadian College of Health Leaders: Ottawa, ON; 2018.
43. Kahneman D. Thinking, fast and slow. New York, NY: Farrar, Straus and Giroux; 2013.
44. Marles K. Distributed leadership: building capacity to maximise collaborative practice in a new teaching research aged care service [Thesis]. Freemantle, WA: University of Notre Dame; 2017. p. 190.
45. Young M. The patients as partners movement and the emerging health leader. Healthc Manage Forum. 2017;30(3):142–5. https://doi.org/10.1177/0840470416678233.
46. KPMG Global Healthcare. Creating new value with patients, careers and communities. KPMG International: Zurich; 2014. https://assets.kpmg/content/dam/kpmg/pdf/2016/07/creating-new-value-with-patients.pdf. Accessed 17 Jul 2019.
47. Berwick DM. What 'patient-centered' should mean: confessions of an extremist. Health Aff (Millwood). 2009;28(4):w555–65. https://doi.org/10.1377/hlthaff.28.4.w555.

Seeing with Two Eyes: Indigenous Leadership and the LEADS Framework

14

Alika Lafontaine, Caroline Lidstone-Jones, and Karen Lawford

> It is time for a renewed, nation-to-nation relationship with First Nation Peoples. One that understands that the constitutionally guaranteed rights of First Nations in Canada are not an inconvenience, but rather a sacred obligation.
>
> The Right Honourable Justin Trudeau, Prime Minister of Canada [2]

Current evidence suggests that building transformational leadership capacity is a precursor for the transformational changes required to deliver on the sacred obligations of the Government of Canada to First Nations [2–4]. As health systems across Canada seek to make transformational challenges to achieve better health outcomes for Indigenous peoples, we would agree that leadership capacity is of paramount importance. This chapter is intended to complement other perspectives on health leadership provided in this book. It will: (1) identify why Indigenous health leadership differs from leadership in non-Indigenous health; (2) provide context to health

Alika Lafontaine is an Indigenous physician of Cree, Anishnaabe, Metis and Pacific Islander descent; past President of the Indigenous Physicians Association of Canada; and an Associate Clinical Professor in the Department of Anesthesia and Pain Medicine at the University of Alberta. He co-led the Indigenous Health Alliance in Canada (2013–2017). Caroline Lidstone-Jones is a member of the Batchewana First Nation and currently works as a senior consultant for Better Together Health Solutions. Prior to this she was Chief Quality Officer and Operating for Weeneebayko Area Health Authority. Karen Lawford, Ph.D., is an Aboriginal Midwife Namegosibiing (Trout Lake, Lac Seul First Nation, Treaty 3), a Registered Midwife (Ontario), and an Assistant Professor in the Department of Gender Studies at Queen's University.

A. Lafontaine (✉)
University of Alberta, Edmonton, AB, Canada

C. Lidstone-Jones
Weeneebayko Area Health Authority, Ontario, ON, Canada

K. Lawford
Queen's University, Kingston, ON, Canada

© Springer Nature Switzerland AG 2020
G. Dickson, B. Tholl (eds.), *Bringing Leadership to Life in Health: LEADS in a Caring Environment*, https://doi.org/10.1007/978-3-030-38536-1_14

leaders who excel in other areas of transformational change struggle in Indigenous health systems; and (3) highlight how three aspects of the LEADS framework (Lead self, Engage others, and Develop coalitions) provide a roadmap to critically assess and predict health leaders' success to affect organizational change in Indigenous health.

While it should be understood that Indigenous cultures are not homogeneous, what this really means is often a challenge for health leaders. The Government of Canada has constitutionally recognized Indigenous peoples as three distinct groups: First Nation, Inuit, and Métis [5]. The government perspective is that each Indigenous group is entitled to certain rights, although these recognized rights often do not align with Indigenous nations' own perception of treaty and entitlement [6]. To appreciate how rights flow from these treaties begins by understanding there are two definitions of what it means to be Indigenous: (1) a constitutional definition, and (2) Indigenous nations and peoples definitions of themselves. The second definition recognizes that self-determinations of Indigenous identities and their cultures are not homogenous, but are plural and complex. Recognizing this is necessary in developing a personal awareness of Indigenous people's experiences in Canada. Generalizations about Indigenous nations and peoples often lead to superficial insights.

Etuaptmumk [Mi'kmaq], Two-Eyed Seeing

Two-Eyed Seeing is a conceptual framework applied in many education settings. The formal research application of Etuaptmumk is attributed to the work of Mi'kmaq Elders Murdena and Albert Marshall, with the assistance of Dr. Cheryl Bartlett [7]. This framework has been used in many academic settings, including health care [8–10]. Two-Eyed Seeing postulates that leadership is enhanced when different perspectives are acknowledged and valued, leading toward new, holistic paths to change [11]. In practice, however, Two-Eyed Seeing can be difficult to define and challenging to implement. It requires leadership to reflect on their limited perspectives and personal experiences necessary to provide holistic health system delivery. Indeed, anthropologist and University of Alberta health researcher Nancy Gibson says, in her study of tuberculosis in Indigenous communities, that it is important to "honour the life circumstances of people we are working with... guided by mutual respect and appropriate confidentiality" and that we need to "be sensitive and responsive to the values, culture and priorities of the individuals and communities" we serve [12].

LEADS in a Caring Environment Capabilities Framework

The LEADS framework has five domains: Lead self, Engage others, Achieve results, Develop coalitions and Systems transformation. The focus of this chapter is to link three of the domains (Lead self, Engage others, and Develop coalitions) with

Two-Eyed Seeing and transformational leadership for Indigenous health improvement. What follows is our own personal advice regarding the barriers and challenges in moving from this first step to applying components of the LEADS framework in Indigenous cultural contexts, which are derived from our own experiences in Indigenous health. We hope to inspire others to think differently and creatively so they can meaningfully engage with Indigenous people and reframe perceived barriers in working together as self-motivated leaders. We also encourage others to begin discussing uncomfortable leadership challenges related to Indigenous health issues and concerns so that true transformation can be achieved.

Lead Self: Unconscious Bias and "A World Out There We Don't See"

Visual acuity may seem an eclectic place to begin our discussion of the first domain of the LEADS framework, Lead self, but there is a lot our eyes can teach us about perception. As light passes through our pupil, it covers the retina positioned at the back of our eye. The retina is covered with light-sensing proteins, which transfer visual information to the optic nerve which then carries the visual information to our brain. The optic nerve lies in the field of the retina itself, meaning that in each eye there is an area of visual acuity that cannot receive information. Medically, these are called scotomas, or blind spots. Our two eyes rely on each other to fill in these blind spots with information. Most people can live their whole lives without realizing these blind spots exist.

In the same way, cognitive blind spots exist in perception, comprehension, and world views. Specific to health, perceptions and cognition often differ in considerable ways between providers, academics, policy makers, administrators, and patients. To address these cognitive blind spots, many health systems have moved towards a dyad system of leadership wherein clinicians and administrators work together in teams. In some systems, patients are integrated into leadership structures as advisory groups.

Whether explicitly or implicitly, these approaches acknowledge there is an inability for individuals to see a comprehensive picture when defining problems, articulating solutions, and effectively implementing solutions. The cognitive blind spots are made visible with the inclusion of many experiences and perspectives, which is important to the leadership and provision of health care services.

Lead self can be an area of frustration for many health leaders due to these cognitive blind spots, which are often assumed to be in the areas of history, culture, or language. In reality these blind spots are more likely due to a difference in the personal value system that informs an individual's leadership style, which may not align with the value systems of Indigenous nations and peoples health leaders and the mainstream health system serve.

Without patients, the health system and health leaders would have no purpose.

Dr. Alika Lafontaine

Value systems are often interpreted as the means by which we assign value, but for Indigenous health, the more pressing question may be much narrower: Do we value each other, our relationships, and communities? If health systems exist for the purpose of serving patients and health leaders exist to ensure those systems optimize health services, patients are the lifeblood of health systems. That makes patients the only immutable aspect of system design, because without patients, the health system and health leaders would have no purpose.

Despite this reality, many acknowledge health systems have become overly institutional and provider centric. As we rethink how to rebalance our efforts to centre on our north star, consider that patients have always mattered, even if their role has been sometimes minimized or disregarded. For Indigenous patients, however, experiences in health care are influenced by discrimination, systemic racism, accessibility and stereotypes, to name but a few.

As a health leader, have you ever thought that Indigenous patients are not your responsibility? Have you ever excused a failure in providing similar services to Indigenous and non-Indigenous patients as a result of provincial versus federal jurisdiction issues? Applying Lead self means confronting these personal biases or beliefs. These cognitive blind spots have been acquired through the Canadian experience over many decades, which is the same as millions of other Canadians. In your personal journey to Lead self, the responsibility is not in what you have inherited, but instead, in what you choose to propagate as a health care leader.

Engage Others: Cultural Teachings

Indigenous Peoples use culture to establish a sense of identity and community. Culture is expressed through a connection with the land and environment, language, and kinship. Mother Earth provides us with daily lessons as we progress along our path to understanding and happiness. Mother Earth is the model system, with individual parts working together to ensure balance and harmony with the physical, mental, emotional, and spiritual elements of life.

While these specific lifecycle teachings pertain to Anishinabeg culture, each Indigenous nation has its own creation story that illustrates how every community member, at every age, has a role to play in achieving balance and harmony. The four aspects of self—physical, mental, emotional, and spiritual—may develop at different rates, but there is a need to be rebalanced and progress at every stage of life. By applying the model of Mother Earth, we can understand that leadership does not have to be overt, aggressive, and obvious. Rather, it is process based upon self-evident, reflective understanding of one's role and the role of others. It results in leadership that may appear passive and quiet, when it really is introspective, responsive, and patient.

Contrast can be made between the hierarchical models commonly placed upon Indigenous peoples and communities and the pre-contact models we see emerging as Indigenous nations reconnect with their teachings. In hierarchical models, power and authority are consolidated at high-level decision-making tables. Leadership is often synonymous with authority and enforcement. Value in this type of system is derived from the ability to enforce a decision and conformity is a major driver of decisions.

In leadership models more aligned with Indigenous teachings, power and authority are decentralized, with decision-making being enabled at the points of impact. Leadership becomes synonymous not with authority and enforcement, but with responsibility and impact. Value in this type of system is derived from the ability to act toward achieving an outcome. Personal autonomy and choice are the major drivers of decisions and are balanced with family and community needs. We believe the LEADS framework, with its emphasis on leading from where you are and who you are, is consistent with these Indigenous teachings.

> The teachings in the Ojibwe culture have been traditionally passed down from generation to generation orally through stories and ceremonies. Historically, this has been done by the elders that carry with them the stories and traditions. Today, the oral traditions are being shared by those who carry the knowledge of such things [13].

The teachings of all Aboriginal cultures encompass the morals, values, structures, ceremonial practices and spiritual beliefs of the group. These teachings also ensured the survival of the people. For the Ojibwe people, the teachings vary from nation to nation, because of the geographical placement of each group. However, the Ojibwe teachings commonly come from the same root and share a similar message.

> Of all the North American Indigenous teachings, the seven Grandfather Teachings are the most commonly shared from coast to coast. Many Aboriginal organizations and communities have adopted the seven guiding principles, in one form or another, as a moral stepping-stone and cultural foundation. There are stories of the origins of the seven Grandfather Teachings in all communities. Each community has adapted the teachings to suit their community values. Despite where the teachings may have originated, they share the same concepts of abiding by a moral respect for all living things…[13].

All health leaders should be aware that not all Indigenous people, communities, and nations fully apply pre-contact approaches to leadership; however, differences between hierarchical and Indigenous styles of leadership can lead to misunderstandings of what actions and impact mean for different stakeholders. Recognizing these potential differences can help you avoid leadership assumptions about community engagement. For example: not every community follows Indigenous ways of being and ceremonies; ceremonies differ among regions; cultural teachings are rooted in the experiences of those communities and their members; and some communities follow both Christian and Indigenous spiritualities. These variations require health leaders to actively listen and actively make space for communities to lead as you become engaged.

> *"As Traditional Knowledge Keepers, we have to make our knowledge available to society — that's engagement."*
>
> The Wîcîhitowin Conference Committee, 2017

Indigenous nations acknowledge leaders by placing them in positions of influence. Leadership qualities often include being charitable, inclusive and community centred. Elders who are recognized by their communities bring wisdom, love and spirituality. Often, Elders are also seen as healers, who offer guidance, counsel, and mentorship. They may have historical, technical, medical and political knowledge, which allows them to not only teach leadership principles but also provide community context. Communities respect Elders as a source of great strength and positivity. "Elders also need help to remain strong. We must keep them free from harm and provide quality care. It is a time to pass their knowledge to the youth since they have been considered to master the meaning of joy and sorrow and many trials and tribulations encountered over the course of their existence" [14]. When Indigenous peoples speak about knowledge keepers, these are some of the individuals being referred to.

Contextual Leadership and Intersectionality

As has become clear throughout this book, all leadership is a function of context and culture. Intersectionality was developed Kimberlé Crenshaw, Ph.D., a Black woman, civil rights activist and legal scholar who examines racism, sexism, and the sociolegal systems that intersect synergistically to effect Black women in the USA [15]. In Canada, and in other colonized countries, Indigenous health is negatively affected by colonialism, racism and sexism at the individual and collective levels, which explains why apparently successful approaches to transformational change are difficult to transpose into Indigenous health.

We hope by this point, health leaders are beginning to see that the issues in Indigenous health are unlike leadership challenges in other areas of health. By appreciating the tenets of intersectionality, we can take the preceding concepts and introduce the idea that the sequence and density of these issues layer one upon the other and cause these barriers to act synergistically. For example, many Indigenous nations experience intergenerational trauma as a result of Indian Residential Schools. In these schools, physical, psychological, and sexual abuse were commonplace [16]. For example, at the St. Anne's residential school run by the Catholic church, Indigenous children were put in "a homemade electric chair used for punishment and sport." [17] Children were taught to deny their languages and cultures, which devalued their family and community identity. Indian Residential Schools imposed a rigid hierarchical structure: children learned a top-down approach to decision making that was reinforced through aggressive and harmful physical punishment. In many residential schools, persons were dehumanized. What would be the expected emotional, mental, physical and spiritual consequences of such an experience?

Now add the layers of known stereotypes and discrimination against Indigenous peoples, some of which are documented in inquests, such as Brian Lloyd Sinclair [18] and academic reports such as First Peoples, Second Class Treatment [19]. Add another layer of being an Indigenous woman or a Two Spirit person [20]. Finally, include additional determinants of health like low socio-economic status, limited health access because of geographic disadvantage, crowded housing not meeting standards and undrinkable water. Imagine these layers magnifying the impacts of Indian Residential Schools, for example.

It must be acknowledged that any individual, family, or community exposed to these experiences would react negatively. The importance of survival for many Indigenous people is evident in their resiliency and their ability to adapt. While all Indigenous peoples do not experience the same kinds and amounts of trauma, intergenerational and community experiences with colonial mechanisms of power, oppression, exclusion, and devaluation create an ongoing risk to Indigenous people even before they engage with the health system. Consequently, we argue that unless health care systems are prepared to understand Indigenous patient behaviour and mitigate the friction that can arise as sensitized patients enter provider- and system-centric models of care, propagation of Indigenous health disparities will remain.

Develop Coalitions: Indigenous Health Alliance and the ALIGN Model

The Indigenous Health Alliance [21] is a prime example of how articulating and unwinding these conflated layers led to measurable change across disparate stakeholders. By bringing together Indigenous territorial and provincial organizations representing more than 150 First Nations, the Indigenous Health Alliance sought to introduce a community-centred definition of health transformation into Indigenous health systems that included quality improvement, adherence to safety standards, and patient-centred care.

In fall 2018, the Indigenous Health Alliance successfully lobbied [22] for community-led health transformation supported by a $68 million dollar funding commitment from the Federal Government. For four years, these Indigenous provincial and territorial organizations worked with researchers to develop a narrative reflecting community experiences. The result was the ALIGN model, articulated and published by Lafontaine and Associates and Alignment by Design Labs [23]. Applying the ALIGN model allows communities to take ownership of health transformation and move forward on their own terms and with their own understandings.

The ALIGN model begins with articulating the profound consequences of slow or ineffective reconciliation in Indigenous health systems contributing to:

- Widening health disparities.
- Progressive patient morbidity and mortality.
- Devastating human costs to families, communities, and nations.
- Loss of economic and educational opportunities for Indigenous patients and their families.
- Escalating health care costs and burden of chronic disease.
- Expanding health system bureaucracy.
- Ongoing fiscal and legal liability of health systems, providers and governments.
- Impact on other priority policy areas requiring engagement of Indigenous peoples, including energy and economic development, among others [23].

From a community perspective, it is evident that Indigenous health systems are not achieving the same outcomes as non-Indigenous health systems. As health leaders we should be asking why. Instead of focusing on greater efficiency and increased resourcing as the primary solutions to poor health outcomes, community perspectives must be used to redesign existing health systems around Indigenous communities. Redesign should explicitly identify disparate priorities between Indigenous communities, providers, administrators, regulators and governments. Investing greater fiscal and human resources into misaligned health systems where the priorities of providers, administrators, regulators and governments have overwhelmed the priorities of Indigenous communities in ways incongruent with best practices in non-Indigenous health systems, usually leads to worsening misalignment. Over time this misalignment can become normalized in processes and actions. Abnormal norms remain abnormal regardless of whether they are within the Indigenous or non-Indigenous context.

Furthermore, colonialism relied upon the extinguishment of inherent Indigenous rights towards land, resources, health and wellbeing. As such, the outcomes of current Indigenous health systems better align with colonial outcomes and make misalignment a neccessary state of colonial health systems. Patients cannot remain in communities due to lack of health access and leave their inherent rights when they relocate. Patients cannot exercise their inherent rights to land if they are suffering from high burdens of chronic disease due to physical limitations. Higher rates of mortality mean potential inherent rights holders cannot exercise their rights due to death. Because health care systems are designed around colonial outcomes, as long as those designs perpetuate, they will continue to achieve these outcomes. Regardless of our personal and professional leadership goals, we are part of the health care system and we have inherited and heretofore propagated, substantial health care inequities for Indigenous peoples in Canada.

These inequities are reflected in a common anecdote among Indigenous health leaders: Indigenous health transformation is like "driving a bus that's on fire, down a road that's in the process of being built." So if health leaders are responding to perpetual crises with little to no time of recovery, why do we keep approaching Indigenous health transformation in the same way? Asked more broadly, would health leaders ever accept this reality in their own health systems? Or would systemic change become a fully resourced priority?

We also posit that perpetual crises in health care systems are an integral part of the lived experience of many Indigenous people, communities, and nations. While crises are common in non-Indigenous health systems (limited human resources, fiscal restrictions, jurisdictional challenges, aging infrastructure, etc.) perpetual crises are very different. With each crisis, the resiliency of a system is challenged. Often, a crisis pushes a system past its threshold of viability and poor patient outcomes occur. Non-Indigenous health systems have mechanisms to study, act, plan and implement; quality improvement uses these steps to operationalize aims, identify measures and enable system change. But when serial crises occur, which is often the situation in health systems that serve Indigenous people, there is little or no time or resources to assist in the recovery. Health systems that are unable to recover and meet subsequent crises eventually "break" and enter into a state of perpetual crises. The ALIGN model articulates how communities can move forward from perpetual crises in overwhelmed Indigenous health systems. Once perpetual crises have been resolved and a resiliency plan is in place, misalignment can be addressed. Once an aligned system has been achieved, greater efficiencies and resourcing will have the intended effect of improved health outcomes. These objectives do not need to be sequential, but a targeted strategy must be in place for each.

Coming Full Circle: LEADS and Traits of Indigenous Leadership

This brings us full circle through the three LEADS steps that we focused on: Lead self, Engage others and Develop coalitions. Health care leaders can only understand Indigenous communities and their health care needs if they truly understand our own ways of valuing each other using shared leadership tools, like those described by Lead self. Engagement requires giving space to Indigenous communities to co-define problems, co-articulate solutions and co-design implementation, which is described in Engage others. Health care leaders can only achieve results by Developing coalitions, because health care systems were not designed to guide Indigenous Peoples, communities, and nations to health. We now outline the leadership traits of Indigenous people and how those traits help understand the five domains of LEADS in an Indigenous context. Figure 14.1 shows the overall framework. We then explain each domain separately.

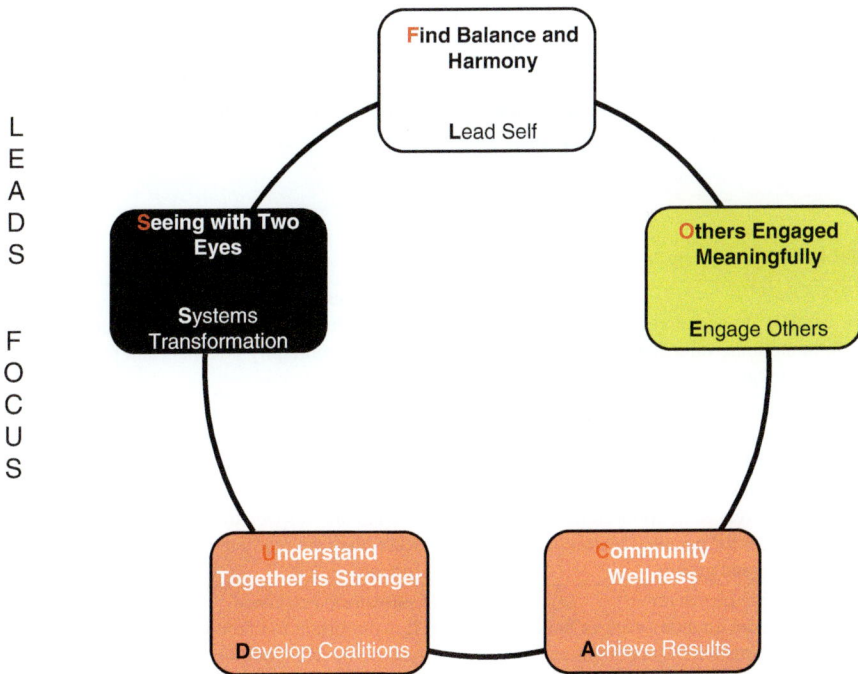

Fig. 14.1 LEADS as expressed in Indigenous culture

It has been our experience that building our relationships with Indigenous health leaders is a circular process. As relationships develop, we are constantly re-evaluating previous steps so our work can more closely align with holistic approaches reflecting all five domains of the LEADS framework: Lead self, Engage others, Achieve results, Develop coalitions and Systems transformation.

Lead Self: Find Balance and Harmony (Table 14.1)

Genuineness and Respect: Leading from a Place of Passion

Leaders need to be trusted and genuine. People in the community need to believe in what leaders are saying. Leaders who are not genuine and who demonstrate a lack of decorum when communicating their ideas will be voted out at community elections or communities will make strong statements by withdrawing their support. For example, councillors will walk away from council and demand a new election if they feel their chief is speaking from a place that does not respect their community and its members. Although this is an uncommon practice it does display how strongly community members feel about the best interests of their community.

Resiliency and Cultural Ties

Experiencing serial trauma has helped to reinforce the importance of recognizing Indigenous identity and cultural knowledges because this is what grounds us as a people. It is important to know who we are, where we are from and to be proud of that grounding. Consequently, you can only lead others successfully if you feel comfortable in your own shoes. If someone has lost their way, it is a community responsibility to wrap them in a circle of care. This circle of care recognizes that each person in the system carries a leadership role at some point in their lives regardless of age, stature or occupation.

Table 14.1 Mapping Indigenous leadership traits to Lead self

Self aware	*Genuine, respectful and passionate*
• Leaders are aware of their own assumptions, values, principles, strengths, and limitations	• Leaders must be genuine and gain the respect of their community members and peers
Manage themselves	*Respect cultural roots*
• Leaders take responsibility for their own performance and health	• Leaders must be comfortable in their own shoes
Develop themselves	*Cultural revitalization*
• They actively seek opportunities and challenges for personal learning, character building, and growth	• A solid and respected leader understands when they are ready to pass knowledge forward
Demonstrate character	*Demonstrate resilience*
• They model qualities such as honesty, integrity, resilience, and confidence	• It is important to know who you are, where you come from, and being proud of that grounding. It is your identity

The use of humour is also a critical component of leadership in Indigenous health. The ability to laugh together fosters wellness. It is a natural healing response and an Indigenous form of healing because it teaches us that life is not always serious. It can also be a coping mechanism and can bring comfort to variety of situations.

Revitalizes Indigenous Cultures and Knowledge

Knowledge of the land, history, culture, and language is vital. In order to successfully implement Lead self, we need to take back what was lost and reinforce these as important components of being and self-identity. This commitment is also of great importance to next generations. It is significant to recognize where you are on your wellness path or healing journey because your core needs to be strong in order to successfully lead others. A solid and respected leader also understands when they are ready to pass knowledge forward, which is often an ongoing process and not a singular event. Some people are ready for this sooner rather than later and others develop leadership sharing as they experience more in life. The road may be rocky, but leaders know when this happens because individual community members go to them for advice and guidance.

This process appears to less formal than attaining a position like CEO, executive director, manager, or director, for example because leadership is often given by community members, who seek you out for knowledge and assistance. For example, we know someone advances to an Elder when the community gives them this title, which is earned and is based on how these individuals interact in the community. Indigenous leaders demonstrate caring and compassion for others; they feel good in their shoes, they feel good about themselves and where they have been; and they accept that they have knowledge to offer. Becoming an Indigenous leader tends to evolve responsively and often aligns with their own journey to wellness.

Engage Others: Meaningful Support and Engagement (Table 14.2)

Community Leadership

Community leadership tends not to be individual focused. Chiefs and council members aim to make decisions collectively and as a team. They want to hear the information firsthand and they want time to digest what they are hearing. Often personal and community experiences and stories are told during information sharing, so there is quite a bit of time spent listening and asking questions. When establishing relationships with Indigenous peoples, communities, and their leadership, listening is the most important skill and is a key ingredient when developing a relationship. Community leaders want to ensure their community needs are being heard and validated. They want to understand the commitments being made and have the opportunity to gain assurances they will have positive effects for their community. Conversations with Indigenous leadership and community members must be genuine, come from a good place, demonstrate transparency, and clearly articulate the positive outcomes of engagement.

Table 14.2 Mapping Indigenous leadership traits to Engage others

Foster the development of others	Foster community leadership
• Leaders support and challenge others to achieve professional and personal goals	• Leadership is fostered across the community
Contribute to the creation of healthy organizations	Contribute to collective decision-making
• They create engaging environments in which others have meaningful opportunities to contribute and ensure resources are available to fulfill expected responsibilities	• They want to hear the information first-hand and they want time to digest what they are hearing
Communicate effectively	Listen Actively and Hear Stories
• They listen well and encourage an open exchange of information and ideas using appropriate communication media	• They listen more, talk less, and ask questions then demonstrate actively listening • They let the community take the lead
Build teams	Support community driven processes
• They facilitate environments of collaboration, and cooperation to achieve results	• They want to understand the commitment being made and be assured it will have a positive effect for their community

Oral Tradition (Storytelling) and Active Listening

Storytelling is a significant part of Indigenous peoples' cultures and knowledge transmission. It is a way of activating a teaching and the associated lessons. Beginning in childhood, Indigenous people are taught how to listen and absorb information from their Elders and their peers. Talking less and listening more are important and so is asking questions to pass knowledge between generations.

> *I think back to a time when I was working as the chief quality officer at Weeneebayko Area Health Authority (WAHA) and we established a partnership with the Northeast Specialized Geriatrics Centre (NESGC). The partnership was structured so that seniors in the James and Hudson Bay region can be screened, assessed and have care plans developed specific to their needs. Part of the comprehensive individualized assessment included a mental wellness checklist to help determine if a senior was showing signs of depression, delirium or dementia. One of the questions in the assessment included:*
>
> *Please identify what season it is right now?*
>
> *When one of our seniors was asked this question, they specified the season as freeze up. The person conducting the assessment identified that the senior was not able to identify what season it was, and this affected their assessment outcome.*
>
> *Typically, everyone would think there are only four answers to this question: summer, fall, winter and spring. But there are six seasons for the Cree living along the James and Hudson Bay: Winter; Spring; Break-up; Summer; Fall and Freeze Up. This knowledge stems from understanding seasonal cycles and identifying their critical importance to the lifelines of the communities (examples are hunting and trapping cycles and winter roads).*
>
> *This misinterpretation was caught when WAHA staff and NESGS were doing integrated case reviews for care plan development. Subsequently we were able to provide some cross-cultural education to the geriatrics team coming in.*
>
> *What did this experience teach us? Both the WAHA and NESGS teams realized the importance of talking together. We needed to share knowledge among each other first so that we were on the same page before providing care to our patients. This is part of practicing cultural safety and humility. We as organizations both had a role to play in fostering this.*

What did we do the next time? We collaboratively reviewed all the assessment materials and amended where necessary, and we included our cultural and language translators in the reviews. We customized the materials so that it made sense for the clients we were serving.

Caroline Lidstone-Jones

Achieve Results: Community Wellness (Table 14.3)

Decision-Making

Often being elected as the chief is based on your ability to listen to others the best, and to act for the collective and not for single individuals. It is not a position for the attainment of individual notoriety or power. The locus of control is shared with council and community members because leadership is about having discussions and thinking about the potential consequences of those decisions.

Sharing the floor for discussion is also a common practice in communities. This creates a space where everyone has an opportunity to speak and learn from each other, which generates information that is considered in community decision making processes. So Indigenous leadership strives to create a safe space for community members to voice their concerns and provide input into community decisions.

Jurisdictional Clarity

Leaders need to work in an environment where ownership of change is essential, because it also supports self-governance. Communities cannot continue to be caught in the jurisdictional challenges between federal and provincial governments.

Table 14.3 Mapping Indigenous leadership traits to Achieve results

Set direction	*Foster community ownership*
• Leaders inspire vision by identifying, establishing, and communicating clear and meaningful expectations and outcomes	• The community sets the direction
Strategically align decisions with vision and values and evidence	*Seek community input*
• Leaders integrate organizational missions and values with reliable, valid evidence to make decisions	• Creates a space where everyone has an opportunity to speak and learn from each other regardless of who they are
Take action to implement decisions	*Promote community-centred care*
• Leaders act in a manner consistent with organizational values to yield effective, efficient public-centred service	• Cultural safety is more than a history lesson, it is about application; it is about opening dialogue channels to have conversations with many different people about wellness • The leader supports the environment for this dialogue and joint learning to take place
Assess and evaluate	*Ensure jurisdictional clarity*
• Leaders measure and evaluate outcomes, compare the results against established benchmarks, and correct the course as appropriate	• Leaders need to have the appropriate environment where ownership becomes essential and supports self-governance

Instead, environments must allow for the authority to make decisions. With this autonomy, responsibility is learned because the results of your decisions are made evident, which establishes true learning.

This raises the question: who is taking leadership of health at the community level? The health director provides direction at the service level, a band council member is appointed to hold the health portfolio; the chief is the community spokesperson, and in addition, many communities have a health board and/or social services board to assist with strategic planning efforts. Leadership becomes a collective effort because many people feed into the process at varying levels of influence. It is also expected knowledge keepers will be brought into conversations when needed to better inform a decision-making process. This type of community engagement helps to create balance between Indigenous and Western approaches of decision making. It facilitates capacity building at the community level, which serves to assist with decision implementation. It is one thing to lead a process, but in true testament to leadership, when people can witness and experience inclusion in decision making, determined outcomes are contextually derived. This engaged leadership model thus further supports why any model of leadership and engagement must be flexible to fit in to each community, and that all processes must be community driven and led.

Community-Centred Care

Community-centred care is based on the belief that every single person plays a leadership role in the wellness path. For example, British Columbia's First Nations Health Authority's "role is to be a partner to every BC First Nations person on their health and wellness journey by meeting them where they are at and supporting them to get to where they want to be" [24]. Building on this statement, we assert health care is based on a series of interactions with many different types of providers and that human contact is a basic need to human development, despite the introduction of artificial intelligence in health care. The harmony in the old and the new is still being established in Indigenous health and in Indigenous communities because technology is still very new; these relationships need to be developed with people, communities and nations over time and as they gain capacity to harness this technology.

We are also mindful that cultural safety is more than a history lesson. It is about appreciation, application and open dialogue with many different people about various pathways to health and wellness. The health leader supports an environment for this dialogue and joint learning, to give people the confidence to seek out the services they need. The more that people seek out their identified services, the more outreach, use of the service, and the more trusted the services become. This is a benchmark for performance in health systems. For Indigenous peoples, trust is something that is not easily given and it must be earned. Consequently, it takes time to engage with an Indigenous person and in their wellness goals. Unfortunately, children who attended Indian Residential Schools were taught not to question authority and to submit to every violence and atrocity at these genocidal institutions. Their options were to follow authority or be punished for not following direction. This is but one of many examples where the ability to take care of self was removed, thus reinforcing care systems that served to harm Indigenous peoples.

By implementing community-centred care models, leaders can create safe environments that circulate around positive, reciprocal, and transparent relationship building. Health leaders must, therefore, facilitate and encourage people to ask questions, support small talk and get to know who they are caring for so the people getting care know who they are. This helps to level the playing field and situates everyone as people so relationships with leaders are not based on authority alone. Instead, everyone starts from the understanding that everyone has something to offer.

Develop Coalitions: Understand Together Is Stronger (Table 14.4)

Relationships Cannot Be Rushed and Must to Be Nurtured Over Time

Contemporary business principles and ways of engaging with presumed stakeholders do not align with Indigenous ways of knowing and being. Many Indigenous people, communities, and nations are very uncomfortable with pressure to make quick decisions, so their responses often demonstrate hesitation. Unfortunately, the lack of immediate endorsement or movement can be viewed as laziness and lack of capacity. Tentative responses and hesitancy should, however, be understood in broader efforts of civilization and assimilation legislation and policies, such as: Indian residential schools; Indian hospitals; the 60s Scoop, boarding schools and forced, coerced, and involuntary sterilization. This is especially true for non-Indigenous people who come into the community without a pre-established relationship; community radar will go

Table 14.4 Mapping Indigenous leadership traits to Develop coalitions

Purposefully build partnerships and networks to create results • Leaders create connections, trust, and shared meanings with individuals and groups	*Develop community trust* • The community needs to trust what you are saying is genuine
Demonstrate a commitment to customers and service • Leaders facilitate collaboration, cooperation, and coalitions among diverse groups and perspectives aimed at learning to improve service	*Foster community satisfaction* • They get to know the people in the community so that a better understanding of how the community operates is developed • They also nurture relationships over time. They do not expect to go into a community once, but rather, are dedicated to long term relationships
Mobilize knowledge • Leaders employ methods to gather intelligence, encourage open exchange of information, and use quality evidence to influence action across the system	*Engage Knowledge Keepers* • They pass forward information and knowledge • They protect the wisdom of the past and use it to educate the future • They recognize knowledge can come from many different sources
Navigate socio-political environments • Leaders are politically astute, and can negotiate through conflict and mobilize support	*Respect treaty right to health* • They acknowledge the respect of historic agreements and their key places in Indigenous history as foundational to many conversations

up and people will proceed with caution, which is a natural response. If community leadership and their members are not comfortable, they will err on the side of caution and not move forward, or they will ask for more information.

As a leader in health, it is important to remember that sometimes the issue that matters most to you might not represent the burning issue for the community. To help address this miscommunication, leaders in health must gain an understanding of each community's priorities and integrate them into the conversation. Gaining an appreciation of community needs will help develop trust and build relationships more quickly. Remember, communities and nations are made up of many individuals. Get to know the people in the community you are hoping to work with so you develop a better understanding of how the community operates. Also, nurture relationships over time. Do not expect to go into a community once and complete your task. Decision making is very community driven, even when certain people, like a chief, speak on behalf of full community. These are core tenets we offer to guide relationship building.

Systems Transformation: Seeing with Two Eyes (Table 14.5)

What is important to remember as a leader is sometimes the pressing platform for someone coming into the community might not be the burning issue for the community.

Caroline Lidstone-Jones, Batchewana First Nation

Table 14.5 Mapping Indigenous leadership traits to Systems transformation

Demonstrate systems/critical thinking • Leaders think analytically and conceptually, questioning and challenging the status quo, to identify issues, solve problems and design, and implement effective processes across the systems and stakeholders	*Be respectful of self-governance* • They recognize communities and nations need control over their systems, so they can make decisions for themselves • Leaders are inclusive to all health care providers, Western and Indigenous
Encourage and support innovation • Leaders create a climate of continuous improvement and creativity aimed at systemic change	*Be flexible and adaptable* • They allow the community to set the agenda and priorities • They recognize each community is unique, so an approach must be unique for each community; there is no one size fits all
Orient themselves strategically to the future • Leaders scan the environment for ideas, best practices, and emerging trends that will shape the system	*Think seven generations forward* • They realize today's decisions impact the leaders of tomorrow and have impact on the quality of their lives in the future
Champion and orchestrate change • Leaders actively contribute to change processes that improve health service delivery	*Support reconciliation* • They acknowledge health transformation pushes limits to promote required changes • They account for and modify timelines, so community decision making is not rushed

Treaty Right to Health

It is vital to recognize the relationship between the Crown and Indigenous peoples. Acknowledging historic and contemporary agreements is foundational to many conversations. Our Indigenous ancestors were tasked to think beyond the immediate and for our future seven generations. As a result, Indigenous leaders recognize their responsibility to think beyond the immediate and incorporate big picture thinking into their decision-making.

Decision Making

Coming to a decision tends to rely on consensus: take time to talk, get to know one another, and develop a trusting relationship. Often you will hear leaders making decisions for the future seven generations because Indigenous leaders know decisions made today impact our people tomorrow, which affects the quality of our future.

Flexibility and Adaptability

When working with Indigenous people, communities, and nations, leaders in health must be extremely flexible so work can be adapted on the fly. There is no one-size-fits-all approach when it comes to working with Indigenous people, communities, and nations. Each community must set the agenda and priorities, so they can set the pace of their engagement. By remembering each community is unique, it is easy to appreciate and adapt the work that needs to get done.

Summary: What Lessons Have We Learned?

In many ways, the five LEADS domains reflect the same skills needed to be a successful leader when working with Indigenous people, communities, and nations. There are many similarities, but we assert the stakes are higher when working in Indigenous health due to the complexities inherent in current articulations of health care systems.

As discussed above, leadership in health is influenced by experiences of trauma, which Indigenous peoples have been subjected to since contact with white settlers. Navigating health care systems that survive perpetual crises necessitates leadership that deals with the immediate while also preparing for the next crisis, so there is little—to no—room for strategic planning. As such, we assert current articulations of health care systems are not designed to effectively provide the best possible care for Indigenous people, communities, and nations. In fact, many of the health inequities are inherent qualities that are built into health care systems. As we have shown, by seeing through two-eyes to re-articulate the domains and capabilities of LEADS from an Indigenous perspective, leadership behaviour to facilitate health for Indigenous peoples is not the same as in non-Indigenous communities.

To effect meaningful change, we advocate for clear and transparent authorities and accountabilities for those working in Indigenous health as part of health transformation. Health leaders working with Indigenous people, communities, and nations must understand the complex and often convoluted jurisdictional issues that interfere with the provision of appropriate health care.

Revisiting Etuaptmumk (Mi'kmaq), Two-Eyed Seeing

Two-Eyed Seeing requires leaders in health to reflect on their limited perspectives and personal experiences in order to provide holistic health system delivery, which is extremely important when working with Indigenous people, communities, and nations. We live in a world with multiple diversities and different perspectives that must be considered, so we must place greater importance on the importance of culture, history and language when working (for example) with Indigenous people, communities, and nations. As leaders in health, we cannot be blind and judge others. We must be open to all possibilities and to the future because our responsibilities for shaping health systems have to be based on respect, equality, positive outcomes, flexibility and adaptability while also working in true collaborations and partnerships.

Conclusion: The FOCUS Approach

FOCUS (see Fig. 14.2) is explained as follows. Each person needs to acknowledge and understand their past. This step allows you to move forward and generates momentum for the future while also nurturing leadership qualities. We call this F: *finding balance and harmony.*

True engagement must be based on mutual respect, community centred, reflective of community needs, respectful of local protocols and developed over time. We call this O: *others engaged meaningfully.*

Ideas of health cannot be solely based on the Euro-Canadian biomedical model. Health must also incorporate aspects of the physical, mental, emotional, and spiritual well-being. Holistic care involves individuals, their families and their communities. We call this C: *community wellness.*

Operating in silos is not healthy. Strategically aligning sectors in order to eliminate gaps teaches us how to work better together. We call this U: *understanding together is stronger.*

Indigenous people, communities, and nations have many rich, contextual and important perspectives to offer. These perspectives can be applied in multiple settings, including health and health leadership, but the leaders must see the possibilities of using S: *seeing with Two Eyes*. Above all, stay in FOCUS!

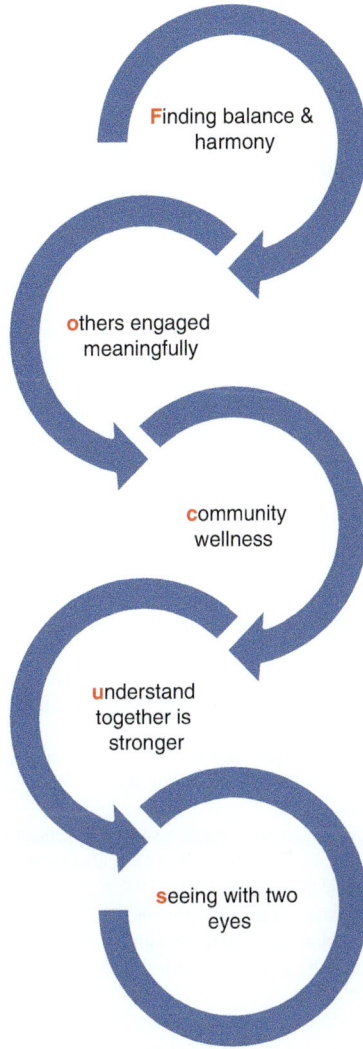

Fig. 14.2 Future Applications: FOCUS

References

1. Trudeau J. Winter assembly of first nations. 2015.
2. Mutwiri B, Witt C, Denysek C, Halferdahl S, McLeod KM. Development and implementation of the Saskatchewan leadership program: leading for health care transformation. Healthc Manage Forum. 2015;29(1):23–7. https://doi.org/10.1177/0840470415617404
3. Dickson G. Transformations in Canadian health systems leadership: an analytical perspective. Leadersh Health Serv (Bradf Engl). 2009;22(4):292–305. https://doi.org/10.1108/17511870910996132.
4. Tremblay K. Health care @ the speed of thought: a digital world needs successful transformative leaders. Healthc Manage Forum. 2017;30(5):246–51. https://doi.org/10.1177/0840470416686975.
5. Constitution Act, 1982. Sec. 35(2) Canada: Justice Laws Website. https://laws-lois.justice.gc.ca/eng/const/page-16.html.

6. Borrows J. Frozen rights in Canada: constitutional interpretation and the trickster. Am Indian Law Rev. 1998;22(1):37–42.
7. Bartlett C, Marshall M, Marshall A. Two-Eyed Seeing and other lessons learned in a co-learning journey of bringing together indigenous and mainstream knowledges and ways of knowing. J Environ Stud Sci. 2012;2(4):331–40.
8. Marsh TN, Cote-Meek S, Toulouse P. The application of two-eyed seeing decolonizing methodology in qualitative and quantitative research for the treatment of intergenerational trauma and substance use disorders. Int J Qual Methods. 2015;14:1–13. https://doi.org/10.1177/1609406915618046.
9. Greenwood M, Lindsay N, King J, Loewen D. Ethical spaces and places: indigenous cultural safety in British Columbia health care. AlterNative. 2017;13(3):179–89. https://doi.org/10.1177/1177180117714411.
10. Hutt-MacLeod D, Rudderham H, Sylliboy A, Sylliboy-Denny M, Liebenberg L, Denny JF, et al. Eskasoni First Nation's transformation of youth mental health care: partnership between a Mi'kmaq community and the ACCESS Open Minds research project in implementing innovative practice and service evaluation. Early Interv Psychia. 2019;13(Suppl 1):42–7.
11. Whiting C, Cavers S, Bassendowski S, Petrucka P. Using two-eyed seeing to explore interagency collaboration. Can J Nurs Res. 2018;50(3):133–44. https://doi.org/10.1177/0844562118766176.
12. Gibson N, Cave A, Doering D, Ortiz L, Harms P. Socio-cultural factors influencing prevention and treatment of tuberculosis in immigrant and Aboriginal communities in Canada. Soc Sci Med. 2005;61(5):931–42.
13. The seven grandfathers teachings. Uniting three fires against violence; 2019. www.unitingthreefiresagainstviolence.org/services/the-seven-grandfather-teachings/. Accessed 25 Aug 2019
14. Life cycle teachings. Equaywuk; n.d. http://www.equaywuk.ca/HFHNDVT/LifeCycleTeachings.pdf. Accessed 30 Aug 2019.
15. Crenshaw K. Demarginalizing the intersection of race and sex: a black feminist critique of antidiscrimination doctrine, feminist theory and antiracist politics. Univ Chic Leg Forum. 1989;140:139–67.
16. National Centre for Truth and Reconciliation. Truth and Reconciliation Commission of Canada reports. Winnipeg: National Centre for Truth and Reconciliation; 2015. http://nctr.ca/reports.php. Accessed 30 Aug 2019.
17. Barrera J. Ottawa initially fought St. Anne's residential school electric chair compensation claims. CBC News. 2 Dec 2017. https://www.cbc.ca/news/indigenous/st-annes-residential-school-electric-chair-compensation-fight-1.4429594. Accessed 3 Aug 2019.
18. In the Provincial Court of Manitoba in the matter of: The Fatality Inquiries Act, and in the matter of: Brian Lloyd Sinclair, deceased. Winnipeg: Provincial Court of Manitoba. 2014. http://www.manitobacourts.mb.ca/site/assets/files/1051/brian_sinclair_inquest_-_dec_14.pdf. Accessed 30 Aug 2019.
19. Allen B, Smylie J. First peoples, second class treatment: the role of racism in the health and well-being of indigenous peoples in Canada. Toronto, ON: Wellesley Institute; 2015. https://www.wellesleyinstitute.com/wp-content/uploads/2015/02/Summary-First-Peoples-Second-Class-Treatment-Final.pdf. Accessed 23 Aug 2019.
20. Brotman S, Ryan B, Jalbert Y, Rowe B. Reclaiming space-regaining health: the health care experiences of two-spirit people in Canada. J Gay Lesbian Soc Serv. 2008;14(1):67–87.
21. Dr. Alika Lafontaine (Project chair, Indigenous Health Alliance) at the Natural Resources Committee. Openparliament.ca; 2016. https://openparliament.ca/committees/natural-resources/42-1/12/dr-alika-lafontaine-1/only/. Accessed 23 Aug 2019.
22. Indigenous Services Canada (2018, September 6). Government of Canada investing nearly $68 million over three years to support First Nations-led health transformation [Press release]. Retrieved from https://www.canada.ca/en/indigenous-services-canada/news/2018/09/government-of-canada-investing-nearly-68-million-over-three-years-to-support-first-nations-led-health-transformation.html.
23. Lafontaine AT, Lafontaine CJ. A retrospective on reconciliation by design. Healthc Manage Forum. 2019;32(1):5–19. https://doi.org/10.1177/0840470418794702.
24. Gallagher J. Indigenous approaches to health and wellness leadership: a BC First Nations perspective. Healthc Manage Forum. 2019;32(1):5–10. https://doi.org/10.1177/0840470418788090.

LEADS and the Health Professions

15

John(y) Van Aerde

This chapter describes how LEADS can serve as an antidote to some of the leadership challenges health professionals experience—including fragmented health care systems, limited engagement and burnout among staff, diversity and equity issues and demand for high quality leadership practice. We focused on physicians and nurses because together they are the majority of clinicians in the health system. We offer specific examples of how LEADS is being used by physicians and nurses as well as ideas for further use of the framework. However, we're not giving prescriptive answers—instead inviting you to explore what you think is possible with LEADS.

This look at LEADS considers four main challenges. First, using LEADS for professionals working in fragmented systems; second, LEADS as an enabler of professional engagement and as a means of supporting professional health and well-being; third, fostering diversity and equity through a LEADS-based distributed leadership model; and fourth, LEADS as a pathway to the development of high quality leadership in the health professions.

Challenge One: Using LEADS for Professionals Working in Fragmented Health Systems

Earlier in the book Canada's health system was described as fragmented [1, 2], Constitutional, geographical and structural silos detract from the quality of patient care. Even in regions—created to link care across institutional boundaries—silos prevent patients from getting the continuity of care they need, whether they are elderly people transitioning between hospitals and hospices, adolescents with mental health issues bounced around among social services, or patients moving from hospital to community or home care. Patients with multiple chronic ailments also

J. Van Aerde (✉)
Canadian Society of Physician Leaders, Ottawa, ON, Canada
e-mail: johny.vanaerde@gmail.com

© Springer Nature Switzerland AG 2020
G. Dickson, B. Tholl (eds.), *Bringing Leadership to Life in Health: LEADS in a Caring Environment*, https://doi.org/10.1007/978-3-030-38536-1_15

struggle to navigate the primary-specialist care continuum, if they can get a primary care physician at all.

At the same time, physicians' attention is fragmented by struggles with electronic records and barrages of emails, by ever-increasing expectations of patients and dwindling resources, and by redefining their professional roles. A final touch of fragmentation may be added by the uniquely legislated role of physicians that makes most of them independent practitioners running businesses based on fee-for-service payments [3], in contrast to other care givers—like nurses—who are employees of organizations. However, in their organizational silos, nurses can also feel disconnected from other parts of the organization that have responsibility for patient care. It should come as no surprise patients become disoriented when they enter our fragmented non-system without a map and little clarity on where services are located.

This structural and functional fragmentation goes hand in hand with professional fragmentation, as an increasing number of subspecialties and programs are created. There are also multiple agencies representing the interests of nurses and doctors. Do they compete with one another for their members and for the attention of politicians? Do they act to protect the status quo of their profession at the expense of needed change? The answer to both questions, more often than not, is yes. It is tempting for professional bodies, health organizations and providers to look after their self-interest and performance, rather than to work in partnership with others for the benefit of all [4].

In both instances—at a micro or patient-care level and in macro systemic reform—LEADS is increasingly seen as an antidote to fragmented leadership across health care. It works in three ways: as a universal vocabulary for leadership action, by embracing distributed leadership for system change and by emphasizing the unifying goal of caring for one another and patients as the goal of health leadership.

LEADS as a Common Vocabulary for Leadership in Prince Edward Island's Health System

In July of 2010, Prince Edward Island formed a single provincial health authority, Health PEI, which assumed the operational services of the government's new Department of Health and Wellness. One board was created, and leadership development was united across silos—all facilities and practice areas. At that time, the LEADS framework was implemented by the senior leaders.

During these changes, a new clinical information system and a shift to a collaborative model of nursing were introduced simultaneously. The IT implementation and the introduction of collaborative care caused a lot of unrest in the system, requiring leadership for the change throughout the system. This example demonstrates that the LEADS framework works best when it is interpreted as a framework for both leadership development and as a model to implement change.

In April of 2018, in keeping with using LEADS as a common leadership vocabulary, the Medical Society of Prince Edward Island kicked off a custom, seven-month run of its Physician Leadership Development Program which is cross referenced with the Canadian College of Health Leaders' LEADS framework and prepares doctors to work with others in PEI's health system [5].

In the case of PEI, LEADS offers a simple and clear vocabulary for leadership that can be shared among clinical, administrative, and technical partners. This helps overcome the fragmented relationship that can exist between physicians and non-physician leaders due to their unique contractual connection to the system, as well as different mental models of each other's roles [6]. If leadership is a force to overcome systemic fragmentation, its language must reflect that. LEADS provides a common vocabulary for people trying to create an organizational culture that engages staff and makes them receptive to change and innovative practices [7].

The story below shows how Alberta Health Services is putting LEADS to work in a professional context to accomplish these goals (see Chap. 12 for further detail).

LEADS as a Common Leadership Language for Distributed Leadership in Alberta

Alberta Health Services (AHS) is the province-wide health authority responsible for delivering service to the population of Alberta. Presently, AHS is designing a leadership development institute based on the LEADS capabilities and adapted for different levels of leadership expertise, some for physicians specifically [8]. Covenant Health, a faith-based health organization, also uses LEADS for its leadership development purposes.

To build synergy with the work of these two delivery systems, the Alberta College of Family Physicians and the Alberta Medical Association decided to embrace LEADS in primary care. In 2016 the college sponsored a LEADS in-house facilitator program offered by LEADS Canada, to prepare 16 individuals—eight of them physicians—to develop leadership development facilitators that could act as a resource for the Alberta Primary Care Network initiative sponsored by the Alberta government.

The facilitators developed LEADS programming to support their colleagues in dealing with the challenges of integrating government policy, primary care physician needs, and the concept of a patient medical home (promoted by The College of Family Physicians of Canada) into primary care networks dedicated to improving patient care. The common language of LEADS helped network leaders engage with other leaders in Alberta Health Services and the ministry in discussing leadership issues.

The facilitators used their knowledge of LEADS to help develop provincial change agents and physician leadership networks to facilitate a number of improvement initiatives for network members. They also supported the networks in developing leadership skills in their teams to implement the Alberta's unique approach to primary care (Terri Potter. Executive Director, Alberta College of Family Physicians. Personal Communication, 5 May 2019).

Distributed leadership, promoted by the LEADS Framework, helps overcome fragmentation by releasing the considerable leadership potential of medical, nursing, and administrative staff [9]. Distributed leadership emphasizes the need for collaborative skills in leaders, and the responsibility of people, in formal and informal leadership roles, to take initiative [10–12]. The collaborative skills are also important for physicians and nurses in the context of patient- and relationship-centred care.

But perhaps the most compelling influence LEADS has against fragmentation is its emphasis on caring. Caring unites the efforts of physicians, nurses, and other health professionals through its appeal based on a common purpose, and each profession's identity. An explicit emphasis on caring can unite professionals across what might otherwise be fragmented scope and practice boundaries. Care is a shared value and strong motivator that binds and connects everybody involved in the health care system (see section below on caring, empathy and burnout).

Challenge Two: LEADS for Professional Engagement and for Wellbeing of Health Professionals

Both doctors and nurses have been central to health care from the beginning, although they took different routes to the roles they play today. Physicians began as independent practitioners in the days of barber-surgeons and barber-apothecaries and weren't integrated into institutions until the mid-twentieth century [13]. Nurses, on the other hand, essentially created health care institutions: hospitals started as hospices where people went to die, and both the nursing and administrative components were offered by religious groups, mainly nuns [14].

Because nursing evolved from that original group of caregivers, nurses have been more engaged in the health care system from the beginning. While the nurses were *caring* inside the hospitals, the physicians were *curing* outside the walls of those institutions. But as more and more complex equipment and technology were needed to diagnose and treat patients, physicians increasingly needed to have a connection with at least one hospital.

It's only in the last few decades that physicians have, somewhat unwillingly, become full participants in the entire health system and they've done so without historical or cultural knowledge of how that engagement might work. From this historical and cultural perspective, it is understandable physicians often perceive their accountability is to the patient first, their profession second, and to the organized health care system third—if at all.

LEADS and Professional Engagement

For centuries physicians were considered leaders by virtue of their profession and standing in their community, but they had no background or training in leadership [15]. Today, in response to the changing demands in the field, medical leadership is undergoing a paradigm shift from its traditional role to one founded on collaborative leadership and administration [16]. At the end of the twentieth century, the medical profession came to a turning point due to two related concepts: quality control and leadership. Evidence shows a link between these two concepts for physicians: studies have found physicians are more likely to become engaged in health system reform if they take on leadership roles in quality improvement initiatives [8, 17, 18].

In Canada, several recent reports have highlighted the importance of physician leadership and engagement for health care reform [7, 19, 20]. According to the Canadian Society of Physician Leaders, physicians have a unique place and responsibility in the delivery of universal health care, and efficient and effective reform cannot happen without their active and willing participation. As a result, leadership development has become a priority [7, 21–23].

Similarly, leadership from nurses is vital in terms of shaping and influencing processes, procedures, and practices for optimal patient care, whether those decisions are made in the corporate office or on the front-line or care delivery: [24, 25] nurses "…must engage with physicians and other health care professionals to deliver efficient and effective care and assume leadership roles in the redesign of the health care system" [26].

Spurgeon and colleagues defined physician engagement as a two-directional social process where the organization must reciprocate the engagement of individual physicians with high quality care by putting in place opportunities and processes for physicians to participate (Fig. 15.1) [27]. This model can be extrapolated to include nurses, although it has not been validated by research in that context.

This model of professional engagement contains two dimensions: individual capacity which reflects skills leading to increased self-efficacy and personal empowerment to tackle new challenges (the horizontal axis of Fig. 15.1), and organizational opportunities reflecting structural, political and cultural conditions that facilitate doctors becoming more actively engaged leadership activities (the vertical

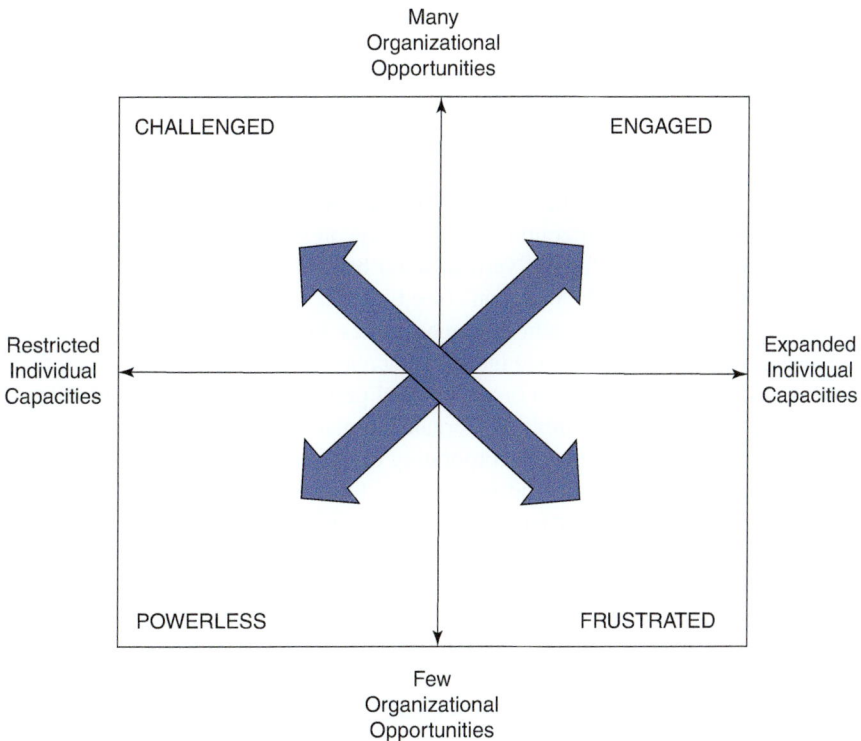

Fig. 15.1 The Spurgeon model to guide improvements in professional engagement [27]

axis of Fig. 15.1). Depending on what conditions are missing, professionals can feel powerless, frustrated or challenged.

Spurgeon's research showed that engaged physicians are positively associated with organizational quality [28]. In the NHS, the introduction of the Medical Leadership Competency Framework [29] together with organizational opportunities to be engaged, has led to improved medical engagement scores and better outcomes, including lower mortality rates and fewer patient safety incidents. Once doctors become engaged throughout the system, the scores for patient experience improve as well, as was seen in Cleveland Clinic [30]. Although studies do not directly use the Spurgeon model in relation to nurses, there is evidence validating the importance of nurses feeling engaged [31, 32].

Learning how to lead is fundamentally important to Spurgeon's construct of developing individual capacity. According to the 70/20/10 concept of blended learning [33], 10% of learning takes place in the classroom by knowledge transfer and formal learning [34], the *knowing* or expertise component of learning leadership. Twenty per cent of learning leadership comes from a variety of activities that include social learning, mentoring and coaching. The 70% share comes from hands-on-experience [35], in the form of challenging assignments [36] comprising the practice and acquisition of skills derived from the classroom knowledge (sometimes in simulated situations) [37].

The LEADS framework, the 70/20/10 approach to learning, and the Spurgeon model can be integrated to explain how to engage physicians and nurses: when everybody who works in an organization has leadership skills and opportunities to use them, true engagement happens. While an individual's ability or capacity increases an individual's 'can do,' organizational opportunities improve personal motivation and the 'want to do.' The LEADS framework provides a set of expectations and standards that can be used both to guide leadership development for individuals (Lead self, the horizontal axis of Spurgeon model) and for organizations (other LEADS domains for the vertical axis) by embedding leadership practices reflective of the framework "in action" (see Fig. 15.2).

By following LEADS practices, opportunities for professionals to engage are enhanced. For example, evidence indicates increasing the percentage of doctors on boards has a positive impact on organizational performance and improving patient experience [37]. Other examples of organizational opportunities include quality improvement initiatives [18] or incorporating professionals in the provincial health care governance structure, as the province of Saskatchewan in Canada has [38]. Embedding opportunities for engagement in organizational structure is important (vertical axis of Fig. 15.2). Professionals who learn LEADS capabilities are also motivated and able to take on organizational opportunities because they have the skills to do so (horizontal axis of Fig. 15.2). When both work together the professional's engagement increases, and more clinicians move into the right upper quadrant of the model.

St. Joseph's Health Care in London, Ontario has LEADS-based leadership development programs for all staff, including nurses and physicians—although for the latter, the leadership development program is a hybrid between the CanMEDS 2015

Many
Organizational
Opportunities

CHALLENGED   ENGAGED

Embeddedness: 70%

Restricted   Expanded
Individual   ←——————— *Expertise & Experience: 30%* ———————→   Individual
Capacities   Capacities

POWERLESS   FRUSTRATED

Few
Organizational
Opportunities

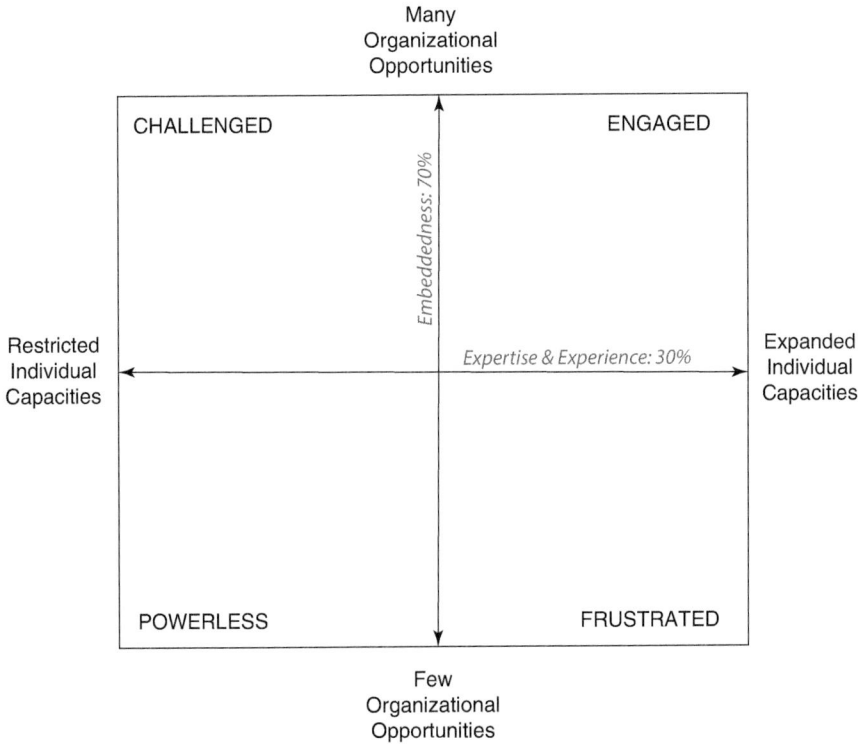

Fig. 15.2 Clinical engagement model and blended learning (Modified from Spurgeon et al., 2008) [27]

role of Leader [39] and LEADS. It's designed for three levels of physician leadership: entry level for newly recruited physicians, mid-career level as part of talent management, and executive level. The following vignette explains the St. Joseph approach in greater detail.

Three Levels of Physician Leadership Program at St. Joseph's Health Care

About 15 years ago, Dr Gillian Kernaghan, President and CEO of St. Joseph's Health Care, helped develop a leadership program in collaboration with Western University, where many physicians have cross-appointments. LEADS capabilities were used to develop performance evaluation tools in order to individualize the development of each physician's leadership skills. As a result, the organization's culture is one of ongoing learning and evaluation: LEADS-based self- and 360-evaluations are used to review goals, strengths and areas for growth, aligned with templates for role descriptions. There are three levels to physician leadership development.

The Foundational Leadership Series (entry level) has to be taken by all newly recruited physicians during their first three years. Its focus is on self-development, knowledge and skills, including running efficient meetings, ethics, career development, finances 101, and working in a unionized environment. To ensure the series meets needs, the content and delivery are tweaked based on feedback to questions like "What do you know now that you wished we would have told you when you started?" This level corresponds to the Lead self, Engage others and Achieve results domains of LEADS.

The Talent Management System (mid-level) runs in collaboration with the university. It is appropriate for site chiefs, divisional leaders, program leaders, associate deans—middle management roles. In talent management, self-awareness and self-management are further explored, along with engaging others through teamwork and collaboration, strategic thinking and planning and systems theory. This level of the leadership development covers all five domains of LEADS. Templates with role descriptions of physician leaders are complemented with a list containing the skills and LEADS capabilities that are required for different leadership roles. St. Joseph Health Care also uses a recruitment tool that maps candidates' LEADS capabilities against the capabilities needed for the position they're applying for.

The Executive Level of the development program is designed for the departmental chairs, Medical Advisory Committee chair, vice-dean and medical directors of large programs. Talent management, including succession planning, and leadership development are all integrated. The self-assessment and 360s are used as part of succession planning—for example, the capabilities of a physician being considered for a job are compared with the LEADS capabilities required for that role. In collaboration with Western University's Ivey School of Business, physicians can do leadership projects, including quality improvement initiatives, in their organizational environment. This approach reflects the vertical axis of the physician engagement Spurgeon model.

Dr. Kernaghan says "LEADS has given our organization a framework for leadership development and physician engagement," adding "A framework is all very good, but it's what you do with the framework and how you embed it in the organization that makes the difference."

Leadership, LEADS, Psychological Well-Being and Burnout

A recent Institute for Health Improvement paper on well-being at work emphasized that workers are unlikely to become engaged if they don't feel psychologically safe in their workplace [40]. Figure 15.3 shows a continuum of psychological states from engagement and leadership at the top to burnout at the bottom. Without trust or psychological safety health care workers won't engage, instead descending into change fatigue and moral distress, ultimately leading to moral injury and burnout.

As the evidence makes clear, burnout is a growing problem: physicians, nurses, pharmacists, residents, and medical students are increasingly struggling with high levels of stress, which is a key precursor to burnout [41–46]. Burnout reduces work effort by professionals [47] and leads to more mistakes and lower quality of care. Burned-out doctors order more unnecessary tests, prescribe more unnecessary drugs, have a negative impact on team satisfaction, and provide less empathetic care [51].

Physicians' wellness also suffers when they can't provide the quality of care they want to because of system limitations [48]. While personal characteristics like perfectionism were originally identified as the main reasons for burnout, more recently organizational and systemic factors are getting the blame [49]. The main causes of burnout are embedded in the structure and culture of

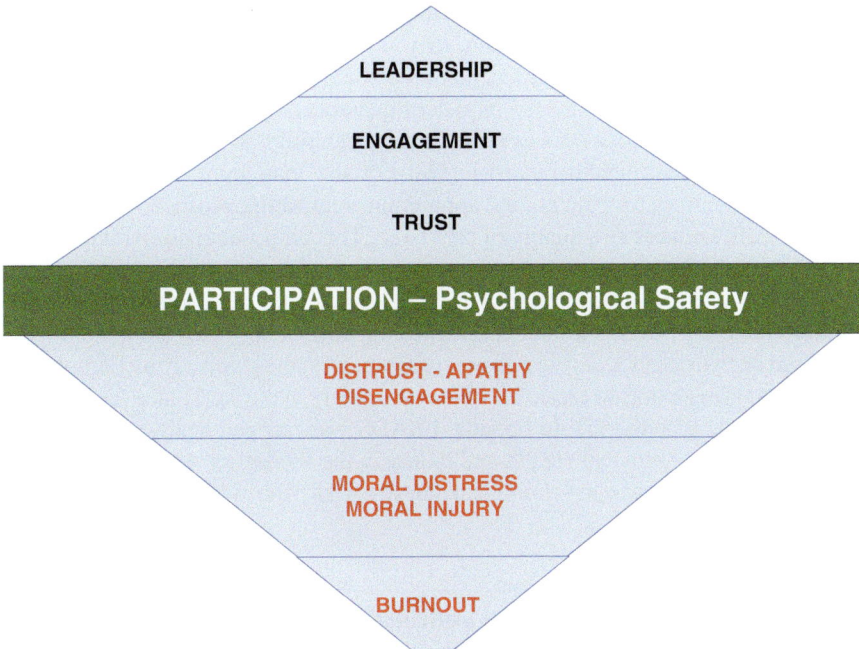

Fig. 15.3 Degrees of engagement and psychological stress in the health care system

organizations. That in turn creates conditions that clash with the personal and professional values of physicians and nurses. Trying to care for people in the face of increasing limits on resources results in a demoralizing misalignment between professional values and meeting patients' needs, for reasons that are beyond an individual professional's control [49]. Paradoxically, the introduction of electronic health records, which were supposed to improve patient care, has led to widespread complaints from physicians that they reduce the quality of physician-patient interaction, leading to less satisfaction and more burnout [50].

Chen and Chen identified leaders' ineffectiveness and lack of emotional intelligence as a major contributor to nurses' burnout. Contrarily, leadership effectiveness and positive emotional intelligence reduce burnout [51].

Two specific LEADS capabilities should help leaders to deal with the burnout raging through health care. The Lead self domain calls for leaders to model self-care by taking responsibility for their own health, which is as important for employees to see as it is for the benefit of the individual leader. One of the Engage others capabilities is to contribute to the creation of healthy organizations; i.e., changing so people have the resources they need to do their jobs encourages engagement [52].

Other suggestions for supporting the mental health of physicians include work from the Massachusetts Medical Society, the Massachusetts Health and Hospital Association, together with Harvard's School of Public Health and Global Health Institute. They suggest organizations should, in the short-term, improve access to staff support offices which provide health and mental health assistance and resilience learning [53–55]. Medium term, they say, organizations can increase physician engagement in design, implementation and customization of electronic health records and promise to reduce the burden of documentation and measurement they place on physicians (LEADS has been used successfully in the design and implementation electronic health records) [56]. For the long term, they recommend improving resources for patients and appointing chief wellness officers to study and monitor staff wellness as a quality of care issue. This proposal to use individual and systemic tools for wellness resembles the horizontal and vertical axes of the Spurgeon model for embedding leadership and leadership development throughout the system, using LEADS as an instrument (Fig. 15.2).

Based on two decades of research in organizations in the U.S.A., Amy Edmondson has created frameworks to create psychological safety in the workplace for learning, innovation and growth [57]. In Canada, LEADS was mapped against the National Standard for Psychological Health and Safety in the Workplace and can be used as a framework to improve psychological safety for all who work in the health care system [58].

Challenge Three: Distributed Leadership to Foster Diversity and Equity in the Health System

Equity and diversity inside and outside health care are receiving increasing attention recently, including issues of gender, inclusion of patients and their advocates, ethnicity, and age [59–62]. All affect the professions but this section focuses on gender challenges for leaders in health professions, including creating equity among professions and roles through distributed leadership. Generally, gender issues in professional communities focus on female nurses and doctors struggling to be well-represented in leadership roles [63–68]. One 2018 literature review found gender discrimination limits women's potential for seniority and leadership and said gender gaps in modern health organizational leadership are driven by stereotypes, discrimination, power imbalance and privilege [69]. Carolyn's story, below, speaks to gender issues faced when female nurses move into leadership roles.

Challenging Stereotypes: A Nurse's Story

Carolyn Pullen is the chief executive officer of the Canadian Cardiovascular Society with a Ph.D. in nursing. This is her story of challenges with diversity.

> *My early experience in formal leadership was as a young adult leading extended canoe trips in the high Arctic. I grew into this summer job naturally, coming up the ranks in Canada's tradition of summer camps and gaining the required skills, certifications and experience. However, leading self-sufficient groups of high-paying customers on northern rivers characterized by challenging white water, extreme weather conditions, and an*

abundance of bears is typically seen as a role for males. When corporate clients disembarked from float planes at the headwaters of a wild river, I imagined their reaction would be "Where's the larger-than-life, burly, hairy, six-foot guy in whom I will place my trust and safety?"

To address this self-imposed credibility problem, I felt I needed to demonstrate traits I perceived as more typically male: boundless confidence, strength, and bravado. In short, I tried to act like a guy. I tried on personas that told brave tales and bawdy jokes. I carried loads across portages that weighed more than I did. Before long, I realized I felt uncomfortable playing an inauthentic role, and I got a really sore back!

Furthermore, I overlooked the fact that no one—not the clients, my male colleagues, or my employers—expected me to be anything other than what I was: a collaborative, capable young leader. I was slow to realize it was my differences they valued: a calculated approach to managing risk, strong interpersonal and team-building skills, expertise in northern flora and fauna, etc.

In addition, the company owner and longest-serving guide was a woman—a diminutive, calm, solid leader. She subtly suggested she understood my position and would share insights and model ways to lead from the seat I occupied: a female leader with unique strengths who enhanced the diversity of her team. She shared tips for doing the physical aspects of the job in a way that didn't require herculean strength (e.g. finesse over brawn). She demonstrated confidence in her abilities and her role and was effective and thoroughly acceptable to our high-adventure clients. She helped me understand that, in a stereotypically male role, it is fine to be a female and be yourself. I went on to be among the longest-serving guides for the company, leading dozens of high Arctic expeditions, often as the solo guide.

This learning translated well into my career in health care. As a developing leader, nurse leader and new CEO I have found support and sponsorship from female and male leaders alike. It is the connectors, collaborators and strong communicators, regardless of gender, who embody highly effective leadership. I believe in drawing fully from a broad cross section of perspectives and styles to leverage diversity across genders, generations and geography to develop and bring the most talent to tackling our wicked problems in health care. Today, I strive to intentionally lead highly collaborative and inclusive teams and I have those northern trips to thank for this insight.

Carolyn's story emphasizes the mental shifts required to realize one's potential to be a leader. She needed to be aware of her own assumptions, as the first capability of the Lead self domain says. If she had not challenged her own notion of who is a leader and who is a follower, she would not have recognized her own leadership. Similar changes in thinking are required to confront equity and diversity challenges in the professions. An effective multidisciplinary team, for example, needs leadership to be distributed amongst the professions [9]. West et al showed teams that share responsibilities decrease age-standardized deaths after emergency surgery by 275 per 100,000 [70]. But effective teamwork can't be achieved unless the stereotype of physicians as leaders and nurses as followers is eradicated (see Chap. 2: Build teams).

There's also an equity issue in the views administrators and physicians have of each other. It's common for doctors to see administrators as getting in the way of their care for patients, while administrators often see doctors as impediments to system change. Essentially physicians see themselves as advocates for each patient's care, while administrators advocate for all patients [6, 71]. Solving this requires the two groups to share their talents in a distributed leadership model, which could be helped by more emphasis on dyad models where physicians and administrators are paired to work together [72]. Efforts to distribute leadership on teams can benefit from the Lead self, Engage others and Achieve results domains, while the work between physicians and administrators requires the capabilities of all five domains of LEADS.

Leader-follower similarities can also be seen in the doctor-patient relationship, which has evolved from profession-centred to patient-centred, and which will have to evolve into relationship-centred care, focused on the relationship between patients and the teams that care for them [12]. Because the primary purpose of the health care system is to respond to the needs of the patient, the process of real engagement of patients and citizens for their care in the system can only occur through relationship-centered care based on distributed leadership and effective follower-ship. This is a delicate dance between all engaged partners.

One of the prime leadership functions of LEADS is to address issues around integration of care. Use your knowledge of LEADS to analyze how distributed leadership and effective followership could have resolved the disconnected care that led to the disastrous and unfortunate death of Greg Price [73], described in the following Learning Moment.

Learning Moment: Greg's Wings
Greg Price was in his early thirties when he died following a series of health care mishaps, mainly caused by poorly coordinated communication and no continuity of care. As a result, instead of being cured of testicular cancer that was detected early, he died two years later. It was a prime example of a complete lack of continuity of care or shared leadership.

In the first six months after his death, Greg's father and his family connected with the Health Quality Council of Alberta (HQCA), an organization designed to measure, monitor and survey the health system in Alberta. Following the study by the HQCA, Dr. Ward Flemons, the lead on the report approached the Price family about turning Greg's story into an educational film, with the intent of using the finished product to reinforce the importance of teamwork, shared leadership, effective followership, and communication in the health care system.

Falling Through the Cracks: Greg's Story [73] explores Greg's journey through the health care system, noting the lapses in communication and breaks in the continuity of his care. The movie has won several awards. It is not just shown to people inside the health care system, but also to the public across the country; more than one hundred times in the first year alone. It stresses the importance of public engagement when it comes to effecting change in the health care system. In a relationship-centred context, patients want greater involvement in their care, they want to participate in making decisions about that care and they want to know that things are moving along at a reasonable pace.

Greg's Wings, the non-profit organization behind the movie, has demonstrated two things that relate to shared leadership:

1. Greg's death is an example of failed continuity of care due to an inadequate information system and lack of distributed leadership or effective followership.
2. By engaging people inside and outside the health care system, the Price family and Dr. Flemons demonstrates how patients, the public and the health care workers can change relationships with the health system. By practising the delicate dance between shared leadership and effective followership, the Price family and the health care workers alternate roles toward the common goal of optimizing continuity of care.

LEADS was not part of Greg's care, but his story shows the possibilities of distributed leadership and effective followership.

EXERCISE: Reflect on how the LEADS domains might have influenced what happened before and after Greg's death.

Challenge Four: LEADS as a Pathway to Develop Professional Leaders

How can LEADS be used to embed life-long leadership learning for physicians, nurses and other health professionals into the structure and culture of organizations and the health system? Efforts by physician- and nursing-education bodies in the UK, Australia and in Canada (using LEADS) are models for developing leadership in the professions.

Blended Learning Approaches to Leadership Development

Earlier, the concept of 70/20/10 model of blended learning was mentioned as an essential part of developing individual capacity. The model combines formal learning with workplace and informal learning opportunities. The following story shows how the Holland Bloorview Kids Rehabilitation Hospital put LEADS to work through that kind of blended approach.

Putting LEADS to Work in Leadership Development

The Holland Bloorview Kids Rehabilitation Hospital in Toronto, which employs about 1,000 people, has developed a 90-minute session for each of the twenty LEADS capabilities. Because resources, particularly time, are limited, participants have welcomed the 90-minute sessions at the hospital. Knowledge, relevance and potential application are explored for each capability in an integrated real-life way, to make them easier to translate into the workplace. This is where many leadership training programs stop—staff go back to work, where the culture doesn't make using their new skills easy, and the effort is soon dropped.

However, Holland Bloorview follows up the training sessions with real-time coaching and 360 evaluations to help leadership learners try out and develop each capability on the job.

If education and training are about the *what* of leadership, then the 70% is about *how* to lead. That 70% should take place in the organization through action learning such as day-to-day activities and problem solving [34, 35] (Fig 15.2).

Talent management and succession planning are part of the structure and culture of a learning organization and should be integrated into the development of professional leaders [12]. Adopting LEADS would make talent management and succession planning consistent across organizations and indeed an entire system.

Using LEADS to Increase the Quality of Leadership in the Professions

With the release of *To Err is Human: Building a Safer Health System* by the Institute of Medicine in 1999 [74] (which estimated between 44,000 and 98,000 people died annually in the U.S.A. from medical errors), physicians had no choice but to become engaged in quality control and leadership. That drove medical leadership to leave behind the traditional autocratic role physicians played and shift to more collaborative clinical and administrative leadership. Many were not ready for the change: physicians traditionally did not get any leadership or management training because they were automatically considered leaders by virtue of their profession. But without evidence-based best models of effective leadership, the evolution has been "anything goes!" Doctors learn by observing others or on the job [15].

To counter this phenomenon in 2015, Canada's Royal College of Physicians and Surgeons changed the CanMEDS manager role into a leader role [39, 75]. This has given rise to LEADS-based physician leadership development both in Canada and abroad.

LEADS in the Nursing Profession

The LEADS framework has been adopted by the Royal College of Physicians and Surgeons and the College of Family Physicians of Canada, which is developing a curriculum to align the competencies of the CanMEDS 2015 role of leader with the LEADS framework.

The Physician Leadership Institute under the umbrella of the Canadian Medical Association, and with the support of the Canadian Society of Physician Leaders, organizes its professional development leadership courses according to the LEADS framework (Fig. 15.4).

There's also a Canadian Certificate for Physician Executives, awarded by the Society of Physician Leaders based on achieving certain educational requirements

Physician Leadership Institute (PLI) courses / LEADS capabilities	Self-aware	Manage themselves	Develop themselves	Demonstrate character	Foster development of others	Contribute to healthy organizations	Communicate effectively	Build teams	Set direction	Strategically align decisions with vision, values and evidence	Take action to implement decisions	Assess and evaluate	Purposefully build partnerships and networks to create results	Demonstrate commitment to customers and service	Mobilize knowledge	Navigate socio-political environments	Demonstrate systems/critical thinking	Encourage and support innovation	Orient themselves strategically to the future	Champion and orchestrate change
									LEAD SELF			ENGAGE OTHERS				ACHIEVE RESULTS			DEVELOP COALITIONS	SYSTEMS TRANSFORMATION
Insights Discovery*: Understanding your Personality Preferences	•	•	•	•			•	•												
Leading with Emotional Intelligence	•	•	•	•			•	•												
Personal Leadership: Identifying your Core Values & Vision	•	•	•	•			•	•												
Leadership Begins with Self-awareness	•	•	•	•																
Leadership for Medical Women		•	•	•																
Physician Leadership Focus: Managing workplace distractions to increase productivity	•	•	•	•		•	•													
Professionalism and Ethics	•	•	•	•			•	•												
Navigating your career: essential skills for the modern physician	•	•	•	•	•															
Building and Leading Teams					•	•	•	•						•						
Engaging Others	•	•			•	•	•	•												
Managing Disruptive Behaviour	•	•	•		•	•														
Managing People Effectively					•	•	•	•												
Facilitating Meetings					•	•	•	•	•	•	•	•								
Coaching for Excellence					•	•	•	•												
Maximizing your patient relationships	•			•		•	•	•						•						
Dollars and Sense									•	•	•	•								
Leading High Performance Culture					•		•		•	•	•	•	•	•						
Quality Measurement for Leadership and Learning									•	•		•							•	•
Strategic Thinking for Results									•	•							•	•	•	•
Talent Management for Exceptional Leadership					•				•		•									
Conflict Management and Negotiation	•	•				•	•			•		•		•	•	•				
Leadership Strategies for Sustainable Physician Engagement					•	•	•						•	•	•					
Developing and Leading System Improvement									•	•	•			•			•	•	•	•
Developing Strategic Influence													•			•				•
Leading Change						•				•							•	•		•
Social Systems Leadership: Thriving in Complexity													•				•	•	•	•

CORE

PLI courses that have been identified as essential training for physicians interested in or engaged in a position of leadership. These courses may be taken in any order.

Fig. 15.4 LEADS as a foundation for Physician Leadership Institute courses (Used with permission from the Physician Leadership Institute, Ottawa, 2019 Sep 19)

and senior leadership experience (which must include all LEADS capabilities) [76]. *The certificate must be renewed every five years through the same rigorous process.*

 The shift from manager to leader has also spurred changes in medical education. For example, the Association of the Faculties of Medical Education in Canada [77] *states: "Medical leadership is essential to both patient care and the broader health system. Faculties of Medicine must foster medical leadership in faculty and students, including how to manage, navigate, and help transform medical practice and the health care system in collaboration with others."*

 LEADS is also being introduced into the curriculum for nurses, as the following example shows:

 The Canadian Academy of Nursing was established in 2019 by the Canadian Nurses Association (CNA) as the first pan-Canadian organization dedicated to identifying, educating, supporting, and celebrating nursing leaders across all the regulated categories and all domains of practice. The Academy will build a comprehensive Canadian hub designed to educate, empower and support nurses to lead, advocate, innovate, influence public policy and create sustainable change.

 The LEADS framework — and along with principles of Strengths-Based Nursing Leadership, will serve to ground the work of the Academy. All CNA staff participated in one-day Bringing LEADS to Life team development sessions (2012) and the LEADS Capability Framework is used currently in personal performance measurement for the chief executive officer.

 As the Academy activity ramps up in 2020, we will reference LEADS in spearheading the development of core capabilities and competencies for nursing leadership in Canada, including capabilities in diverse domains such as nursing administration, informatics and policy. In addition, the Academy will serve as a repository for a comprehensive roster of leadership development programs for nurses including post graduate degree programs in universities, certificate programs and professional development initiatives offered across Canada and beyond.

 As of 2020, the Academy of Canadian Executive Nurses and the highly successful Dorothy Wylie Health Leaders Institute both sit within the Academy. The Dorothy Wylie residential program delivers a concentrated program of study of leadership principles, models, behaviours, skills and tools that align strongly with key capabilities of the LEADS framework. The CNA's popular workshops focused on policy leadership and change management also speak to key capabilities under the LEADS framework and will be offered through the Academy going forward.The Canadian Academy of Nursing was established in 2019 by the Canadian Nurses Association (CNA) as the first pan-Canadian organization dedicated to identifying, educating, supporting, and celebrating nursing leaders across all the regulated categories and all domains of practice. The Academy will build a comprehensive Canadian hub designed to educate, empower and support nurses to lead, advocate, innovate, influence public policy and create sustainable change.

LEADS can also be useful for feedback and accountability, both for learning and in organizations. The Health Standards Association of Canada, which runs Canada's accreditation processes, calls LEADS a guide to assist organizations in developing the standards of leadership assessed for accreditation [78].

International Examples of Professionalizing Physician Leadership

A great example of how LEADS can be integrated in resident education is Sanokondu [79], a non-profit, international collaboration of health leadership educators and organizations with interest in health leadership development. A set of modules portraying real clinical scenarios was developed for residents and preceptors, based on the five domains of LEADS and several of the CanMEDS 2015 roles, mainly Leader. Sanokondu has made those modules available free of charge online [80].

The two-year fellowship program from the Royal Australasian College of Medical Administrators in Melbourne, Australia is one of the best examples of a professionalized leadership degree for physicians [81]. According to Karen Owen, the organization's immediate-past CEO, "When the role of leader was introduced in parallel to that of manager one decade ago, LEADS was used as the framework and it allowed [us] to articulate the curriculum and courses for the role of leadership" (Personal communication, 2019 Mar 27).

Progress toward professionalization is also being made in England where the Faculty of Medical Leadership and Management has developed Leadership and Management Standards for Medical Professionals [82]. The standards are articulated as a set of core values and behaviour designed to work across all career levels. Interestingly, the standards are strongly related to the LEADS framework outlined in Chap. 3. The Faculty of Medical Leadership and Management believes an effective medical leader is defined by how and what they do, underpinned by why they do it. The faculty has introduced a fellowship program it hopes is the beginning of a professionalized leadership learning program. Younger doctors are particularly interested in taking the program, which they see more and more as part of their clinical work and career development.

To take a final example, the LEADS framework and the PLI program structure have also been influential in shaping the National Physician Leadership Training Program in Israel. After exploring the American and Canadian program structures, and after two years of consultation and dialogue with physicians, the Israeli project team chose the Canadian framework. Israel's five core competencies are similar to the LEADS capabilities: e.g. "team engagement" correlates with Engage others; "from vision to workplan" corresponds with Achieve results; and "forming collaborations" aligns with Develop coalitions. They don't yet have a module dealing solely with System transformation, but the capabilities are being introduced into other training modules. "The LEADS framework will definitely continue to serve as a compass for the continued development of of our directors' training program", says Dr. Oren Tavor, Project Director (Personal Communication, 2019, Sept 11).

In conclusion, LEADS can provide a set of standards for guiding development that will professionalize leadership in the health care system, for the individual and for organizations. Just as CanMEDS 2015 provides a framework to standardize professional competencies for medicine, LEADS can serve as a similar model to standardize leadership capabilities.

Summary

In Canada, many health care organizations, including medical, nursing and administrative organizations, have endorsed LEADS. As a common vocabulary and a set of leadership standards, LEADS can provide many benefits to health professionals in general and to the physician and nurse communities specifically. By working together and using LEADS as a common framework, health organizations can embed leadership development in the structure and culture of the Canadian health system. LEADS provides a simple entry point to understanding the research and evidence base behind best practices of leadership. It can help unite stakeholders with a collectively accepted understanding of leadership and encourage adoption of the leadership behaviour needed for health system sustainability and transformation. Finally, LEADS can be used to improve wellbeing and reduce burnout among all health professionals.

References

1. Van Aerde J, Dickson G. Accepting our responsibility: a blueprint for physician leadership in transforming Canada's health care system Canadian Society of Physician Leaders; 2017. https://physicianleaders.ca/assets/whitepapercspl1003.pdf.
2. Lewis S. A system in name only – access, variation and reform in Canada's provinces. NEJM. 2015;372(6):497–500.
3. Science Daily. Doctors should be paid by salary, not fee-for-service, argue behavioral economists. Science News; 9 May 2017. https://www.sciencedaily.com/releases/2017/05/170509121934.htm. Accessed 2 Aug 2019.
4. Lazar H. Why is it so hard to reform health-care policy in Canada? In: Lazar H, Lavis J, Forest P, Church J, editors. Paradigm freeze. Montreal, QC: McGill-Queens' University Press; 2013.
5. Vilches S, Fenwick S, Harris B, Lammi B, Racette R. Changing health organizations with the LEADS leadership framework: report of the 2014–2016 LEADS impact study. Fenwick Leadership Explorations, the Canadian College of Health Leaders, & the Centre for Health Leadership and Research, Royal Roads University; 2016. https://leadscanada.net/document/1788/LEADS_Impact_Report_2017_FINAL.pdf.

6. Bujak J. How to improve hospital-physician relationships. Front Health Serv Manage. 2003;20(2):3–21.
7. West M, Eckert R, Collins B, Chowla R. How compassionate leadership can stimulate innovation in health care. London: The King's Fund; 2017. www.kingsfund.org.uk/publications/caring-change.
8. Van Aerde J. Physician leadership development. Alberta Health Services: Edmonton, AB; 2013. https://www.albertahealthservices.ca/assets/info/hp/phys/if-hp-phys-physician-leadership-development-report.pdf. Accessed 27 Mar 2019.
9. Spurgeon P, Clark J. Medical leadership: the key to medical engagement and effective organisations. London: CRC Press; 2017.
10. Rydenfalt C, Johansson G, Odenrick P, Akerman K, Larsson P. Distributed leadership in the operating room: a naturalistic observation study. Cogn Technol Work. 2015;17(3):451–60.
11. VanVactor J. Collaborative leadership model in the management of healthcare. J Bus Res. 2012;65(4):555–61.
12. Van Aerde J. Relationship-centred care: toward real health system reform. Can J Phys Leadersh. 2015;1(3):3–6. https://cjpl.ca/assets/cjplwinter_2015.pdf
13. Simpson J. Chronic condition. Toronto, ON: Allen Lane; 2012.
14. Picard A. The path to health care reform. The Conference Board of Canada: Ottawa, ON; 2013. https://www.conferenceboard.ca/e-library/abstract.aspx?did=5863.
15. Perry J, Mobley F, Brubaker M. Most doctors have little or no management training, and that's a problem. Harv Bus Rev. 2017;15:15.
16. Sonnino R. Health care leadership development and training: progress and pitfalls. J Healthc Leadersh. 2016;8:19–29.
17. The King's Fund. Leadership and engagement for improvement in the NHS: together we can. Report from The King's Fund Leadership Review. London: The King's Fund; 2012. http://www.kingsfund.org.uk/sites/files/kf/field/field_publication_file/leadership-for-engagement-improvement-nhs-final-review2012.pdf.
18. Vaillancourt L, Mondoux C. Gaining physician involvement in quality improvement initiatives: an organizational perspective. Healthc Q. 2018;21(3):71–6.
19. Dickson G, Tholl B, Baker G, Blais R, Clavel N, Gorley C. Partnerships for health system improvement, leadership and health system redesign: cross-case analysis. Ottawa, ON: Royal Roads University, Canadian Health Leadership Network, Canadian Institutes of Health Research, Michael Smith Foundation for Health Research; 2014. http://chlnet.ca/wp-content/uploads/PHSI-Cross-Case-Analysis-Report-2014.pdf. Accessed 25 Jun 2019.
20. Naylor D, Girard F, Mintz J, Fraser N, Jenkins T, Power C. Unleashing innovation: excellent health care for Canada. Report of the Advisory Panel on Health Care Innovation. Ottawa, ON: Health Canada; 2015. http://tinyurl.com/qx2cf8z. Accessed 12 Jul 2019.
21. Matlow A, Chan MK, Bohnen JD, Blumenthal M, Sanchez-Mendiola S, de Camps Meschino D. Collaborating internationally on physician leadership education: first steps. Leadersh Health Serv (Bradf Engl). 2016;29(3):220–30.
22. Spurgeon P, Barwell F, Mazelan P. Developing a medical engagement scale (MES). Int J Clin Leadersh. 2008;16:213–23.
23. Denis JL, van Gestel N. Medical doctors in healthcare leadership: theoretical and practical challenges. BMC Health Serv Res. 2016;16(S2):158. https://bmchealthservres.biomedcentral.com/track/pdf/10.1186/s12913-016-1392-8.
24. Kirk H. Nurse executive director effectiveness: a systematic review of the literature. J Nurs Manag. 2008;16(3):374–81. https://doi.org/10.1111/j.1365-2834.2007.00783.x.
25. Player K, Burns S. Leadership skills: new nurse to nurse executive. Nurse Lead. 2015;13(6):51–43. https://doi.org/10.1016/j.mnl.2015.09.008.
26. Robert Wood Johnson Foundation Initiative on the Future of Nursing. The future of nursing: leading change, advancing health. Washington, DC: The National Academies of Sciences Engineering and Medicine: Health and Medicine Division; 2010. http://www.nationalacademies.org/hmd/Reports/2010/The-Future-of-Nursing-Leading-Change-Advancing-Health.aspx. Accessed 27 Mar 2019.

27. Spurgeon P, Mazelan P, Barwell F, Mazelan P. Developing a medical engagement scale (MES). Int J Clin Leadersh. 2008;16:213–23.
28. Spurgeon P, Mazelan P, Barwell F. Medical engagement: a crucial underpinning to organizational performance. Health Serv Manag Res. 2011;24(3):114–20.
29. NHS Institute for Innovation and Improvement & Academy of Medical Royal Colleges. Medical leadership competency framework. 3rd ed. London: NHS England; 2010. https://www.leadershipacademy.nhs.uk/wp-content/uploads/2012/11/NHSLeadership-Leadership-Framework-Medical-Leadership-Competency-Framework-3rd-ed.pdf. Accessed 27 Mar 2019.
30. Merlino J, Raman A. Health care's fanatics. Harv Bus Rev. 2013;91(5):108–16.
31. Malila N, Lunkka N, Suhonen M. Authentic leadership in healthcare: a scoping review. Leadersh Health Serv (Bradf Engl). 2018;31(1):129–46. https://doi.org/10.1108/LHS-02-2017-0007.
32. Regan S, Laschinger H, Wong C. The influence of empowerment, authentic leadership, and professional practice environments on nurses' perceived interprofessional collaboration. J Nurs Manag. 2016;24(1):e54–61. https://doi.org/10.1111/jonm.12288.
33. Rabin R. Blended learning for leadership: the CCL approach. Greensboro, NC: Center for Creative Leadership; 2014. https://www.ccl.org/wp-content/uploads/2015/04/BlendedLearningLeadership.pdf.
34. Duberman T. Developing physician leaders today using the 70/20/10 rule. Phys Exec. 2011;37(5):66–8. https://pdfs.semanticscholar.org/f3a3/7c28f8a2b65cb11625e89547b1ef565033ec.pdf.
35. Kellerman B. Professionalizing leadership. New York, NY: Oxford University Press; 2018.
36. Veronesi G, Kirkpatrick I, Altanlar A. Clinical leadership and the changing governance of public hospitals: implications for patient experience. Public Adm. 2015;93:1031–48.
37. Halligan A. Investing in leadership post-Francis. Health Serv J. 2013. https://www.hsj.co.uk/leadership/investing-in-leadership-post-francis/5054916.article. Accessed 27 Mar 2019.
38. See the Saskatechewan HA's organization chart. https://www.saskhealthauthority.ca/about/Leadership-and-Structure/Documents/Org-Structure-ELT.pdf.
39. Dath D, Chan MK, Abbott C. CanMEDS 2015: from manager to leader. Royal College of Physicians and Surgeons of Canada: Ottawa, ON; 2015. http://www.google.ca/url?sa=t&rct=j&q=&esrc=s&source=web&cd=2&ved=2ahUKEwji0aGkyMvkAhUpHTQIHQ1wAtMQFjABegQICxAE&url=http%3A%2F%2Fwww.royalcollege.ca%2Frcsite%2Fdocuments%2Fcbd%2Fcanmeds-2015-manager-to-leader-e.pdf&usg=AOvVaw35uR-SiTCQjtkmguX9ZaPT. Accessed 27 Mar 2019.
40. Perlo J, Balik B, Swensen S, Kabcenell A, Landsman J, Feeley D. IHI framework for improving joy in work. Cambridge, MA: Institute for Healthcare Improvement; 2017. http://www.ihi.org/Topics/Joy-In-Work/Pages/default.aspx. Accessed 24 Mar 2019.
41. Post S, Roess M. Expanding the rubric of "patient-centered care" to patient and "professional centered care" to enhance provider well-being. HEC Forum. 2017;29:293–302.
42. Shanafelt T, Boone S, Tan L, Dyrbye L, Sotile W, Satele D, et al. Burnout and satisfaction with work-life balance among US physicians relative to the general US population. Arch Intern Med. 2012;172(18):1377–85.
43. Canadian Medical Association. CMA National physician health survey. Ottawa, CA: CMA; 2018. https://www.cma.ca/sites/default/files/2018-11/nph-survey-e.pdf. Accessed 24 Mar 2019.
44. Boudreau R, Grieco R, Cahoon S, Robertson R, Wedel RJ. The pandemic from two surveys of physician burnout in Canada. Can J Commun Mental Health. 2006;25:71–88.
45. Hunsaker S, Chen H-C, Maughan D, Heaston S. Factors that influence the development of compassion fatigue, burnout, and compassion satisfaction in emergency department nurses. J Nurs Scholarsh. 2015;47(2):186–94.
46. McHugh MD, Kutney-Lee A, Cimiotti JP, Sloane DM, Aiken LH. Nurses' widespread job dissatisfaction, burnout, and frustration with health benefits signal problems for patient care. Health Aff (Millwood). 2011;30(2):202–10.

47. Shanafelt T, Mungo M, Smitgen J, Storz K, Reeves D, Hayes S, et al. Longitudinal study evaluating the association between physician burnout and changes in professional work effort. Mayo Clin Proc. 2016;91(4):422–31.
48. Lemaire J, Ewashina D, Polachek A, Dixit J, Yiu V. Understanding how patients perceive physician wellness and its links to patient care: a qualitative study. PLoS ONE. 2018;13(5):e0196888. https://doi.org/10.1371/journal.pone.0196888.
49. Shanafelt T, Noseworthy J. Executive leadership and physician well-being: nine organizational strategies to promote engagement and reduce burnout. Mayo Clin Proc. 2017;92(1):129–46.
50. Shanafelt T, Dyrbye L, Sinsky C, Hasan O, Satele D, Sloan J, West C. Relationship between clerical burden and characteristics of the electronic environment with physician burnout and professional satisfaction. Mayo Clin Proc. 2016;91(7):836–48.
51. Chen S-C, Chen C-F. Antecedents and consequences of nurses' burnout: leadership effectiveness and emotional intelligence as moderators. Manag Dec. 2018;56(4):777–92.
52. Jiminez P, Bregenzer A, Kallus KW, Fruhwirth B, Wagner-Hartl V. Enhancing resources at the workplace with health-promoting leadership. Int J Environ Res Public Health. 2017;14(10):1264.
53. Shanafelt T, Gorringe G, Menaker R, Storz K, Reeves D, Buskirk S, et al. Impact of organizational leadership on physician burnout and satisfaction. Mayo Clin Proc. 2015;90(4):432–40.
54. Shanafelt T, Lightner D, Conley C, Petrou S, Richardson J, Schroeder P, Brown W. An organization model to assist individual physicians, scientists, and senior health care administrators with personal and professional needs. Mayo Clin Proc. 2017;92(11):1688–96.
55. Ashish KJ, Iliff AR, Chaoui AA, Defossez S, Bombaugh MC, Miller YR. A crisis in healthcare: a call to action on physician burnout. Waltham, MA: Massachusetts Medical Society, Massachusetts Health and Hospital Association, Harvard T.H. Chan School of Public Health, and Harvard Global Health Institute; 2019. https://cdn1.sph.harvard.edu/wp-content/uploads/sites/21/2019/01/PhysicianBurnoutReport2018FINAL.pdf. Accessed 12 Mar 2019.
56. Walker R, Kearns G, Janzen T, Jarmain S. Engaging physician leadership in multi-hospital clinical information technology transformation technology. Can J Phys Leadersh. 2017;4(2):50–4.
57. Edmondson A. The fearless organization: creating psychological safety in the workplace for learning, innovation, and growth. Hoboken, NJ: Wiley & Sons; 2019.
58. Dickson G. Transforming healthcare organizations. Healthier workers. Healthier leaders. Healthier organizations. Ottawa, ON: Mental Health Commission of Canada; 2018. https://www.mentalhealthcommission.ca/sites/default/files/2018-11/healthcare_crosswalk_eng.pdf. Accessed 23 Aug 2019.
59. Bandiera G. Mind the gap: thoughts on intergenerational relations in medical leadership. Can J Phys Leadersh. 2018;5(2):74–9.
60. John J. What patients want: care that is human as well as advanced. Can J Phys Leadersh. 2018;5(2):80–2.
61. Puddester D. LGBTQ2S+ diversity: leading and celebrating pride. Can J Phys Leadersh. 2018;5(2):88–91.
62. Soklaridis S, Kuper A, Whitehead CR, Ferguson G, Taylor VH, Zahn C. Gender bias in hospital leadership: a qualitative study on the experiences of women CEOs. J Health Organ Manag. 2017;31(2):253–68. https://doi.org/10.1108/JHOM-12-2016-0243.
63. Canadian Medical Association and Federation of Medical Women of Canada. Addressing gender equity and diversity in Canada's medical profession: a review. Ottawa, ON: Canadian Medical Association and Federation of Medical Women of Canada; 2018. https://cma.ca/sites/default/files/pdf/Ethics/report-2018-equity-diversity-medicine-e.pdf. Accessed 19 Feb 2019.
64. Alberta Health Services. Female physician leaders in AHS. Edmonton, AB: AHS; 2018. https://www.albertahealthservices.ca/assets/about/publications/ahs-pub-ahs-female-physician-leaders.pdf. Accessed 19 Feb 2019.
65. Roth VR, Theriault A, Clement C, Worthington J. Women physicians as healthcare leaders: a qualitative study. J Health Organ Manag. 2016;30(4):648–65.
66. Delisle M, Wirtzfeld D. Gender diversity in academic medical leadership: are we moving the needle? Can J Phys Leadersh. 2018;5(1):39–47.

67. Bourgeault I, Yvonne J, Lawford K, Lundine J. Empowering women leaders in health: a gap analysis of the state of knowledge. Can J Phys Leadersh. 2018;5(2):92–100.
68. Elias E. Lessons learned from women in leadership positions. Work. 2018;59(2):175–81. https://doi.org/10.3233/WOR-172675.
69. World Health Organization. Delivered by women, led by men: a gender and equity analysis of the global health and social workforce. Geneva: World Health Organization; 2019. https://www.who.int/hrh/resources/health-observer24/en/. Accessed 1 May 2019.
70. West M, Borrill C, Dawson J. The link between the management of employees and patient mortality in acute hospitals. Int J Hum Resour Man. 2002;13:1299–310.
71. Golden B. Redefining health care, a dialogue on health policy. Strengthening hospital-physician relationships. Ontario Hospital Association: Toronto, ON; 2017. https://www.rotman.utoronto.ca/-/media/Files/Brian-Golden---Designing-for-Hospital-Physician-Alignment.pdf?la=en&hash=0ABB48F424D9A88A99EDF1064103FB8077D4E46B. Accessed 27 Mar 2019.
72. Hewitt T, Tiller-Hewit T. Building effective dyad teams. Mgma Connexion. 2017;17(4):22–4.
73. Falling through the cracks: Greg's story. Greg's Wings; 2019. https://gregswings.ca/fttc-gregsstory/. Accessed 23 Sep 2019.
74. Kohn L, Corrigan J, Donaldson M. To err is human: building a safer health system. Washington, DC: Institute of Medicine, National Academy Press; 1999. https://www.ncbi.nlm.nih.gov/books/NBK225182/pdf/Bookshelf_NBK225182.pdf.
75. Chan MK, de Camps Meschino D, Dath D, Busari J, Bohen J, Samson L, et al. Collaborating internationally on physician leadership development: why now? Leadersh Health Serv (Bradf Engl). 2016;29(3):231–9.
76. Canadian Certified Physician Executive. Your leadership check-up. Ottawa, ON: Canadian Society of Physician Leaders. http://physicianleaders.ca/assets/ccpe-leadership-checkup.pdf. Accessed 27 Mar 2019.
77. The Association of the Faculties of Medical Education in Canada. The future of medical education in Canada (FMEC): a collective vision for MD education. 2017. https://www.afmc.ca/future-of-medical-education-in-canada/medical-doctor-project/collective-vision.php. Accessed 27 Mar 2019.
78. Qmentum program. Ottawa, ON: Health Standards Organization: Accreditation Canada; 2011. https://ontario.cmha.ca/wp-content/uploads/2017/03/accreditation_canada_leadership_standards.pdf. Accessed 27 Mar 2019
79. Sanokondu is an adaptation of "health leadership" in the universal language of Esperanto.
80. Welcome. Sanokondu; 2019. https://sites.google.com/site/sanokondu/. Accessed 2 Aug 2019.
81. Royal Australasian College of Medical Administrators. Fellowship training program. Melbourne (AUS). RACMA; 2019. https://www.racma.edu.au/. Accessed 25 Jun 2019.
82. Faculty of Medical Leadership and Management. Medical leadership and management standards. London: Faculty of Medical Leadership and Management; 2019. https://www.fmlm.ac.uk/individual-standards. Accessed 2 Aug 2019.

Pathway to Professionalization of Health Leadership

16

Graham Dickson and Bill Tholl

> *Do not die in the history of your past hurts and past experiences, but live in the now and future of your destiny.*
>
> Michelle Obama

Michelle Obama's quote could have been about the future of both modern health care systems and of the leaders who will create them. Modern health care systems are full of hurts and difficult experiences and newspaper headlines reflect pressure for change: "Review ordered after Nova Scotia man dies waiting for hospital transfer;" "Researchers aim to find solutions to 'hallway medicine' in hospitals;" and "Ontario inspects health care facilities in 'blitz' to curb workplace violence" [1]. But, as the stories in this book suggest, health care is also full of examples of caring, compassionate and efficient service. Leadership's job is to replace the former with the latter. Achieving the goals of seamless service, healthy workplaces and efficient and effective transformation of health systems is the territory of leadership and the job of leaders. Therefore, instead of dwelling on hurtful experiences, and giving up on the job, leaders need to learn from past mistakes while scaling up and spreading successful innovations and stories.

In Chap. 9 we quoted John F. Kennedy saying the essence of leadership in modern society is learning. That was a theme we introduced in Chap. 1 and kept returning to in subsequent chapters. We also emphasized the importance of learning personal and organizational leadership in Chap. 4, advocated for the capability of self-learning in Chap. 5, introduced the four capabilities of Achieve results as an

G. Dickson (✉)
Royal Roads University, Victoria, BC, Canada
e-mail: graham.dickson@royalroads.ca

B. Tholl
Canadian Health Leadership Network, Ottawa, ON, Canada
e-mail: btholl@chlnet.ca

ongoing learning cycle for organizations and systems in Chap. 7 and stressed how coalitions should be used for learning in Chap. 8. In Chaps. 10–15 we outlined what we've learned about LEADS as a change model and invited other authors to share their knowledge of putting LEADS to work in different ways in different contexts.

In this, the final chapter, we share macro lessons we gained writing this book. And since the point of learning is to understand the world around us better and appreciate its beauty and challenges more, it's our job as leaders to use what we've learned to improve our world. We're concluding by summarizing the steps we as leaders can take to improve our leadership—and subsequently the health and wellness of the public we serve.

Lessons About Health Leadership, LEADS and Making a Better System

Leadership in health care is about accomplishing three key functions: integrating care for patients and families, creating healthy and productive workplaces and changing the system to respond to environmental pressures and population needs. Leadership is not the person or the position: it is a responsibility shared by those who choose to lead. We lead from where we are and who we want to be.

We defined leadership earlier as "the collective capacity of an individual or group to influence people to work together to achieve a common constructive purpose: the health and wellness of the population we serve." This definition, when operationalized in context, in Canada, became the LEADS in a Caring Environment capabilities framework.

This second edition of our book has five themes: the importance of learning to effective life-long leadership; how LEADS has been put to work in Canada and Australia; the importance of caring as a driving force of health leadership (including equity, diversity and inclusion), how context fundamentally affects leadership, and the significant advances made in leadership and leadership development as chronicled in the research literature and grey literature: i.e., in Canada, Australia, England, Scotland and New Zealand.

A review of the chapters considering these five themes highlights five key lessons for us. They are:

1. LEADS works.
2. Caring leadership is gaining ascendancy in modern health systems.
3. Context shapes leadership.
4. The speed of change demands a culture of leadership.
5. It's time to professionalize health leadership.

LEADS Works

The reader is not likely to be surprised we make this claim. After all, the purpose of the book was to provide a five-year retrospective on ways the LEADS in a Caring Environment capabilities framework (and its Australian counterpart) have been put to work to deal with service integration, healthy workplaces and meaningful health reform. The stories and the vignettes interspersed throughout and the chapters, where leaders of all stripes testify to how LEADS can contribute to their leadership and to developing others, testify to that.

We've looked at LEADS being put to work at different levels of responsibility, ranging from deputy ministers, board members, chief executives and front-line leaders, to informal caregivers. The construct and face validity of LEADS have been independently reaffirmed in Canada and in other jurisdictions. But we cannot assume the framework is inviolate; we must always be open to adapting it to changes in context and circumstance.

LEADS works, we think, for three main reasons. First, the effort to use it has been a collaborative effort, engaging many leaders in shaping how it can and should be used. By emphasizing leadership without ownership and ownership by all (distributed leadership), our LEADS work has become an invitation to participate in an important and inclusive project aimed at improving Canada's health system.

The second reason LEADS works is the willingness of leaders to stick with it. A few people who initiated the work have kept promoting it, keeping its values and vision alive and (in the spirit of losing control, discussed in Chap. 9), trusting others to join in. It has helped that organizations have resisted the urge to develop their own frameworks, instead accepting the argument that a common leadership vocabulary will contribute to better integrated health care across the country.

The third reason is the integrity of the LEADS framework and the belief systems behind it. People accept the framework is an expression of the fundamental practices of good leadership and that those practices must reflect the person you are as a leader, and be adapted to the context in which you work.

The Ascendancy of Caring Leadership

The concept of caring leadership—central to the LEADS framework—is spreading, which can be seen in both grey literature (primarily out of the UK), and published leadership literature more broadly. Its impact across Canada is reflected in the LEADS stories we've collected and in the relationship between the LEADS framework's desired leadership practices and the goal of creating healthier workplaces.

In the UK, articles such as "Collaborative and compassionate leadership" [2] and "Caring to change: how compassionate leadership can stimulate innovation in health care" [3] show a growing emphasis on creating healthier workplace cultures; and this emphasis is reflected in efforts by the NHS England and NHS Scotland to support leaders becoming capable champions of creating healthy workplaces. In business, some authors have also emphasized the importance of compassionate and caring leadership [4–7]. The emphasis we put on mindfulness in Chap. 5 resonates with this view of compassionate leadership [8] and recent systematic reviews of leadership theory highlight the growing influence of transformational (empowerment) and moral theories of leadership (distributed, authentic, servant, ethical, spiritual) and their positive impact on workplace cultures and productivity [9–11].

The growth of a caring ethos in health leadership may well be because evidence shows many health workplaces are surprisingly unhealthy, and unhealthy providers cannot provide optimum patient and family care. The discussion of healthy work-places in Chap. 6, the alignment of LEADS to the National Standard for Psychological Health in the Workplace discussed in Chap. 10 and the struggles doctors and nurses have with burnout outlined in Chap. 15, all demonstrate the point.

The emphasis on caring and compassion also fuels a growing desire for greater diversity, equity and inclusion in the ranks of health care leaders, for two reasons. First, it can be difficult to understand a group's needs when you have not experienced its issues. Diverse role models are therefore required—as Nelson Mandela said "if you talk to a man in a language he understands, that goes to his head. If you talk to him in his language, that goes to his heart." Chapter 14, on leadership viewed through the two-eyed seeing of Indigenous culture, underscores just how important it is for non-indigenous leaders to speak the language of the heart—in the spirit of Wichitiwin (working together from the heart).

A second reason for the ascendency of a caring culture across health systems is the value of fairness implicit in caring. Our invited authors and case studies and stories tell us LEADS helps attain the twin goals of fairness and equity. A significant majority of stories and vignettes—highlighting the use of LEADS—feature women leaders. This was not by design, it's just what we found. Clearly LEADS is particularly appealing to women who aspire to leadership roles. Dr. Ivy Bourgeault put it this way:

> LEADS is empowering. The framework helps lift leaders and leadership up. It helps women leaders to lead from where they are and who they are; to effect change from where you and your colleagues are on the ladder of leadership.
>
> Building on the LEADS premise of shared leadership, we have also learned the more you let go (for example in working with Indigenous health leaders), the more you are able to accomplish together.
>
> Because it is strength-based and capabilities-based, rather than competency-based and focused on shoring up weaknesses, I think LEADS has been particularly emancipating for women health leaders across Canada.
>
> I think women are really good at acknowledging and dwelling on their weaknesses and not nearly as good at recognizing and building on their strengths. If a senior leadership job comes open with ten boxes to tick and a woman believes she can't tick all the boxes she is far less likely to apply than a male colleague who realizes he might only tick half the boxes but still applies and then gets the job.

Chapters 13–15 also highlight the need leaders have to understand and care about the perspectives of diverse groups—patients, families and citizens, Indigenous populations, and health care professionals—in order to get them actively engaged in their care and improve the health care organization or system. Chapter 13 featured the patient's perspective, challenging leaders' notions of where organizational boundaries are, and encouraging all of us to expand those boundaries so patients and families can be part of planning and operations, not just recipients of care. If we truly care about the welfare of patients, families and citizens, we will commit to engaging them meaningfully in shaping the health systems of the future. We will also seek to become advocates for those who do not have a clear voice. In Chap. 8 we feature how we can all be allies in giving voice to the voiceless or the disenfranchised in health care systems. Chapter 14 lays out the raw and deeply disturbing challenge facing leaders trying to improve health conditions in Indigenous communities: having to rebuild trust with peoples who have experienced decades of paternalistic abuse. In this chapter Dr. Alika Lafontaine, Caroline Lidstone-Jones and Karen Lawford describe how LEADS can be translated to hold all of us more accountable for being more culturally responsive. Chapter 15 outlines the need to care for our providers: to recognize their unique needs by creating healthier workplaces, and to invite them—through LEADS—to be real partners in our leadership efforts.

Context Shapes Leadership

Beginning in Chap. 2 and throughout the rest of the book we have emphasized what the recent literature on leadership is telling us: context shapes how leadership is practiced and developed. Context is created by structural and environmental conditions, the mindsets of followers and through broadly shared cultural beliefs [12, 13].

One clear lesson about context is the trend we're seeing in Canada toward amalgamating smaller, more local health care systems and replacing them with single, jurisdiction-wide organizations that oversee both care delivery and health care policy (Chap. 12). The same trend is found in primary care in Australia and NHS England. The tendency to create larger organizations may reduce administrative costs and help avoid silos but it can also create new tensions between the central government and regional delivery systems. As we learned in Chap. 11, each country's constitution shapes how and in what way leaders can act to improve health care. These changes create a need to align accountabilities, authorities and responsibilities between central and de-centralized structures and a concomitant need for leaders to understand how they are supposed to work.

This situation is exacerbated by the rapid rise of technological innovation and demographic demands. We see these tensions at play in Chap. 11, where the authors discuss national systems of leadership talent management; in Chap. 12, where regionalization is in the forefront; and in Chap. 7, when we talk about the growth of accountable care organizations as new models for taking a population health approach to service delivery and financing. Technology enables new models of service delivery, empowering patients and their care providers (including informal caregivers) through instantaneous communication, measurement and sharing of information. These factors fuel the pace of change and create what we called (Chap. 9), a VUCA (volatile, uncertain, complex and ambiguous) context, rife with change.

From the perspective of the leader-follower dynamic, these structural changes require everyone in the health system to change their mindsets, sometimes their belief systems and always their behaviour. Many leaders struggle with issues around equity, diversity and inclusivity but change demands each of us learn new skills and abilities, build new relationships and adopt new practices. We have emphasized these dynamics in all the chapters on LEADS, but especially in Chap. 10 (when we looked at putting LEADS to work as a change model) and in the five invited chapters. How leaders and followers react emotionally and logically defines the people context for change. Learning to navigate context, to pay greater attention to it, is a demand all leaders face.

A final lesson is that today's health leaders are facing a paradox: the growing need to change and the messiness it creates reduces the amount of time available for leaders to support their people. In stable environments, where practices are standardized and understood by all, there is time for human interaction. In VUCA environments—where you are, as our Indigenous authors said, "Driving a bus that's on fire, down a road that's in the process of being built"—it's hard to take your eyes off the road long enough to look at a map. There is less time for human interaction and greater stress as a result. In the context of Indigenous people, the authors called this "perpetual crisis." We sometimes feel endless, rapid change in health care is driving us to a similar state.

We began this section with the title 'Context shapes leadership'. However, we close it by saying that maybe it is also leadership's job to shape context. Context—certainly people context—is not inviolate; nor is structural context. Human beings created the context we work in and therefore human beings can change it. To simply accept what shapes us without in some cases resisting it, or reshaping it, when it is inconsistent with achieving our vision of health and wellness for all, is a diminution of our visionary capabilities. That may be the biggest leadership challenge of all.

The Speed of Change Demands a Culture of Leadership

A corollary to the lessons of leadership and context is that the speed of change demands a culture of leadership, so we can shift our approach from managing things to leading people. To shift priorities from tasks to people, we've learned leaders need to support and collaborate with followers to achieve change. To embrace the lesson on embedding caring in our organizational practices, we must make it part of our day-to-day actions, part of who we are.

NHS England [14] and NHS Scotland [15] realized their aspirations by creating caring provider cultures and showing compassion for the caregivers as well as for the recipients of care. To promote widespread adoption of the Mental Health Commission of Canada's Standard for psychologically healthy workplaces we mapped the Standard's 13 factors to the 20 LEADS capabilities [16]. To realize the maximum return on our investment as a society in health care, CHLNet developed and shared a leadership impact assessment tool. But in order to create a caring culture, people must have the skills, willingness and especially the opportunity.

What is a culture of leadership? It is an environment of human interactions in which each person accepts responsibility for initiating action to improve the health and wellness of others. As we said in Chap 2: "Leaders always cross the road first." It requires an organizational climate where the quality of relationships matters, where critical thinking and respectful communication are the norm and where people can disagree without being disagreeable. In a leadership culture, everyone, regardless of background, can contribute their unique attributes to the shared cause. A leadership culture can exist in many contexts—nationally, provincially, regionally or in departments and teams–but unless it also resides in our minds, culture change will not happen. Creating a leadership culture will stretch our limits; yet it is a goal to be pursued not only in our workplaces or for the health care system, but for society.

To create a healthy leadership culture, formal leaders must model the behaviour consistent with it—willing to give up leadership to others when that's the right thing to do so even people who consider themselves followers can step into leadership when needed. The chapters in this book have shown us this is what providers, patients, families and citizens and leaders themselves want. It is our belief and hope the LEADS framework can be a guide to help create and sustain healthy cultures.

It's Time to Professionalize Health Leadership

To close, we suggest it is time to establish a pathway toward professionalizing health leadership. Professionalization is needed to ensure we and others continue to practice what we know works, so our health care systems adapt and adjust to the significant, constant changes today's world demands (and will continue to demand) of those systems. Transforming any vocation into a profession—whether its nursing, law or engineering—is the best way to ensure high-quality practice is consistently maintained in the public interest.

Professionalizing health care leadership will improve many of the aspects of health care we have discussed. It will promote integration of services, healthier and compassionate workplaces, and build systems more resilient in the face of change. It will help us eliminate the situations that led to Greg's Wings in Chap. 15, the Staffordshire crisis in the UK (Chap. 11), the burnout and bullying of clinicians and employees found in many workplaces described in Chaps. 6 and 15, and encourage everyone to take on change with the courage and boldness Canterbury Health exemplified in Chap. 9.

We believe the foundations for professionalizing health leadership are in place in Canada [17], to some degree emulating efforts in medical leadership in Australia and the UK. For a vocation to become a profession many factors need to be present. According to Barbara Kellerman [18], in medicine and law, the markers associated with professional status are:

- Generally accepted body of knowledge.
- Extended education and training.
- Required continuing education and training.
- Clear criteria for evaluation and for (re)certification.
- Clear demarcation of those in the profession and those without.
- Explicit commitment to the public interest and to a code of ethics.
- Professional organization with the power and authority to monitor the status of the profession and the conduct of its members.

The body of knowledge underpinning LEADS—as testified by the content of this book—and its acceptance in a broad-base of leadership communities, suggests we have a generally accepted body of knowledge for health leadership in Canada. This knowledge, moreover, reflects similar frameworks in the Faculty of Leadership and Management in the UK (Chaps. 3 and 11) and the Royal Australasian College of Medical Administrators (Chap. 15) and much of the content in the UK's National Health Service's Leadership Framework. Canada has the added benefit of that body of knowledge being accepted as a common vocabulary across professions and jurisdictions through LEADS.

It's also true, as we've shown in this book, there are extended education and training offerings for LEADS across Canada, including many universities and colleges offering graduate degrees in health leadership or health administration. Continuing education and training are not required yet, but it is available through many organizations in the health care system (for example LEADS Canada, the Physician Leadership Institute, and CHA Learning). Criteria for evaluation and certification in LEADS practice are also available (Chaps. 11 and 15). There is no clear demarcation between those in the profession and those outside it but the recognition in the various clinical professions of leadership as a function rather than a person or position is encouraging people to identify themselves as health leaders.

What we need is for purveyors of education and programming, of certification and of voluntary leadership associations to band together to define the scope and breadth of who is a health leader, make it official that health leadership is an explicit calling and design a professional organization with the power and authority to monitor the status of the profession and the conduct of its members.

Professionalizing health care leadership may even be a *necessary* condition for health care systems to respond to the challenges of integrating service, creating healthy workplaces, and generating productive change. In this context David Johnston, the former governor general of Canada said "Professions serve vital functions that help hold a society together. When trust in a profession erodes, this glue dissolves and society is weakened. To mix my metaphors, professions also serve as grease that help societies function more smoothly. When trust in the profession dissolves, friction results" [19]. A health leadership profession could be both the glue and the grease to accomplish the daunting goals our society desperately needs fulfilled.

Summary

The landscape of leadership is in constant flux, like health care itself. Indeed, in the five years since the first LEADS book, we have seen advances in our understanding of leadership and its application in the health sector that are almost overwhelming in breadth and scope. There appears to be a greater awareness among health leaders and the clinical professions that better leadership will lead to healthier workplaces and thus to healthier citizens.

Frameworks like LEADS, like Health LEADS Australia, the NHS' Healthcare Leadership Model, NHS Scotland's dimensions of leadership in Project Lift, the

UK's Faculty of Medical Leadership and Management standards, the New South Wales Leadership Framework, and the Royal Australasian College's leadership model are all proof of our need to define the qualities of leadership. These frameworks enable people in both formal and informal roles to know what it takes to practice their craft at the highest level. While all these frameworks are aspirational, they represent the best of leadership practice as defined by research and are what those being led are looking for. How they are used, promoted, and supported is important for practice change to occur.

It's clear that while many pockets of success exist, the challenge of being a better leader eludes many because the changes required to be one are so prodigious. The conditions that demand the exercise of good leadership can undermine our own ability to meet our leadership aspirations. Only by learning the lessons of LEADS—of caring, of context, of large-scale change, and of professionalism, and putting those lessons into practice will we succeed in leading our modern health system into its next incarnation. To develop better leadership in tomorrow's leaders, and to practice it, remains our goal and our hope (for further tools and connections related to the content of this book, go to the LEADS Global website at: http://www.leads-global.ca/).

Our lives begin to end the day we become silent about things that matter.
—Martin Luther King, Jr.

References

1. The Medical Post. Selected healthcare headlines. Canadian Healthcare Manager; 2019. http://mail.canadianhealthcarenetwork.ca/portal/public/ViewCommInBrowser.jsp?Sv4%2BeOSSucxeZyGIGtgdMpWt5UwH8UX0vq%2BlapQvZdJa09b64KaqBh8Xg41Wb3%2FaeOShWnMQRt%2FDzCor8Wib5w%3D%3DA. Accessed 29 Aug 2019.
2. The King's Fund. Michael West: collaborative and compassionate leadership. London: The King's Fund Leadership Summit; 2017. https://www.kingsfund.org.uk/audio-video/michael-west-collaborative-compassionate-leadership. Accessed 27 Jul 2019.
3. West M, Collins B, Eckert R, Chowla R. Caring to change: how compassionate leadership can stimulate innovation in health care. London: The King's Fund; 2017. https://www.kingsfund.org.uk/publications/caring-change?gclid=CjwKCAjwkqPrBRA3EiwAKdtwk5vAyD-T7Tu7J6TcUjGzyxwwJPeUShHYvffJOT7lL-hIVn8SvIg1_BoCnHkQAvD_BwE. Accessed 30 Aug 2019.
4. Hougaard R, Carter J, Beck J. Assessment: are you a compassionate leader? Brighton, MA: Harvard Business Review; 2018. https://hbr.org/2018/05/assessment-are-you-a-compassionate-leader. Accessed 30 Aug 2019.
5. Poorkavoos M. Compassionate leadership: what is it and why do organisations need more of it? Horsham: Roffey Park Institute; 2016. https://hbr.org/2015/05/why-compassion-is-a-better-managerial-tactic-than-toughness. Accessed 30 Aug 2019.
6. Warrell M. Compassionate leadership: a mindful call to lead from both health and heart. New York, NY: Forbes Media; 2019. https://www.forbes.com/sites/margiewarrell/2017/05/20/compassionate-leadership/#d0a280b5df91. Accessed 30 Aug 2019.
7. Seppala E. Why compassion is a better managerial tactic than toughness. Harvard Business Review: Brighton, MA; 2015. https://hbr.org/2015/05/why-compassion-is-a-better-managerial-tactic-than-toughness. Accessed 30 Aug 2019.

 8. The Dalai Lama with Rasmus Hougaard. The Dalai Lama on why leaders should be mindful, selfless, and compassionate. Harvard Business Review: Brighton, MA; 2019. https://hbr.org/2019/02/the-dalai-lama-on-why-leaders-should-be-mindful-selfless-and-compassionate. Accessed 30 Aug 2019.
 9. Dinh J, Lord R, Gardner W, Meuser J, Liden R, Hu J. Leadership theory and research in the new millennium: current theoretical trends and changing perspectives. Lead Q. 2014;25(1):36.
10. Malila N, Lunkka N, Suhonen M. Authentic leadership in healthcare: a scoping review. Leadersh Health Serv (Bradf Engl). 2018;31(1):129–46. https://doi.org/10.1108/LHS-02-2017-0007.
11. Spano-Szekely L, Clavelle J, Quinn Griffin MT, Fitzpatrick JJ. Emotional intelligence and transformational leadership in nurse managers. J Nurs Adm. 2016;46(2):101–8.
12. Sharma P. Moving beyond the employee: the role of the organizational context in leader workplace aggression. Lead Q. 2018;29(1):203–17. https://doi.org/10.1016/j.leaqua.2017.12.002.
13. Zacccaro SJ, Green JP, Dubrow S, Kolze M. Leader individual differences, situational parameters, and leadership outcomes: a comprehensive review and integration. Lead Q. 2018;29(1):2–43. https://doi.org/10.1016/j.leaqua.2017.10.003.
14. NHS England. Building and strengthening leadership: leading with compassion. London: NHS England; 2014. https://www.england.nhs.uk/wp-content/uploads/2014/12/london-nursing-accessible.pdf. Accessed 30 Aug 2019.
15. NHS Scotland. Project Lift. Edinburgh: NHS Scotland; 2019. https://www.projectlift.scot/. Accessed 31 Jul 2019.
16. Dickson G. Transforming health care organizations. Mental Health Commission of Canada: Ottawa, ON; 2019. https://www.mentalhealthcommission.ca/sites/default/files/2018-11/health-care_crosswalk_eng.pdf. Accessed 30 Aug 2019.
17. Dickson G, Tholl B, Van Aerde J. Pathway to professionalizing health leadership in Canada: the two faces of Janus. Healthc Manage Forum. 2020;33(1):25–9.
18. Kellerman B. Professionalizing leadership. New York, NY: Oxford Univ Press; 2018.
19. Johnston D. Trust: twenty ways to build a better country. Toronto, ON: McClelland and Stewart; 2018.

Index

Dialogue, 110–113
Dispositional/trait theories, 30
Distributed leadership, 25, 26, 31, 301

E
Effective leadership, 266
e-leadership, 12
Emotional intelligence, 83, 84
Engagement
    and diversity, 101, 102
    communication
        deep listening, 110
        dialogue, 110–113
        social media, 113
    decision making, 106
    definition, 99
    employee's abilities, 103
    follower-centred approach, 103
    in context, 100, 101
    mental health and wellness, 104
    narcissistic/abusive behaviour, 106
    staff satisfaction and self-reported
        health, 104
    style of leadership, 107, 109
    team building, 114
    unhealthy workplaces, 104
Ethical leadership, 36
Executive leadership, 246
Executive Level, of development
        program, 306

F
Follower-centric leadership, 30
Followership theories, 30
Foundational leadership series, 305

G
Gandhi, 12

H
Health professionals, fragmented
        health systems
    clinical engagement model and blended
        learning, 305
    diversity and equity, 308
    professional engagement, 303
    role of physicians, 300
Health Standards Organization in
        Canada and Accreditation
        Canada, 263

I
Implicit leadership theory, 28
Indigenous communities, 325
Indigenous health
    ALIGN model, 285, 286
    community engagement, 283
    contextual leadership and
        intersectionality, 284
    hierarchical models, 282
    lead self, 281, 282
    pre-contact models, 282
    sense of identity and community, 282
Indigenous leaders, 289
Indigenous leadership
    decision making, 294
    decision-making, 291
    flexibility and adaptability, 294
    jurisdictional clarity, 292
Indigenous people
    communities and nations, 294
    community-centred care, 292
    storytelling and active listening, 290
Informal leaders, 267
Information processing, 29

K
Kids Health Alliance, 151
King, Martin Luther, 22

L
Lead self, 288–289, 309
    indigenous peoples, 281
    moral character
        emotional intelligence, 92
        resilience, 92, 93
    personal mastery, 88, 89
    self-awareness
        components, 80–82
        emotional intelligence, 83, 84
        mindfulness, 80
        mindset, 84, 86
        personal responsibility and
            accountability, 86, 87
        self-management, 82
    strengths-based approach, 90
    value systems, 282
Leader and follower cognition theory, 28
Leader emergence, 35
Leader–member exchange(LMX), 29
Leadership and information processing
        theories, 28
Leadership and leader